Renal Function

Mechanisms Preserving Fluid
and Solute Balance in Health

Renal Function

Mechanisms Preserving Fluid and Solute Balance in Health

Second Edition

Heinz Valtin, M.D. Andrew C. Vail Professor and Chairman of Physiology, Dartmouth Medical School, Hanover, New Hampshire

Little, Brown and Company : Boston/Toronto

The cover design, representing two kidneys on a background of the world, is based on the official emblem of the V International Congress of Nephrology, Mexico City, 1972. The symbol is used with the kind permission of Dr. Herman Villarreal, President of the Congress.

To
Nancy
and
Tom and Alison

Preface to the First Edition

With the advent of new curricula, virtually every medical educator has had to try to define the basic material in his particular discipline. This book represents my view of the essential elements in renal, fluid, and electrolyte physiology, which every medical student should master. These are necessarily personal choices, and thus most teachers in this field may find some fault with them or, what is more likely, will point out omissions.

Problems. Many chapters are supplemented by one or more quantitative problems that amplify the material in the text. The answers — as well as explanations of how the answers were obtained — are given in the section Answers to Problems following the text.

A note to students. This textbook has been prepared with a certain amount of hesitation, for fear that its concise style may tend to underplay the importance of mastering basic scientific principles. I firmly believe that the basic sciences are the foundation of excellence in medicine. The references at the end of each chapter are meant to underscore this conviction by encouraging those individuals whose curiosity has been aroused to read further. In selecting the references, I have tried to fulfill three purposes: (1) to list some classic contributions; (2) to cite original experiments, especially when their results conflict with those of other studies; (3) to list review articles in which many further references can be located. As a result, these reference lists, although selective, are somewhat long, and I advise students to enlist the help of their instructors in selecting the particular works that are appropriate to their purpose.

A request for critique. I shall appreciate suggestions from any reader — be he student or teacher — on how this text might be improved.

H.V.

Preface to the Second Edition

The wide acceptance of this book by both students and teachers has been most gratifying. While I realize that, by the usual standards, a second edition has been long overdue, I take solace from what Robert Pitts wrote in the second edition of his textbook: "What a student needs to know in 1968 is not especially different from what he needed to know in 1963." The same may be said for the decade of the 1970s. This is not to say, of course, that much of the elegant work being published is unimportant; only, that most such work deals with refinements of concepts, not with new principles that form part of the fundamentals of a field. Lest my colleagues be insulted by this view, let me point out that one of the major changes in this second edition is the extensive updating of the bibliographies at the end of each chapter. The list of references has been lengthened mainly to aid teachers in locating the information on which the text is based.

Major additions of concepts include the following: nephron heterogeneity, especially in regard to salt and water reabsorption; dependence of glomerular filtration on glomerular plasma flow and on the electrostatic barrier; secondary active transport and cotransport; tubuloglomerular feedback; newer views on isosmotic reabsorption; and the passive model of countercurrent multiplication. Also added were appendixes on the renin-angiotensin-aldosterone system and on the cellular action of vasopressin. Deletions involved matters of detail, not of changes in concept.

In preparing this second edition, I have tried to follow several guiding principles: (1) Part of the success of the first edition lay in its brevity. Therefore, for everything that I have added to the text, I have tried to remove something of equal length. (2) Problems with extensive answers were a popular feature of the first edition. This second edition contains many more problems. (3) Again, I have tried to present all topics in the context of the function that they subserve. There is thus no chapter on, say, "hormones and the kidney"; rather, renin-angiotensin-aldosterone is discussed as part of Na^+ balance; the antidiuretic hormone as part of H_2O balance; the prostaglandins as part of hemodynamics; and so on. (4) Quantitative treatment of data has been emphasized throughout. In order to aid that process, an array of normal values, useful for calculations, has been assembled in the Appendix to Chapter 1.

A request for critique. Suggestions about the first edition from students and teachers have been very helpful, and most of them have been incorporated into this second edition. Again, therefore, I invite comments.

H. V.

Acknowledgments

If the material in this second edition is accurate and up to date, it is largely because every chapter was read by one or two experts in the topic of that chapter. I have asked this help of very busy people, whom I thank not only for their time and effort but also for their indulgence with my audacity. As I name them here, I live in fear of having forgotten someone; only that individual will spot the inadvertent oversight, and he or she will do me a great favor in bringing the omission to my attention so that I can correct it: C. Craig Tisher, Reinier Beeuwkes III, Lise Bankir, John V. Taggart, Norman S. Lichtenstein, Howard S. Frazier, Luis G. Navar, Brian R. Edwards, Gerhard H. Giebisch, F. John Gennari, Thomas H. Maren, Adrian Spitzer, Fred S. Wright. In addition, I have benefited greatly from on-the-spot advice of many colleagues at Dartmouth Medical School, especially: Gilbert H. Mudge, Brian R. Edwards, Paul Stern, Roy P. Forster, Eugene E. Nattie, Donald Bartlett, Jr., S. Marsh Tenney, Allan U. Munck, William G. North, Hilda W. Sokol, Kirk P. Conrad, and Matthew P. Longnecker.

I am grateful to many authors and publishers for permission to reproduce their work, especially for many striking photographs. I have tried to acknowledge this debt in the legends to the figures.

Special thanks are due to the following: the very able, kind, and sensitive staff in the Medical Division at Little, Brown & Company, especially Lin Richter Paterson, Fred Belliveau, Clifton Gaskill, and Elizabeth M. Welch; Ethel B. Garrity, Mary L. Kenyon, Teresa I. Mitchell, and Jane Ballinger for secretarial and editorial assistance; Sally D. Whitlock and Valma and Henry Page for diligent help with illustrations and photography; the librarians at the Dana Biomedical Library at Dartmouth and the Radcliffe Science Library at Oxford for expert help; and Charles G. Phillips and John F. Morris of the Department of Human Anatomy at the University of Oxford for providing a most hospitable atmosphere in which this task could be completed.

H. V.

Contents

Renal Function

Mechanisms Preserving Fluid
and Solute Balance in Health

1 : Components of Renal Function

The lay view of renal function is that the kidneys remove waste liquids and potentially harmful end products of metabolism, such as urea, uric acid, sulfates, and phosphates. While this is true, it should be emphasized that an equally important function is the conservation of substances that are essential to life. Such substances include water, sugars, amino acids, and electrolytes such as sodium, potassium, bicarbonate, and chloride. Therefore, the kidneys should be viewed as regulatory organs that selectively excrete and conserve water and numerous chemical compounds and thereby help to preserve the constancy of the internal environment.

A castaway at sea may survive for three weeks without drinking water, and a man lost in the desert may survive from two to four days without water or salt. Conversely, a healthy individual frequently tolerates dietary excesses of fluid and salt. The reason that such extreme conditions can be endured lies primarily in the renal control of salt and water excretion and conservation. It is obvious that the renal adjustments must be relatively rapid if they are to preserve life. In fact they are brought into play within minutes or at most a few hours after the individual has been subjected to the environmental challenge.

Anatomy

The major gross anatomical features of the mammalian kidney are illustrated in Figure 1-1. The kidney consists of cortical and medullary substances and a pelvis that connects with the ureter. The medullary substance is divided into an outer and an inner portion (Fig. 1-2), the latter, or inner, medulla having one or more papillae (tips), depending on the species. The outer medulla is further subdivided into an outer and an inner stripe (Fig. 1-2). The renal artery enters the kidney alongside the ureter, branching to become progressively the interlobar artery, the arciform or arcuate artery, the interlobular artery, and then the afferent arteriole that leads to the glomerular capillary network. The venous system has subdivisions with similar designations, terminating in the renal vein, which also courses beside the ureter.

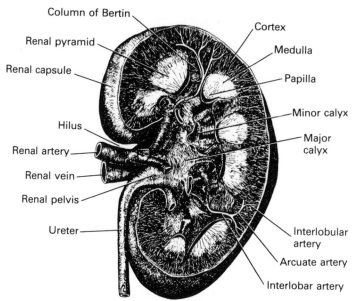

Fig. 1-1

A. Sagittal section of a human kidney, showing the major gross anatomical features. The renal columns are extensions of cortical tissue between the medullary areas. Not shown is the adrenergic nerve supply, not only to the large renal vessels but also to the vascular and tubular components of the nephron. Redrawn and very slightly modified from Braus, H. *Anatomie des Menschen,* Vol. 2. Berlin: Springer, 1924.

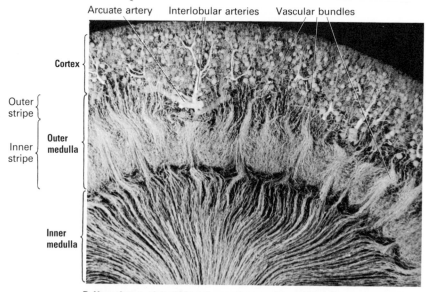

B. Vasculature of the kidney from a desert rodent (*Meriones*), showing: the cortex with numerous glomeruli; the outer medulla, containing capillary networks, and vascular bundles with vasa recta; and the inner medulla, containing vasa recta. (For further orientation, see Fig. 1-2B.) The vessels were filled with silicone rubber (Microfil) by arterial injection. Courtesy of Lise Bankir.

By *renal blood flow* (RBF), we mean the total amount of blood that traverses either the renal artery or the renal vein per unit time. The difference between flow in the renal artery and flow in the vein is the urine flow, which is negligibly small compared to the total blood flow. In adult humans about 1,300 ml of blood (i.e., about 25% of the cardiac output) flows through the two kidneys each minute, even though they constitute less than 0.5% of the total body weight. About 1,299 ml of blood leaves through the renal veins each minute, so a normal urine flow is about 1 ml per minute. *Renal plasma flow* (RPF) refers to the amount of plasma that traverses either the renal artery or the renal vein per unit time. Obviously, if the hematocrit (Hct) is 45%, RPF constitutes 55% of RBF.

The Nephron

The nephron, or functional unit of the kidney, consists of a glomerular capillary network that is surrounded by Bowman's capsule, a proximal tubule, a loop of Henle, a distal tubule, and a collecting duct (Fig. 1-2A). Each of the tubular parts can be sub-divided as shown in Figure 1-2A. Together, the adult human kidneys comprise roughly two million such functional units, which provide tremendous reserve. At rest, one can survive on about one-tenth this amount of functioning renal tissue, and be able to continue an active life even though about 75% of the tissue has been destroyed.

OUTER CORTICAL AND JUXTAMEDULLARY NEPHRONS. Two types of nephron have been described (Fig. 1-2A and B). The outer cortical nephron arises in the more superficial parts of the cortex, it has a short loop of Henle that reaches varying distances into the outer medulla, and its efferent arteriole branches into the peritubular capillary network that surrounds the tubular segments belonging to its own and other nephrons. This capillary network nourishes the tubular cells, picks up substances that have been reabsorbed from the tubules, and brings substances to the tubules for secretion.

The juxtamedullary nephron arises from the deep cortical regions. Its glomerulus is larger than that of an outer cortical nephron, and its loop of Henle extends varying distances into the inner medulla, sometimes all the way to the papilla. Its efferent arteriole continues not only as a peritubular capillary network but also as a series of vascular loops called the vasa recta. The vasa recta descend in bundles to varying depths in the inner medulla. There they break up into capillary networks that surround the collecting ducts and ascending limbs of Henle. The blood then returns to the cortex in ascending vasa recta that run within the vascular bundles. The ratio of outer cortical to juxtamedullary nephrons varies with the species of mammal. In humans, about

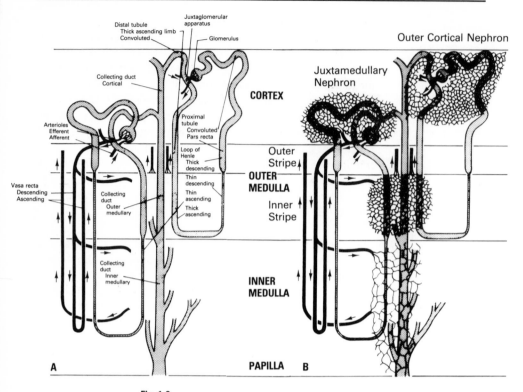

Fig. 1-2

A. Outer cortical and juxtamedullary nephrons, and their vasculature. The glomerulus plus the surrounding Bowman's capsule are known as the "renal corpuscle." There is some overlapping nomenclature; for example, the loop of Henle consists of the pars recta, the descending and ascending thin limbs, and the ascending thick limb, even though the first and the last parts are also considered to belong to the proximal and distal tubules, respectively. The beginning of the proximal tubule — the so-called urinary pole — lies opposite the vascular pole, where the afferent and efferent arterioles enter and leave the glomerulus. The ascending thick limb of the distal tubule is always closely associated with the vascular pole belonging to the same nephron; the juxtaglomerular apparatus is located at the point of contact (see also Fig. 1-3).

B. Capillary networks have been superimposed on the nephrons illustrated in (A). Both diagrams are highly schematic (for a more accurate portrayal, see Beeuwkes, R., III, and Bonventre, J. V. *Am J. Physiol.* 229:695, 1975), and they do not accurately reflect some relationships that probably have functional meanings. In the rat, for example, long thin descending limbs of Henle are located next to collecting ducts, and short thin descending limbs are closely associated with the vascular bundles made up of descending and ascending vasa recta in the outer medulla. The drawings are based mainly on Kriz, W. *Am. J. Physiol.* 241 (Regulatory Integrative Comp. Physiol. 10):R3, 1981.

100 μm   Peritubular capillaries

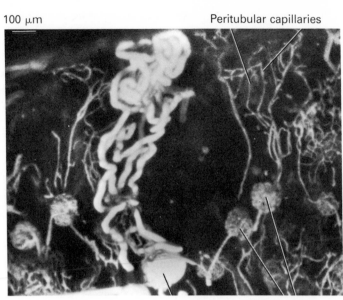

C   Renal corpuscle   Glomeruli

C. The cortex of a dog kidney (photomicrograph) illustrating the highly convoluted course of the proximal tubule. A micropipet (white streak at the lower
left) was inserted into Bowman's space, and the convolutions were filled with a
silicone rubber compound (Microfil). Other glomeruli, as well as peritubular
capillaries, were partially filled with Microfil through an intra-arterial injection.
Photograph courtesy of R. Beeuwkes and A. C. Barger.

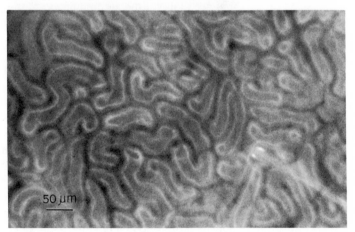

50 μm

D

D. The surface of a rat kidney as seen during micropuncture. The so-called bag
of worms consists mainly of segments of proximal convolutions as they re-
peatedly rise to the surface. A few segments of distal convolutions are also vis-
ible, but glomeruli are not usually found at the surface of a mammalian kidney.
Each tubular segment is surrounded by peritubular capillaries. The light, linear
streak in the lower right is a micropipet that has been inserted into a tubular
segment. The pipet is out of focus because its shaft lies above the renal surface. Photograph courtesy of J. Schnermann.

seven-eighths of all nephrons are outer cortical and one-eighth are juxtamedullary.

ULTRASTRUCTURAL DIFFERENCES OF VARIOUS NEPHRON SEGMENTS. Epithelial cells lining the various nephron segments differ in many respects, such as size, number and length of microvilli at the apical (mucosal) surface, number of mitochondria, number and extent of basal infoldings, and others. The major differences are shown in Figure 1-3; many fruitful correlations between structure and function have been drawn, and these will be referred to when appropriate.

The Juxtaglomerular Apparatus (JGA)

This apparatus (Fig. 1-3) consists of specialized epithelial cells in the thick ascending limb (the so-called macula densa cells), of lacis cells, and of specialized secretory or granular cells at the vascular pole where the afferent and efferent arterioles enter and leave the glomerulus. The JGA thus is a combination of specialized tubular and vascular cells. The macula densa cells come into contact with the lacis cells as well as with the granular cells of the afferent and efferent arterioles belonging to the same nephron; this is the result of embryonic development, not of some magic process whereby the distal tubule seeks out its own glomerulus. The JGA secretes renin, which is involved in the formation of angiotensin and ultimately in the secretion of aldosterone. It has been postulated that the JGA may be part of a feedback system that accounts for the autoregulation of the glomerular filtration rate and the renal blood flow, a topic that is considered further in Chapter 6.

Processes Involved in the Formation of Urine

The anatomical arrangement of the nephron permits several theories of function; these were hotly debated until the true picture emerged about 60 years ago. In 1842, William Bowman proposed that the glomerular capillaries secrete water, which flushes out solutes secreted by the renal tubules, a view elaborated about 40 years later by Heidenhain. In 1844, Carl Ludwig stated that urine is formed by ultrafiltration of plasma at the glomerulus, and that it merely passes down the nephron without further alteration save for concentration of its solutes by passive reabsorption of water. In 1917, Arthur Cushny modified Ludwig's view by proposing that not only water but also solutes are reabsorbed by the tubules, in "proportions, which are determined by their normal values in the plasma." Cushny denied the possibility of selective tubular secretion because he thought it was a process that would require vitalistic discrimination. It was not until 1923 that E. K. Marshall, Jr., proved that tubular secretion occurs.

We now know that the formation of urine involves a combination of ultrafiltration at the glomerulus, followed by selective tubular

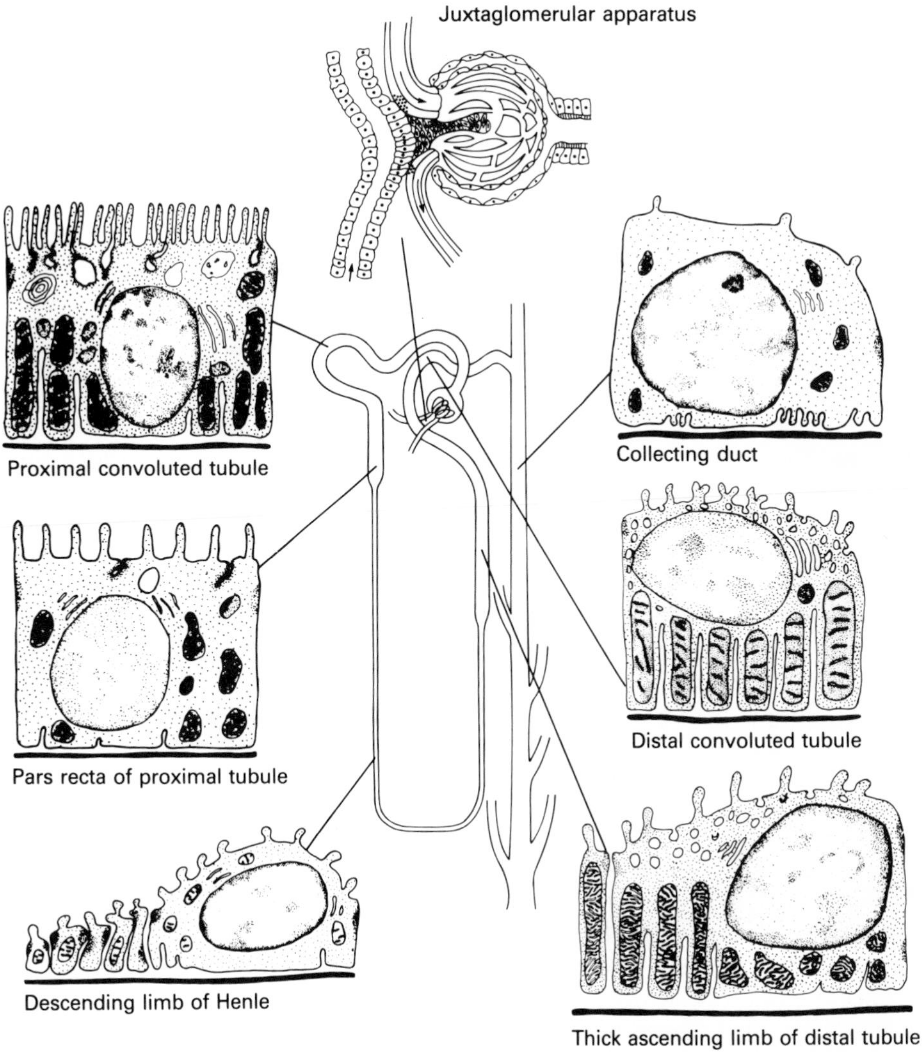

Fig. 1-3 : Diagrams illustrating some of the ultrastructural differences of the major parts of the nephron. Each part can be subdivided into segments, on the basis of ultrastructural and functional features. Also shown is the juxtaglomerular apparatus, which lies at the point of contact between the ascending thick limb of the distal tubule and the vascular pole of its own glomerulus. Not indicated here is so-called *heterogeneity* of nephrons — i.e., the fact that the anatomical (and functional) features of analogous parts of a nephron (say, the descending limb of Henle) may differ in an outer cortical nephron from those in a juxtamedullary nephron, or that the features may differ within a given component of a nephron, such as the proximal or distal tubule (see Reabsorptive Events Along Proximal Tubules. Heterogeneity, Chap. 7). Adapted from Rhodin, J. *Int. Rev. Cytol.* 7:485, 1958.

Table 1-1 : Daily renal turnover of H_2O, Na^+, HCO_3^-, and Cl^- in an adult human.

		Filtered	Excreted	Reabsorbed	Proportion of Filtered Load That Is Reabsorbed (%)
H_2O	L/day	180	1.5	178.5	99.2
Na^+	mEq/day	25,000	150	24,850	99.4
HCO_3^-	mEq/day	4,500	2	4,498	99.9+
Cl^-	mEq/day	18,000	150	17,850	99.2
Glucose	mM/day	800	≈0.5	799.5	99.9+

reabsorption of water and solutes, and selective tubular secretion of solutes. The subject of renal physiology deals primarily with defining what substances are filtered, reabsorbed, and secreted, in what amounts, in which parts of the nephron, by what mechanisms, and to what purpose.

Magnitude of Renal Function

The tremendous amounts of water and of certain solutes that are handled by the kidneys every day are illustrated in Table 1-1. The quantities that are filtered become even more astonishing when one considers that the total amount of water in an adult human is about 42 liters, and the pool of readily exchangeable sodium about 3,000 mEq. This disparity between total availability of essential substances and the rates at which they are filtered points up the necessity for their conservation through reabsorption. Since the examples listed in Table 1-1, as well as many others, are critical components of the internal environment, it is not surprising that they are reabsorbed so avidly. What may be surprising is that the kidneys should operate in such a seemingly inefficient manner as to filter the substances in the first place. The answer to this apparent paradox probably lies in the evolution of renal function.

Evolution

One possible scheme for the evolution of the kidney is depicted in Figure 1-4. The prochordate ancestor of the vertebrates, such as the acorn worm, may have evolved in the Cambrian Sea about 550 million years ago. These animals drank the sea water, bathed their tissues in it, and then expelled the residue through a simple ciliated conduit, which may be the forerunner of the kidney. The Cambrian Sea may have had a relatively high NaCl concentration similar to that of present-day mammalian extracellular fluid (Fig. 2-2). As protovertebrates migrated into fresh water, they retained an internal environment of high salinity, so that their body fluids had a higher osmolality than the freshwater surroundings. The consequent osmotic flow of water into these animals (now freshwater fish) could have resulted in fatal swelling unless an organ capable of high rates of water excretion had been evolved through natural selection. This organ was the

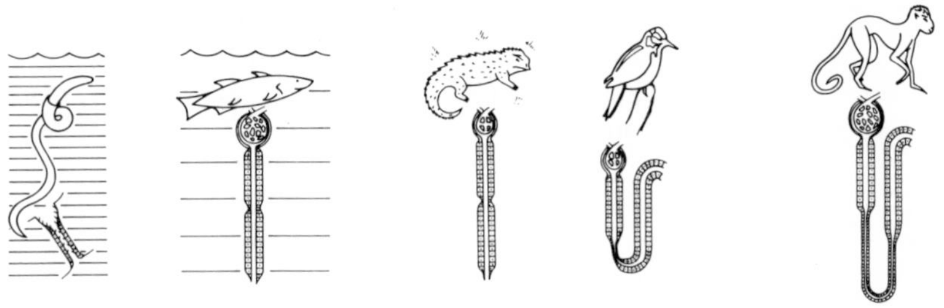

	Prochordates	Freshwater Fish	Reptiles	Birds	Mammals
Environmental problem		Osmotic uptake of water, and swelling	Desiccation	Desiccation	Desiccation
"Evolutionary solution"		High glomerular filtration of plasma water. Reabsorption of plasma crystalloids With water in proximal tubules Virtually without water in distal tubules	Degeneration of glomeruli Excretion of uric acid	Small glomeruli Excretion of uric acid Conservation of filtered water through counter-current system: first appearance of loops of Henle	Conservation of filtered plasma water through countercurrent system involving loops of Henle

Fig. 1-4 : One possible scheme for the evolution of the vertebrate kidney. Modified from Pitts, R. F. *Physiology of the Kidney and Body Fluids* (3rd ed.). Chicago: Year Book, 1974; and Smith, H. W. *The Evolution of the Kidney.* Porter Lectures, Series IX, Lawrence: University of Kansas Press, 1943. Pp. 1–23. It should be noted that J. D. Robertson, among others, does not agree with this scheme. He has proposed that glomerular kidneys may have existed in marine protoverte-brates, and that they thus may have been a useful preadaptation for life in fresh water. Evidence is in fact accumulating that the original habitat of fish was in the sea, and their origin probably goes farther back (by some 40 million years) than is depicted here.

glomerulus, promoting the ultrafiltration of large amounts of plasma, about 92% of which is water. The filtered plasma, how-ever, also contained essential small solutes (often referred to as crystalloids), such as sodium, chloride, bicarbonate, sugars, and amino acids. These essentials were reabsorbed in the proximal tubules, along with osmotically obligated water. The need to expel water may have been so great that a new structure evolved, namely, the distal tubule, in which the small molecules could be reabsorbed to the virtual exclusion of water.

When the vertebrates migrated onto land, they faced the oppo-site problem of the freshwater fish: desiccation. The consequent need to conserve water was apparently solved in two ways: In reptiles, the process of filtration was reduced through evolution-ary degeneration of the glomerulus, and uric acid became the excretory end product of protein catabolism. In contrast to urea, which is the main nitrogenous end product of mammals, uric acid can exist in highly supersaturated solutions and can thus be excreted with minimal amounts of water. In mammals, on the other hand, glomeruli of high filtering capacity were retained, as was the ability to recover essential small molecules mainly in the proximal tubules. In addition, selective forces apparently led to the development of loops of Henle, which promote the avid conservation of water through the countercurrent system (Chap. 8). It is of considerable interest that birds exhibit both solutions, excreting uric acid and also having some nephrons without loops of Henle and some nephrons with such loops.

Not all experts agree with this scheme. An alternative view, which places the origin of fish in the sea, is mentioned in the legend to Figure 1-4.

Summary

The kidneys are regulatory organs that help to maintain constancy of the internal environment in regard to both its volume and composition. They accomplish this purpose through ultrafiltration of plasma at the glomerulus, selective reabsorption of water and solutes, and selective tubular secretion of solutes. The objective of renal physiology is to understand the mechanisms, both within and outside of the kidneys, by which the renal regulation of fluid and solute balance is accomplished. Many special features of renal function, such as the very high rate of blood flow in relation to its size, the difference in both structure and function of the nephron depending on its location within the kidney, and the apparent inefficiency of concurrent, high rates of filtration and reabsorption, may be understood through the evolutionary forces that selected for ability to preserve water and solute balance.

Problem 1-1

Note: The answers to this and subsequent problems are given in a special section at the end of the text.

Additional problems — most of them based on clinical histories — can be found in: Valtin, H. Renal Dysfunction: Mechanisms Involved in Fluid and Solute Imbalance. Boston: Little, Brown, 1979.

Given the following additional data, show how the values for Na^+ listed in Table 1-1 were obtained: plasma concentration of Na^+ (P_{Na^+}) = 139 mEq/L; urine flow ($\dot{V}$) = 1.1 ml/min; urinary concentration of Na^+ (U_{Na^+}) = 95 mEq/L (see Table 11-A). Some of the numerical values will be slightly different from those listed in Table 1-1 because the latter were rounded off.

Problem 1-2   A solution of 0.9% NaCl is commonly used in clinical practice. How many equivalents of Na^+ does 1 liter of this solution contain? How many equivalents of Cl^- does 1 liter contain? What is the osmolality (mOsm/kg H_2O) of this solution? What is the osmolality of a solution of 0.9% NaCl if 5 g of glucose is added to each 100 ml? How many milliequivalents of calcium and how many milliequivalents of chloride are contained in 1 mMole of $CaCl_2$? How many milliosmoles are contributed by 1 mMole of $CaCl_2$?

Appendix   **Normal Values**

There are a number of normal values that one should have readily at hand, especially for calculating problems. These are given in Tables 1-2, 1-3, 1-4, and 1-5. Normal values for urine can be found in the Answer to Problem 11-1, at the end of the book.

Table 1-2 : Normal plasma, serum, or blood concentrations in adult humans.

Substance	Range	Average Value Usually Quoted	Comments
Bicarbonate	24 to 30 mM/L[a]	24 mEq/L[b]	[a]Venous plasma [b]Arterial plasma, which is commonly sampled in patients with problems of H^+ balance
Calcium	4.5 to 5.5 mEq/L	10 mg/100 ml	Approximately 50% is bound to serum proteins
Chloride	96 to 106 mEq/L	100 mEq/L	
Creatinine	0.7 to 1.5 mg/100 ml	1.2 mg/100 ml	
Glucose	70 to 100 mg/100 ml	80 mg/100 ml[c]	[c]Determined in the fasting state; so-called fasting blood sugar (FBS)
Hematocrit (Hct)	40 to 50%	45%	Also called packed cell volume (PCV)
Hydrogen ion concentration [H^+] (arterial)		40 nEq/L	Note that units are nanoequivalents per liter
Osmolality	280 to 295 mOsm/kg H_2O	287 mOsm/kg H_2O[d]	[d]A value of 300 is often used because it is a round figure that is easy to remember. This approximation does not introduce important quantitative error in most computations for evaluation of fluid and solute balance

Pco_2 (arterial)	37 to 43 mm Hg	40 mm Hg	
Po_2 (arterial)	75 to 100 mm Hg	—	While breathing room air. Value varies with age
pH (arterial)	7.37 to 7.42	7.40	
Phosphate[e]	2 to 3 mEq/L	3.5 mg/100 ml	[e]Measured as phosphorus. The exact concentration of phosphate in milliequivalents per liter depends on pH of plasma
Potassium	3.5 to 5.5 mEq/L	4.5 mEq/L	
Protein (total)	6 to 8 g/100 ml	7 g/100 ml	
Sodium	136 to 146 mEq/L	140 mEq/L	
Urea nitrogen (BUN)	9 to 18 mg/100 ml	12 mg/100 ml[f]	[f]Measured as the nitrogen contained in urea. Since urea diffuses freely into cells, values for serum, plasma, or whole blood are nearly identical (BUN = blood urea nitrogen). Average value varies with diet; BUN of 18 mg/100 ml may be normal or may reflect considerable reduction in renal function

Adapted from Valtin, H. *Renal Dysfunction: Mechanisms Involved in Fluid and Solute Imbalance.* Boston: Little, Brown, 1979.

Table 1-3 : Some useful miscellaneous normal values for adult humans.

	Average Value	Comments
Cerebrospinal fluid (CSF)		
pH	7.29 to 7.32	
$[HCO_3^-]$	20 to 24 mM/L	
P_{CO_2}	45 to 50 mm Hg	
pK'	6.13	For application of Henderson-Hasselbalch equation to CSF
Chloride		
Total body	2,400 mEq	Refers to total amount of Cl^- present in the body
Exchangeable	2,000 mEq	Refers to the amount of Cl^- that is readily miscible with ingested or administered Cl^-
Fluid volumes		
Total body water (TBW)	60% of body weight	
Intracellular water (ICW)	40% of body weight	Often abbreviated as ICF (intracellular fluid)
Extracellular water (ECW)	20% of body weight	Often abbreviated as ECF (extracellular fluid)
Plasma	4% of body weight	
Interstitial fluid	16% of body weight	
Glomerular filtration rate (GFR)	125 ml/min	
pK		
Acetic acid	4.7	
Acetoacetic acid	3.8	
Ammonia	9.2	At 25°C
β-hydroxybutyric acid	4.8	
Creatinine	5.0	
Deoxygenated hemoglobin	7.9	
Lactic acid	3.9	
Oxyhemoglobin	6.7	
Phosphoric acid	6.8	Refers to $HPO_4^{2-}:H_2PO_4^-$; phosphoric acid has two other pKs
Potassium		
Total body	3,500 mEq	Same meaning as listed for Chloride
Exchangeable	3,000 mEq	
Sodium		
Total body	5,000 mEq	Same meaning as listed for Chloride
Exchangeable	3,000 mEq	Much of the nonexchangeable Na^+ is in bone
Water content of tissues		
Bone	25%	
Fat	20%	
Muscle	80%	
Plasma	92%	

Adapted from Valtin, H. *Renal Dysfunction: Mechanisms Involved in Fluid and Solute Imbalance.* Boston: Little, Brown, 1979.

Table 1-4 : Average daily balance (amount per day) for water and some major solutes. Data for an adult human under normal environmental conditions who is eating a normal diet containing protein.

Substance	Intake		Output		
	Oral	Metabolic	Urinary	Fecal	Insensible
Water (ml)					
As fluid	1,200	300	1,500	100	900
In food	1,000	—	—	—	—
Sodium (mEq)	155	—	150	2.5	2.5
Potassium (mEq)	75	—	70	5	—
Chloride (mEq)	155	—	150	2.5	2.5
Nitrogen (g)	10	—	9	1	—
Acid (mEq)					
Nonvolatile	—	50	50	—	—
Volatile	—	14,000	—	—	14,000

Reproduced from Valtin, H. *Renal Dysfunction: Mechanisms Involved in Fluid and Solute Imbalance.* Boston: Little, Brown, 1979.

Table 1-5 : Some useful atomic and molecular weights.

Substance	Symbol	Atomic or Molecular Weight*
Albumin	—	60,000
Aluminum	Al	27
Bromine	Br	80
Calcium	Ca	40
Carbon	C	12
Chlorine	Cl	35
Chromium	Cr	52
Citric acid	—	192
Copper	Cu	64
Creatinine	—	113
Ethanol	—	46
Glucose	—	180
Hydrogen	H	1
Inulin	—	$\approx 5,000$
Iodine	I	127
Iron	Fe	56
Lactic Acid	—	90
Lithium	Li	7
Magnesium	Mg	24
Manganese	Mn	55
Mannitol	—	182

Table 1-5 (continued)

Substance	Symbol	Atomic or Molecular Weight*
Mercury	Hg	201
Nitrogen	N	14
Oxygen	O	16
p-Aminohippuric acid (PAH)	—	194
Phosphorus	P	31
Potassium	K	39
Sodium	Na	23
Sulfur	S	32
Urea	—	60
Uric acid	—	158

*Rounded off at least to nearest unit.
Reproduced from Valtin, H. *Renal Dysfunction: Mechanisms Involved in Fluid and Solute Imbalance.* Boston: Little, Brown, 1979.

Selected References

Note: Additional references — especially ones pertinent to clinical nephrology — can be found in: Valtin, H. Renal Dysfunction: Mechanisms Involved in Fluid and Solute Imbalance. *Boston: Little, Brown, 1979. In addition, I agree with the advice given by Dr. Vander [in Vander, A. J.* Renal Physiology *(2nd ed.). New York: McGraw-Hill, 1980], that a good way to stay up to date is to read the reviews (often called editorial reviews), editorials, and symposia that are published in the following journals:* American Journal of Physiology: Renal, Fluid and Electrolyte Physiology; Kidney International; Hospital Practice; New England Journal of Medicine; Lancet; *and* Federation Proceedings. *More exhaustive reviews appear in:* Annual Review of Physiology; Physiological Reviews; *and* Handbook of Physiology.

General

Andreoli, T. E. (Ed.). Renal and electrolyte physiology. *Annu. Rev. Physiol.* 43:567, 1981.
This section includes six authoritative and useful articles on the many interactions of both intrarenal and extrarenal hormones with the kidneys.

Bergeron, M., et al. (Eds.). *Proceedings VII International Congress of Nephrology.* Basel: Karger, 1978.
These volumes, published every three years, provide a succinct, up-to-date résumé of the state of the art.

Boyarsky, S., Gottschalk, C. W., Tanagho, E. A., and Zimskind, P. D. (Eds.). *Urodynamics: Hydrodynamics of the Ureter and Renal Pelvis.* New York: Academic, 1971.

Bradley, S. E. (Ed.). Symposium on hormones and the kidney. *Kidney Int.* 6:261, 1974.

Brenner, B. M., and Rector, F. C., Jr. (Eds.). *The Kidney* (2nd ed.). Philadelphia: Saunders, 1981.

Brenner, B. M., and Stein, J. H. (Eds.). *Contemporary Issues in Nephrology.* New York: Churchill Livingstone, 1978.
Authoritative, up-to-date reviews. Each bound volume is devoted to a major topic.

Chasis, H., and Goldring, W. (Eds.). *Homer William Smith: His Scientific and Literary Achievements.* New York: New York University Press, 1965.

DiBona, G. F. (Ed.). Symposium on neural control of renal function. *Fed. Proc.* 37:1191, 1978.

Earley, L. E., and Gottschalk, C. W. (Eds.). *Strauss and Welt's Diseases of the Kidney* (3rd ed.). Boston: Little, Brown, 1979.

Edelman, I. S. Receptors and effectors in hormone action on the kidney. *Am. J. Physiol.* 241 (Renal Fluid Electrolyte Physiol. 10):F333, 1981.

Fisher, J. W. (Ed.). *Kidney Hormones.* New York: Academic, 1971.

Forster, R. P. Kidney Cells. In J. Brachet and A. E. Mirsky (Eds.), *The Cell. Biochemistry, Physiology, Morphology.* New York: Academic, 1961.

Forster, R. P. Comparative Vertebrate Physiology and Renal Concepts. In J. Orloff and R. W. Berliner (Eds.), *Handbook of Physiology,* section 8,

Renal Physiology. Washington, D.C.: American Physiological Society, 1973.

Giebisch, G. H., and Purcell, E. F. (Eds.). *Renal Function.* New York: Josiah Macy, Jr. Foundation, 1978.

Giebisch, G., Tosteson, D. C., and Ussing, H. H. (Eds.). *Membrane Transport in Biology,* vols. IVA and IVB, *Transport Organs.* New York: Springer-Verlag, 1979.

Katz, A. I., and Lindheimer, M. D. Actions of hormones on the kidney. *Annu. Rev. Physiol.* 39:97, 1977.

Klahr, S., and Massry, S. G. (Eds.). *Contemporary Nephrology,* vol. 1. New York: Plenum, 1981.
The first in a series of bound volumes.

Massry, S. G. (Ed.). Kidney and hormones. *Nephron* 15:161, 1975.

Maxwell, M. H., and Kleeman, C. R. (Eds.). *Clinical Disorders of Fluid and Electrolyte Metabolism* (3rd ed.). New York: McGraw-Hill, 1979.

Orloff, J., and Berliner, R. W. (Eds.). *Handbook of Physiology,* section 8, Renal Physiology. Washington, D.C.: American Physiological Society, 1973.

Peart, W. S. The kidney as an endocrine organ. *Lancet* 2:543, 1977.

Pitts, R. F. *Physiology of the Kidney and Body Fluids* (3rd ed.). Chicago: Year Book, 1974.

Ross, B., and Guder, W. G. (Eds.). Biochemical aspects of renal function. *Int. J. Biochem.* 12:1, 1980.
The proceedings of this symposium, held in honor of H. A. Krebs, have also been published in book form by Pergamon Press.

Schwartz, M. M., and Venkatachalam, M. A. Structural differences in thin limbs of Henle: Physiological implications. *Kidney Int.* 6:193, 1974.

Smith, H. W. *Lectures on the Kidney.* Lawrence: University of Kansas Press, 1943.

Smith, H. W. *The Kidney: Structure and Function in Health and Disease.* New York: Oxford University Press, 1951.

Stephenson, J. L. Case studies in renal and epithelial physiology. *Lect. Appl. Math.* 19:171, 1981.

Takács, L. (Ed.). Kidney and Body Fluids. Vol. II of *Advances in Physiological Sciences.* Budapest: Akadémiai Kiadó, 1981.
This volume of the Proceedings of the XXVIII International Congress of Physiological Sciences deals with a wide range of topics in renal physiology.

Thurau, K. (Ed.). Kidney and urinary tract physiology. *Int. Rev. Physiol.* 6:1, 1974; *ibid.* 11:1, 1976.
This excellent series, published by University Park Press, Baltimore, appears in book form every two to three years.

Vogel, H. G., and Ullrich, K. J. (Eds.). *New Aspects of Renal Function.* Amsterdam: Excerpta Medica, 1978.

Wesson, L. G. *Physiology of the Human Kidney.* New York: Grune & Stratton, 1969.

Anatomy and Development

Andrews, P. M., and Porter, K. R. A scanning electron microscopic study of the nephron. *Am. J. Anat.* 140:81, 1974.

Barajas, L. The ultrastructure of the juxtaglomerular apparatus as disclosed by three-dimensional reconstructions from serial sections: The anatomical relationship between the tubular and vascular components. *J. Ultrastruct. Res.* 33:116, 1970.

Beeuwkes, R., III. The vascular organization of the kidney. *Annu. Rev. Physiol.* 42:531, 1980.

Beeuwkes, R., III, and Bonventre, J. V. Tubular organization and vascular-tubular relations in the dog kidney. *Am. J. Physiol.* 229:695, 1975.

Bulger, R. E. Kidney Morphology. In L. E. Earley and C. W. Gottschalk (Eds.), *Strauss and Welt's Diseases of the Kidney* (3rd ed.). Boston: Little, Brown, 1979.

Bulger, R. E., Siegel, F. L., and Pendergrass, R. Scanning and transmission electron microscopy of the rat kidney. *Am. J. Anat.* 139:483, 1974.

Bulger, R. E., Tisher, C. C., Meyers, C. H., and Trump, B. F. Human renal ultrastructure: II. The thin limb of Henle's loop and the interstitium in healthy individuals. *Lab. Invest.* 16:124, 1967.

Christensen, J. A., Meyer, D. S., and Bohle, A. The structure of the human juxtaglomerular apparatus. A morphometric, lightmicroscopic study on serial sections. *Virchows Arch.* [Pathol. Anat.] 367:83, 1975.

Fourman, J., and Moffat, D. B. *The Blood Vessels of the Kidney.* Oxford: Blackwell, 1972.

Gorgas, K. Struktur und Innervation des juxtaglomerulären Apparates der Ratte. *Adv. Anat. Embryol. Cell Biol.* 54 (Fasc. 2):5, 1978.

Gottschalk, C. W. Renal nerves and sodium excretion. *Annu. Rev. Physiol.* 41:229, 1979.

Huber, G. C. On the development and shape of uriniferous tubules of certain of the higher mammals. *Am. J. Anat.* 4 (Suppl. 1):1, 1905.

Kaissling, B., and Kriz, W. Structural analysis of the rabbit kidney. *Adv. Anat. Embryol. Cell Biol.* 56:1, 1978.

Knepper, M. A., Danielson, R. A., Saidel, G. M., and Post, R. S. Quantitative analysis of renal medullary anatomy in rats and rabbits. *Kidney Int.* 12:313, 1977.

Kriz, W. Der architektonische und funktionelle Aufbau der Rattenniere. *Z. Zellforsch.* 82:495, 1967.

Kriz, W. Organization of Structures Within the Renal Medulla. In B. Schmidt-Nielsen (Ed.), *Urea and the Kidney.* Amsterdam: Excerpta Medica, 1970.

Kriz, W., Barrett, J. M., and Peter, S. The renal vasculature: Anatomical-functional aspects. *Int. Rev. Physiol.* 11:1, 1976.

Maunsbach, A. B., Olsen, T. S., and Christensen, E. I. (Eds.). *Functional Ultrastructure of the Kidney.* New York: Academic, 1980.

von Möllendorff, W. Der Exkretionsapparat. In W. von Möllendorff (Ed.), *Handbuch der Mikroskopischen Anatomie des Menschen,* vol. VII, part 1. Berlin: Springer, 1930.

Myers, C. E., Bulger, R. E., Tisher, C. C., and Trump, B. F. Human renal ultrastructure: IV. Collecting duct of healthy individuals. *Lab. Invest.* 15:1921, 1966.

Oliver, J. *Nephrons and Kidneys: A Quantitative Study of Developmental and Evolutionary Mammalian Architectonics.* New York: Harper & Row, 1968.

Orloff, J., and Berliner, R. W. (Eds.). *Handbook of Physiology,* section 8, Renal Physiology. Washington, D.C.: American Physiological Society, 1973.
The first three chapters deal with the ultrastructure of all parts of the nephron.

Osathanondth, V., and Potter, E. L. Development of human kidneys as shown by microdissection. (This is a series of five papers by these authors, all published in *Arch. Pathol. Lab. Med.,* as follows: I. 76:271, 1963; II. 76:277, 1963; III. 76:290, 1963; IV. 82:391, 1966; V. 82:403, 1966.)

Peter, K. *Untersuchungen über Bau und Entwickelung der Niere.* Jena: Fischer, 1909.

Potter, E. L. *Normal and Abnormal Development of the Kidney.* Chicago: Year Book, 1972.

Rollhäuser, H., Kriz, W., and Heinke, W. Das Gefäss-system der Rattenniere. *Z. Zellforsch.* 64:381, 1964.

Rouiller, C., and Muller, A. F. (Eds.). *The Kidney,* vol. 1. New York: Academic, 1969.

Rytand, D. A. The number and size of mammalian glomeruli as related to kidney and to body weight, with methods for their enumeration and measurement. *Am. J. Anat.* 62:507, 1938.

Sperber, I. Studies on the mammalian kidney. *Zool. Bid. Fran. Uppsala* 22:249, 1944.

Spinelli, F., Wirz, H., and Brücher, C. *Fine Structure of the Kidney Revealed by Scanning Electron-Microscopy.* Basel: Ciba-Geigy, 1972.

Thoenes, W., and Langer, K. H. Relationship Between Cell Structures of Renal Tubules and Transport Mechanisms. In K. Thurau and H. Jahrmärker (Eds.), *Renal Transport and Diuretics.* New York: Springer, 1969.

Thurau, K., and Mason, J. The intrarenal function of the juxtaglomerular apparatus. *Int. Rev. Physiol.* 6:357, 1974.

Tisher, C. C. Anatomy of the Kidney. In B. M. Brenner and F. C. Rector, Jr. (Eds.), *The Kidney* (2nd ed.). Philadelphia: Saunders, 1981.

Tisher, C. C., Bulger, R. E., and Trump, B. F. Human renal ultrastructure: I. Proximal tubule of healthy individuals. *Lab. Invest.* 15:1357, 1966.

Tisher, C. C., Bulger, R. E., and Trump, B. F. Human renal ultrastructure: III. The distal tubule in healthy individuals. *Lab. Invest.* 18:655, 1968.

Trump, B. F., and Bulger, R. E. Morphology of the Kidney. In E. L. Becker (Ed.), *Structural Basis of Renal Disease.* New York: Harper & Row, 1968.

Valtin, H. Structural and functional heterogeneity of mammalian nephrons. *Am. J. Physiol.* 233 (Renal Fluid Electrolyte Physiol. 2):F491, 1977.

Walker, L. A., and Valtin, H. Biological importance of nephron heterogeneity. *Annu. Rev. Physiol.* 44:203, 1982.

Wright, F. S., and Briggs, J. P. Feedback control of glomerular blood flow, pressure, and filtration rate. *Physiol. Rev.* 59:958, 1979.
The first part of this article is a thorough and critical review of the anatomy of the juxtaglomerular apparatus.

Historical

Bowman, W. On the structure and use of the malpighian bodies of the kidney, with observations on the circulation through that gland. *Philos. Trans. R. Soc. Lond.* 132:57, 1842.

Cushny, A. R. *The Secretion of Urine.* London: Longmans, Green, 1917.

Gottschalk, C. W. Dr. A. N. Richards and kidney micropuncture. *Ann. Intern. Med.* 71 (Suppl. 8):28, 1969.

Heidenhain, R. Die Harnabsonderung. In L. Hermann (Ed.), *Handbuch der Physiologie,* vol. V, part 1. Leipzig: Vogel, 1883.

Huber, G. C. The morphology and structure of the mammalian renal tubule. *Harvey Lect.* 5:100, 1910.

Ludwig, C. Nieren und Harnbereitung. In R. Wagner (Ed.), *Handwörterbuch der Physiologie.* Braunschweig: Vieweg, 1844.

Marshall, E. K., Jr., and Vickers, J. L. The mechanism of the elimination of phenolsulphonphthalein by the kidney — proof of secretion by the convoluted tubules. *Johns Hopkins Bull.* 34:1, 1923.

Smith, H. W. Renal Physiology Between Two Wars. In *Lectures on the Kidney.* Lawrence: University of Kansas Press, 1943. Pp. 65–82.

Smith, H. W. De Urina. *Kaiser Found. Med. Bull.* 6:1, 1958.
This lecture is reprinted in: Chasis, H., and Goldring, W. (Eds.). Homer William Smith. His Scientific and Literary Achievements. New York: New York University Press, 1965.

Smith, H. W. Renal Physiology. In A. P. Fishman and D. W. Richards (Eds.), *Circulation of the Blood. Men and Ideas.* New York: Oxford University Press, 1964.

Wearn, J. T. Composition of glomerular urine with conclusive evidence of reabsorption in the renal tubules. A vignette. *Physiologist* 23 (No. 5):1, 1980.

Evolution

Braun, E. J., and Dantzler, W. H. Function of mammalian-type and reptilian-type nephrons in kidney of desert quail. *Am. J. Physiol.* 222:617, 1972.

Repetski, J. E. A fish from the upper Cambrian of North America. *Science* 200:529, 1978.

Robertson, J. D. The habitat of the early vertebrates. *Biol. Rev.* 32:156, 1957.

Romer, A. S. *The Vertebrate Body* (4th ed.). Philadelphia: Saunders, 1970. Pp. 350–369.

Smith, H. W. The Evolution of the Kidney. In *Lectures on the Kidney.* Lawrence: University of Kansas Press, 1943. Pp. 3–23.

Smith, H. W. *From Fish to Philosopher.* Boston: Little, Brown, 1953.

Research Techniques

Andreucci, V. E. (Ed.). *Manual of Renal Micropuncture.* Naples: Idelson, 1978.

Gellai, M., and Valtin, H. Chronic vascular constrictions and measurements of renal function in conscious rats. *Kidney Int.* 15:419, 1979.

Gellai, M., and Valtin, H. The Brattleboro Rat and the Trained, Conscious, Chronically Catheterized Rat. In K. Gärtner and H. Stolte (Eds.), *Research Animals and Concepts of Applicability to Clinical Medicine.* Basel: Karger, 1982. Pp. 102–110.

Giebisch, G. (Ed.). Symposium on renal micropuncture techniques. *Yale J. Biol. Med.* 45:187, 1972.

Gottschalk, C. W. Renal tubular function: Lessons from micropuncture. *Harvey Lect.* 58:99, 1963.

Grantham, J. J., Irish, J. M., III, and Hall, D. A. Studies of isolated renal tubules in vitro. *Annu. Rev. Physiol.* 40:249, 1978.

Handler, J. S., Perkins, F. M., and Johnson, J. P. Studies of renal cell function using cell culture techniques. *Am. J. Physiol.* 238 (Renal Fluid Electrolyte Physiol. 7):F1, 1980.

Hillman, R. E., and Rosenberg, L. E. Amino acid transport by isolated mammalian renal tubules: III. Binding of L-proline by proximal tubule membranes. *Biochim. Biophys. Acta* 211:318, 1970.

Jarausch, K. H., and Ullrich, K. J. Zur Technik der Entnahme von Harnproben aus einzelnen Sammelrohren der Säugetierniere mittels Polyäthylen-Capillaren. *Pflügers Arch. Ges. Physiol.* 264:88, 1957.

Kinne, R., and Schwartz, I. L. Isolated membrane vesicles in the evaluation of the nature, localization, and regulation of renal transport processes. *Kidney Int.* 14:547, 1978.

Maack, T. Physiological evaluation of the isolated perfused rat kidney. *Am. J. Physiol.* 238 (Renal Fluid Electrolyte Physiol. 7):F71, 1980.

Morel, F., Chabardès, D., and Imbert-Teboul, M. Methodology for Enzymatic Cyclase. In M. Martinez-Maldonado (Ed.), *Methods in Pharmacology,* vol. 4B, *Renal Pharmacology.* New York: Plenum, 1978.

Orloff, J., and Berliner, R. W. (Eds.). *Handbook of Physiology,* section 8, Renal Physiology. Washington, D.C.: American Physiological Society, 1973.

Chapters 4 through 7 of this authoritative book critically review the major techniques for assessing renal function.

Richards, A. N. Urine formation in the amphibian kidney. *Harvey Lect.* 30:93, 1936.

de Rouffignac, C., Deiss, S., and Bonvalet, J. P. Détermination du taux individuel de filtration glomérulaire des néphrons accessibles et inaccessibles à la microponction. *Pflügers Arch. Eur. J. Physiol.* 315:273, 1970.

Sacktor, B. Transport in membrane vesicles isolated from the mammalian kidney and intestine. *Curr. Top. Bioeng.* 6:39, 1977.

Sakai, F., Jamison, R. L., and Berliner, R. W. A method for exposing the rat renal medulla in vivo: Micropuncture of the collecting duct. *Am. J. Physiol.* 209:663, 1965.

Schafer, J. A., and Andreoli, T. E. Perfusion of Isolated Mammalian Renal Tubules. In G. Giebisch (Ed.), *Transport Organs,* vol. IVB. New York: Springer-Verlag, 1979.

Walker, A., Bott, P., Oliver, J., and MacDowell, M. The collection and analysis of fluid from single nephrons of the mammalian kidney. *Am. J. Physiol.* 134:580, 1941.

Wearn, J. T., and Richards, A. N. Observations on the composition of glomerular urine with particular reference to the problem of reabsorption in the renal tubules. *Am. J. Physiol.* 71:209, 1924.

Windhager, E. E. *Micropuncture Techniques and Nephron Function.* New York: Appleton-Century-Crofts, 1968.

2 : The Body Fluid Compartments

The internal environment that is regulated by the kidneys is a fluid medium, which is distributed in a number of discernible compartments. In this chapter, we shall consider both the size and the distinctive composition of these compartments, as well as some of the factors that maintain these characteristic differences.

Size of the Compartments

Approximate sizes of the major fluid compartments of an adult human are shown in Figure 2-1, where the dimensions have been expressed both as absolute values and as a proportion of the body weight. The latter is important because it is one basis for estimating fluid volumes, both in experimental animals and in patients. It should be emphasized that all percentages refer to the proportion of *body weight,* not of total body water.

About 50 to 70% of the body is composed of water. The main factor that determines whether the lower or higher figure applies is the amount of fatty tissue, which has a low water content compared to other tissues (see Table 1-3). Thus, the lower figure pertains mainly to obese individuals, and to females who have relatively more fat than men.

The total body water (TBW) is distributed between two major compartments, the intracellular (ICW) and the extracellular (ECW). Of these, ICW is the larger, comprising nearly two-thirds of the TBW. The ECW has two further major subdivisions, the plasma and the interstitial, comprising about 4% and 16% of the body weight, respectively. Lymph, constituting 2 to 3% of the body weight, is included in the interstitial volume. Claude Bernard first pointed out that of all the body fluid compartments, the interstitial is probably the true internal environment, since it is the fluid medium that bathes all cells. A more recent point of view, adopted by some, is that intracellular fluid may be the true environment since it is within cells that major processes, such as enzymatic reactions, occur.

The transcellular compartment is a minor subdivision of ECW. It comprises a number of small volumes, such as cerebrospinal,

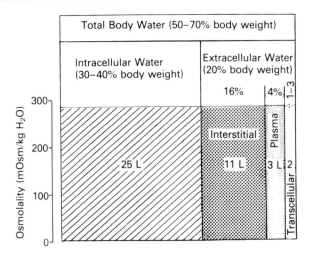

Fig. 2-1 : **Approximate sizes of the major body fluid compartments, expressed both as percentage of body weight and in mean absolute values for an adult human being who weighs 70 kg (154 lb). The ranges of normal among individuals are considerable, and thus no one value should be taken too rigidly; a good rule of thumb is "20, 40, 60," referring to the percentage of the body weight that is constituted by extracellular (ECW), intracellular (ICW), and total body water (TBW), respectively (see Table 1-3). The plasma has a very slightly higher osmolality than the intracellular and interstitial compartments; this small difference can be ignored when dealing with problems of fluid balance.**

intraocular, pleural, peritoneal, and synovial fluids, and the digestive secretions. Unlike interstitial fluid, the transcellular spaces are separated from the blood not only by capillary endothelium but also by epithelium. Except in special circumstances, such as loss of gastrointestinal fluid, the transcellular compartment may be neglected in experimental and clinical problems of fluid balance; the same holds true for the water that is contained in bone (3% of body weight) and in dense connective tissue (4% of body weight).

Relationship of Tissue Water to Tissue Volume

The terms *intracellular, interstitial,* and *plasma "water"* are commonly used interchangeably with the corresponding "fluid" or "volume." Although this is not accurate, in most instances it is permissible for practical purposes, since the vast proportion of each compartment is water. Water constitutes about 92% of the plasma compartment, while for most intracellular spaces the value is 75 to 80%. Bone cells and fat cells, with about 25% and 20% of water, respectively, are notable exceptions.

Measuring the Size of Compartments

TOTAL BODY WATER. These measurements all involve the simple principle of dilution, usually of a substance that can be measured colorimetrically, or of a radioactively labeled compound. For example, TBW can be estimated with a drug, antipyrine, which distributes itself quickly throughout all the major fluid compartments, or with heavy water, D_2O, or tritiated water, HTO. The following is an illustration using tritiated water.

An adult woman who weighs 60 kg is given exactly 1 millicurie (mCi) of HTO intravenously. On the basis of prior experiments in humans, it is known that within 2 hours after the injection, this labeled water will have come into equilibrium with interstitial and intracellular water, and that by this time about 0.4% of the administered dose will have been lost from the internal environment, mainly via the urine. At this time, therefore, a plasma sample is withdrawn and its radioactivity measured by liquid scintillation; it is found to be 0.031 mCi per liter of plasma water. From the relationship:

$$\text{Concentration} = \frac{\text{Amount}}{\text{Volume}} \qquad (2\text{-}1)$$

and knowing that the concentration of HTO in the major compartments will be the same as in plasma, the TBW will therefore be:

$$\frac{0.031 \text{ mCi}}{1{,}000 \text{ ml plasma water}} = \frac{1 \text{ mCi} - (1 \cdot 0.004)}{\text{TBW}}$$

TBW = 32,129 ml, or approximately 32 liters. Thus, the general equation for measuring a volume by the dilution principle is:

$$\frac{\text{Volume of}}{\text{compartment}} = \frac{\text{Amount of substance X given minus}}{\text{Amount of X lost from compartment}} \over \text{Concentration of X in the compartment} \qquad (2\text{-}2)$$

The final volume has been deliberately stated as "approximately" 32 liters because the method may yield an estimate that is high by perhaps 1 liter. The discrepancy arises mainly from exchange of the isotope with hydrogen atoms of organic molecules.

EXTRACELLULAR WATER. The substances and equations used to measure the size of the various compartments are summarized in Table 2-1. There is no ideal test substance for estimating ECW because all substances that diffuse freely from the vascular into the interstitial compartment also in small part penetrate cells; for example, chloride ions enter erythrocytes and are secreted as gastric juice, two losses that are difficult to quantify.

PLASMA. This compartment is measured by the dilution of substances that distribute themselves almost exclusively within the plasma. Radioiodinated serum albumin falls short of the ideal substance in that some albumin crosses the capillary endothe-

Table 2-1 : Substances and equations used to
measure the size of the major body fluid compartments.

Compartment	Substance	Equation
TBW	Antipyrine D_2O HTO	2-2
ECW	Inulin Raffinose Sucrose Mannitol Thiosulfate Radiosulfate Thiocyanate Radiochloride Radiosodium Radiobromide	2-2
Plasma	^{131}I-albumin Evans blue, or T-1824 ^{51}Cr-erythrocytes	2-2
Interstitial	Not measured directly	Interstitial = ECW − Plasma
ICW	Not measured directly	ICW = TBW − ECW

lium into the interstitial space. The same shortcoming applies to the dye known as Evans blue (T-1824), which is bound to serum albumin and thus has the same volume of distribution as the protein. Tagged erythrocytes yield a slightly inaccurate result because erythrocytes do not distribute themselves evenly throughout the plasma; the hematocrit (i.e., the ratio of the volume of blood cells to that of whole blood) is less in fine, peripheral vessels than it is in large, major vessels.

INTERSTITIAL AND INTRACELLULAR WATER. These volumes are not measured directly because there are no known substances that distribute themselves exclusively within these compartments. They are thus calculated as the difference between two compartments that were measured by the dilution technique. The formulas are given in Table 2-1; their derivation is self-evident, or can be deduced from Figure 2-1.

BODY WEIGHT. In many circumstances, changes in body weight provide the most accurate estimate of a change in TBW. As has been mentioned, the measurement of TBW by the dilution technique involves an error of about 1,000 ml in an adult human. The body weight can be determined much more accurately, simply, and cheaply. And in an experimental animal or patient who is eating adequately, an acute (up to 72 hours) change in body weight will be due almost solely to a change in TBW. Of course, this measurement cannot tell us which of the body fluid compartments has lost or gained water, but this additional information can often be surmised from the history of an illness or experimental situation.

The usefulness of measuring body weight in the field of fluid and solute balance cannot be overemphasized. Too many physicians tend to forget that this simple measure frequently yields more accurate and immediate information than do the cumbersome and expensive dilution methods.

Composition of the Compartments

The main solute constituents of the major body fluid compartments are shown in Figure 2-2. Note that these compartments are made up primarily of electrolytes. Although the conveyance by these fluids of nutrients and waste products such as glucose, amino acids, and urea is very important, the nonelectrolytes constitute only a small portion of the total solute.

The concentrations have been expressed as chemical equivalents. Although there is an electrical potential difference (P.D.) at the interface between the compartments (see Gibbs-Donnan Equilibrium, below), the separation of charges is confined to the immediate area of the interface and involves only a minute fraction of the total number of ions. Hence, the bulk of the fluid within a compartment is electrically neutral. The total number of equivalents varies, however, from one compartment to another. As Figure 2-2 shows, this difference is due to the variation in the concentration of proteins. At the pH of body fluids, proteins have multiple negative charges per molecule. Hence intracellular fluid, being relatively rich in proteins, has more total charges than does extracellular fluid. The same explanation applies to the greater total equivalents in plasma as opposed to interstitial fluid.

Sodium is by far the most abundant cation of vertebrate extracellular fluid, and chloride and bicarbonate are the most abundant anions. In contrast, potassium is the most plentiful intracellular cation, and organic phosphates and proteins are the major anions. The similarity in composition between plasma and interstitial fluid is striking, and is explained by the fact that these two compartments are separated by a semipermeable membrane, the capillary endothelium, which allows free diffusion of solutes of low molecular weight (often referred to as "crystalloids").

Explanation for Differences in Composition

The main difference between plasma and interstitial fluid is in the concentration of proteins, which are largely excluded from the interstitial compartment by the capillary endothelium. In conformity with the Gibbs-Donnan relationship (see below), there is a difference of about 5% in the concentrations of diffusible ions between the two compartments. The concentrations of cations

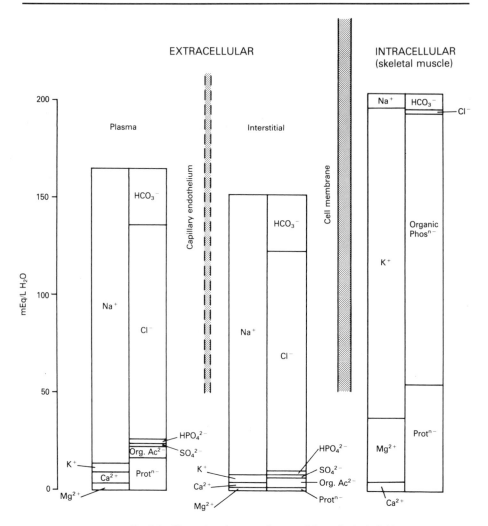

Fig. 2-2 : The main solute constituents of the major body fluid compartments. The concentrations are expressed as chemical equivalents to emphasize that the compartments are made up mainly of electrolytes, and that within any one space the total number of negative charges is neutralized by the positive charges.

The values depicted for intracellular fluid are rough approximations at best. They reflect current estimates for skeletal muscle, but since some cells have unique composition, these estimates are not precisely representative of all intracellular fluid. Furthermore, there is now some evidence that the composition may vary among subcellular compartments, such as the mitochondria, the nucleus, and the cytoplasm. The extent to which some intracellular ions are bound or ionized is not known, so that the equivalences for such ions, as well as for organic phosphates and proteins, are also approximations. Despite these limitations, however, the diagram serves to emphasize important and typical differences between intracellular and extracellular fluid. Organic phosphates include AMP, ADP, and ATP, glycerophosphate, and creatine phosphate. Slightly modified from Gamble, J. L. *Chemical Anatomy, Physiology and Pathology of Extracellular Fluid* (6th ed.). Cambridge: Harvard University Press, 1954.

are slightly greater in plasma than they are in the interstitial fluid; the concentrations of diffusible anions are slightly smaller in plasma than they are in the interstitial fluid. Thus, the differences in composition between plasma and interstitial fluid can be accounted for almost entirely by the unequal distribution of proteins and the resultant Gibbs-Donnan equilibrium. Binding of certain cations, such as calcium and magnesium, to proteins makes a further, small contribution to the differences.

The intracellular compartment is separated from interstitial fluid by the cell membrane (Fig. 2-2). This barrier, unlike the endothelium, has selective permeabilities not only for proteins but also for certain other ions such as the organic phosphates. In addition, the membrane of most cells has a "pump" or pumps that extrude sodium from the cells and move potassium into them. Net movement of these ions across the membrane is called "active" because it requires energy; for example, when a cellular system is exposed to a metabolic poison such as dinitrophenol (DNP), the cells gain sodium and lose potassium (Fig. 2-6). Of course, since most of the intracellular anions are barred from interstitial fluid by the cell membrane, the Gibbs-Donnan effect also applies, and may largely account for the low intracellular concentrations of bicarbonate and chloride. Finally, there is probably considerable binding of certain ions to intracellular proteins and phosphates. Thus, the striking compositional differences between extracellular and intracellular fluids result from the combined effects of selective permeabilities, metabolic pumps, Gibbs-Donnan forces, and ion-binding.

Osmolality in the Major Compartments

It has been shown by a number of experimental techniques that the osmolality of interstitial fluid is equal to that of intracellular fluid (Fig. 2-1). It should be noted that this fact is not in conflict with the differences in total equivalents depicted in Figure 2-2. Osmolality is a function of the *number* of discrete particles in solution (Chap. 7). Thus, a single atom of sodium contributes as much to the osmolality of a solution as does a single molecule of protein, even though the latter weighs perhaps 3,000 times more than the former. But at the pH of body fluids, each molecule of protein contributes several charges to the total equivalence, whereas each atom of sodium contributes only one charge. If the interstitial and intracellular concentrations in Figure 2-2 were expressed as millimoles per liter of H_2O and the colligative properties of each component such as NaCl or $NaHCO_3$ were taken into account (see Answer to Problem 1-2), the resulting osmolalities in the interstitial and intracellular compartments would be equal, as is shown in Figure 2-1.

The osmolality of plasma is very slightly higher than that of interstitial and intracellular fluid. This difference has not been demonstrated directly, since neither interstitial nor intracellular fluid can be sampled; however, according to the Gibbs-Donnan equilibrium (see below), the difference must exist. Its magnitude is not known; it may amount to perhaps 1 mOsm per kilogram H_2O (equivalent to 19 mm Hg hydrostatic pressure), and it can be ignored when dealing with experimental or clinical problems of fluid balance. That is, in solving such problems one treats the plasma *as if* it were in osmotic equilibrium with interstitial and intracellular fluid (see Problem 2-3). This simplification does not introduce serious errors.

Gibbs-Donnan Equilibrium

This equilibrium explains the unequal distribution of diffusible ions on the two sides of a semipermeable membrane if one side contains a nondiffusible or poorly diffusible ion. Let us first consider the initial situation illustrated in Figure 2-3, in which compartments 1 and 2 are separated by a rigid membrane that is permeable to Na^+ and Cl^- but impermeable to protein, Pr^-. The rate at which either diffusible ion moves across the membrane will depend on the frequency with which it collides with the membrane, and that frequency is proportional to the concentration of the ion on each side of the membrane. Since the *difference* in concentration is initially greater for Cl^- than for Na^+, the rate of net movement of Cl^- from compartment 2 to compartment 1 will momentarily exceed that of Na^+. And since Pr^- cannot move across the membrane, a negative charge will be built up at the interface of the membrane. This electrostatic force will enhance the rate of net transfer of Na^+ from compartment 2 to compartment 1, so that in effect the rate of diffusion of both diffusible ions from compartment 2 to compartment 1 will be equal. Furthermore, this electrostatic force permits the buildup of Na^+ in compartment 1 against its concentration gradient, as the

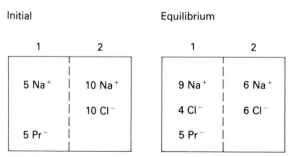

Fig. 2-3 : The attainment of a Gibbs-Donnan equilibrium. The schema assumes that the volumes of compartments 1 and 2 remain constant. Modified from Pitts, R. F. *Physiology of the Kidney and Body Fluids* (3rd ed.). Chicago: Year Book, 1974.

system approaches equilibrium. The work required to move one equivalent of Na^+ up its concentration gradient but down the electrical potential gradient is shown in Equation 2-3:

$$W = R \cdot T \cdot \log \frac{[Na^+]_1}{[Na^+]_2} - F \cdot E \qquad (2\text{-}3)$$

where
$$\begin{aligned}
W &= \text{work} \\
R &= \text{gas constant} \\
T &= \text{absolute temperature} \\
[Na^+]_1 \text{ and } [Na^+]_2 &= \text{concentrations of } Na^+ \text{ in} \\
&\quad \text{compartments 1 and 2, respectively} \\
F &= \text{Faraday} \\
E &= \text{electrical potential difference between} \\
&\quad \text{the compartments}
\end{aligned}$$

The work required to move Cl^- down its concentration gradient but against the electrical potential gradient will be

$$W = R \cdot T \cdot \log \frac{[Cl^-]_1}{[Cl^-]_2} + F \cdot E \qquad (2\text{-}4)$$

At equilibrium, by definition, no net work is performed by the system; hence, the sum of Equations 2-3 and 2-4 must be zero, and

$$\frac{[Na^+]_1}{[Na^+]_2} = \frac{[Cl^-]_2}{[Cl^-]_1} \qquad (2\text{-}5)$$

The equilibrium conditions of the Gibbs-Donnan effect can now be understood, and they are illustrated in Figure 2-3. (1) At equilibrium, the product of the concentrations of diffusible ions in one compartment will equal the product of the same ions in the other compartment (9 · 4 in compartment 1, and 6 · 6 in compartment 2). (2) Within each compartment the total cationic charges must equal the total anionic charges (9 of each in compartment 1; 6 in compartment 2). This requirement for electroneutrality is not in conflict with the existence of a small electrical P.D. across the membrane which, as noted earlier in this chapter, is confined to the interface and involves an insignificant fraction of the ions. (3) The concentration of diffusible cations will be greater in the compartment containing the nondiffusible, negatively charged protein than in the other compartment; and the concentration of diffusible anions will be less in compartment 1 than in compartment 2. (4) The osmolality will be greater in the compartment containing the protein (18 particles per equal volume) than in the other compartment (12 particles). The difference is due not only to the contained protein but also to the fact that the sum of the diffusible ions on the side containing the protein (9 + 4) is greater than the sum of these ions on the other side (6 + 6). The total difference in osmotic pressure that is due to the Gibbs-Donnan effect is known as the *oncotic pressure.*

These conditions hold also for the body fluid compartments, and apply to each of the diffusible ions within them. For example, each compartment is electrically neutral, and diffusible cations such as Na^+ are slightly more concentrated in plasma than in interstitial fluid, whereas the opposite is true of diffusible anions, such as Cl^- (Fig. 2-2). As has been noted, however, the osmolality of the intracellular compartment is actually the same as the interstitial osmolality, mainly because Na^+ is actively removed from cells.

Maintenance of Compartment Size

Importance of Total Solute Content

It follows from Equation 2-1 that for any given solute concentration, the volume or size of a compartment will be a direct function of the total amount of solute within it. The volumes of the main extracellular compartments, plasma and interstitium, depend primarily on the amount of Na^+ and its attendant anions (mainly Cl^- and HCO_3^-) in the body, since these constitute 90 to 95% of the total osmotically active particles in extracellular fluid. Although by weight the plasma proteins have a high plasma concentration — about 70 g per liter — they contribute less than 1% to the total osmolality of plasma.

The effect of adding NaCl to the body is shown in Figure 2-4. Depicted at the top is the distribution of total body water in a healthy adult human, as it was summarized in Figure 2-1. A solution containing 0.9 g of NaCl per 100 ml of solution is then infused intravenously, i.e., into the plasma compartment; this solution has an osmolality of nearly 290 mOsm per kilogram H_2O (see Answer to Problem 1-2). Since the capillary endothelium is highly permeable to Na^+, Cl^-, and H_2O, the infused solution is quickly distributed not only throughout the plasma, but also throughout the interstitial fluid. Although Na^+ will momentarily enter the intracellular space, it will be quickly "pumped out." Thus, there will be no gain or loss of Na^+ from the intracellular space, and since Cl^- follows Na^+, there will be no net change in Cl^-; that is, the solute and hence the H_2O that were added intravenously will be excluded from the intracellular space and will be distributed evenly throughout the extracellular compartment. Accordingly, to the extent that none of the added NaCl solution is lost from the body, the extracellular compartment will be expanded by 2 liters, and the infused solution will be distributed between plasma and interstitial fluid in proportion to their sizes prior to the infusion. Since the infused solution had about the

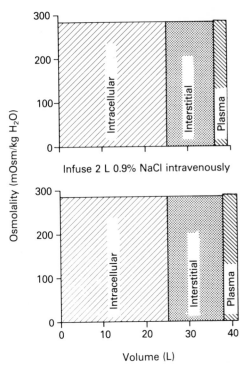

Fig. 2-4 : The effect of an intravenous infusion of NaCl having an osmolality about equal to that of plasma (so-called isotonic saline), on the volume and osmolal concentration of the body fluids. Note that there was no change in the osmolality of any compartment, and that the increase in volume involved only the plasma and interstitial compartments.

same osmolality as the body fluids, there will be virtually no change in the total solute concentration of extracellular fluid and hence no osmotic flow of water in or out of the intracellular compartment.

Maintenance of Plasma and Interstitial Volumes

THE STARLING HYPOTHESIS. Because of the Gibbs-Donnan effect, the plasma has a slightly higher osmolality than does the interstitial fluid. Nevertheless, in the steady (equilibrium) state, the size of each compartment is stable. This is so because the movement of water between the two compartments is governed not solely by osmotic differences but by a balance of all pressures, i.e., of the oncotic and hydrostatic pressures in both compartments.

The forces that determine fluid exchange across the capillary endothelium were outlined by Ernest Starling in 1896. This formulation, known as the Starling hypothesis, is illustrated in Figure 2-5. The major force promoting filtration of fluid out of the capillary into the interstitium is the hydrostatic pressure within the capillaries. This pressure declines along the course of the capillary. A small amount of protein leaks out of the capillaries. Although most of this is returned to the systemic circulation via

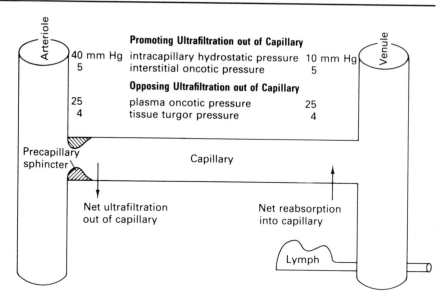

Fig. 2-5 : The Starling hypothesis of fluid exchange between plasma and interstitium. The four factors that determine this exchange are known as "Starling forces."

the lymph channels, some remains, giving rise to a small interstitial oncotic pressure of perhaps 5 mm Hg, which also promotes filtration out of the capillary. These two forces are opposed mainly by the plasma oncotic pressure and a small amount of pressure that is due to the turgidity of the interstitium. The balance of these forces is such that there is net filtration of fluid out of the capillary along slightly more than one-half of the length of the capillary, and net reabsorption of fluid into the capillary as it approaches the venule. The slight excess of fluid that is filtered into the interstitium is returned to the systemic plasma by the lymph channels, so that in the steady state the volumes of the two compartments, plasma and interstitium, remain constant.

Although the principle of opposing forces outlined in Figure 2-5 is correct, it is possible that the main mechanism that ordinarily alters intracapillary hydrostatic pressure is not the resistance along the length of the capillary but rather the activity of the precapillary sphincters. When these relax, hydrostatic pressure throughout the capillary may be sufficiently high to promote net outward filtration along its entire length; when they contract, hydrostatic pressure may be so low that only reabsorption of fluid into the capillary occurs. Furthermore, the rate of fluid flow, $\dot{q}$, across the capillary endothelium is a function not only of the Starling forces, but also of a filtration coefficient, K_f. Equation 2-6 expresses the total relationship:

$$\dot{q} = K_f [(P_c - P_t) - (\pi_p - \pi_t)] \tag{2-6}$$

where $\dot{q}$ = rate of fluid movement across the capillary wall
K_f = the filtration coefficient
P_c = hydrostatic pressure within the capillary
P_t = the tissue turgor pressure
π_p = the plasma oncotic pressure
π_t = the interstitial oncotic pressure

The filtration coefficient is proportional to the total surface area of capillaries, as well as to capillary permeability per unit of surface area. When precapillary sphincters contract, many capillaries are actually shut off from the arterial circulation, so that total capillary surface area is reduced; relaxation of the sphincters during the vasodilator phase has the opposite effect. Thus, activity of the precapillary sphincters, so-called vasomotion, governs fluid flow across the capillary endothelium (Eq. 2-6) by its effect both on the intracapillary hydrostatic pressure, P_c, and on the filtration coefficient, K_f. The balance between the vasodilator and vasoconstrictor phases is such that the net return of fluid to plasma equals its net egress from this compartment (the return via the lymphatics making a very minor contribution).

The above description applies mainly to H_2O, which moves from capillary into interstitium by so-called bulk flow. Solutes, such as glucose and amino acids, move more by diffusion through the aqueous channels of the endothelium than by bulk flow with H_2O. In contrast, lipid-soluble substances, such as O_2 and CO_2, can diffuse across the entire capillary wall, which is made up overwhelmingly of lipids.

EDEMA. Abnormal expansion of the interstitial fluid compartment, known as edema, is one of the most common findings in clinical medicine. It is divided into two forms: *localized* and *generalized*. Localized edema can be explained by changes in one or more variables of Equation 2-6, that lead to an increase in $\dot{q}$. Examples include: inflammation, because an increased vasodilator phase raises both P_c and K_f; obstruction of lymphatic channels, because failure to return proteins to the systemic circulation raises π_t and lowers π_p; and venous obstruction, because of a rise in P_c. Generalized edema, which is seen commonly in cardiac, hepatic, and renal failure, has a more complicated pathogenesis. It probably involves decreased urinary excretion of Na^+, retention of this ion, and expansion of the entire extracellular fluid volume, as follows (at a constant plasma Na^+ concentration) from Equation 2-1.

Maintenance of
Intracellular Volume

Why do cells that have a high oncotic pressure and are freely permeable to water not swell and burst? As noted earlier, the

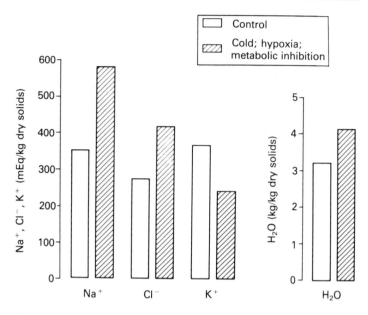

Fig. 2-6 : Effect of depriving cells of metabolic energy, on their content of Na^+, Cl^-, K^+, and H_2O. The heavy intracellular solutes (i.e., proteins) did not change in this experiment. Hence, expressing the data per unit of dry weight makes it possible to interpret the results as content of the measured substances per approximately equal number of cells. Note that during metabolic inhibition, the loss of K^+ is less than the gains in Na^+ and Cl^-; this net entry of solute is followed by movement of H_2O into cells. The example is from cells of the renal cortex, which do not have the extremely low Na^+ and Cl^- concentrations and the high K^+ concentrations that skeletal muscle cells have (see Fig. 2-2). But even in renal cortical cells, the concentrations of these ions differ greatly from those in extracellular fluid. Data from Leaf, A. *Am. J. Med.* 49:291, 1970.

reason is that the distribution of Na^+ between the intracellular and interstitial compartments is not governed simply by the Gibbs-Donnan forces; rather, Na^+ is actively pumped out of cells. That this process requires metabolic energy is shown in Figure 2-6. When cells are deprived of such energy, as by exposing them to cold, or hypoxia, or metabolic inhibitors, they gain Na^+ and Cl^-, and with these solutes, water; that is, when the higher oncotic pressure of intracellular fluid is not opposed by the additional force of active Na^+ movement into the interstitium, cells do in fact swell and frequently burst. The fact that intracellular K^+ decreases when the cell is deprived of energy constitutes part of the evidence that the relatively high intracellular concentration of K^+ in control conditions is to some degree maintained by an active pump.

More than one-third of the metabolic energy of most cells is expended in transporting Na^+, thereby maintaining cellular volume. The question might well be asked why such an inefficient system has been invoked when the simpler expedient of a rigid, thick cellular membrane that excludes Na^+ from the cell interior might solve the problem as well. As was the case for general renal function (Chap. 1), so once again the answer probably lies in evolutionary selection, in this instance for a system that allowed great mobility, and that therefore required pliable cells with a large surface area to permit rapid diffusion of metabolic substrates.

Summary

Total body water, which comprises from 50 to 70% of the body weight, is distributed among three major compartments: (a) intracellular; (b) plasma; and (c) interstitial. The last two are the major subdivisions of extracellular fluid. Each compartment has a characteristic and stable size and composition. Sodium and its attendant anions are the major solutes in extracellular fluid. The main difference between plasma and interstitial fluid is the higher protein content in the former. The relative impermeability of the capillary endothelium to protein sets up a Gibbs-Donnan effect, which accounts for the slight differences in distribution of diffusible ions between plasma and interstitial fluid.

Organic phosphates and proteins are the major anions in most cells, and potassium is the main intracellular cation. The characteristic composition of intracellular fluid results from selective impermeabilities mainly for organic phosphates and proteins, the resulting Gibbs-Donnan equilibrium, binding to nondiffusible compounds, and active transport of sodium out of cells and potassium into them.

The volume of each compartment is fixed by the total solute within it. The steady size of the plasma and interstitial compartments is determined by the balance of Starling forces: (a) intracapillary hydrostatic pressure and (b) interstitial oncotic pressure favoring fluid movement out of the capillary, and (c) plasma oncotic pressure and (d) tissue turgor pressure favoring movement of fluid in the opposite direction.

Active "pumping" of sodium out of cells offsets the oncotic pressure of nondiffusible organic phosphates and proteins, and thereby ordinarily prevents swelling and bursting of cells.

Problem 2-1

A woman weighing 60 kg is given 10 mg of T-1824 dye (Evans blue) intravenously. Ten minutes later, a blood sample is obtained from another vein, and colorimetric analysis of the plasma shows the presence of 0.4 mg of T-1824 per 100 ml of plasma.

Assume that the administered dye was evenly distributed throughout the plasma compartment by the end of the 10 minutes, and that no dye was lost from the plasma during this interval; then calculate the woman's plasma volume.

If the blood corpuscles, mainly erythrocytes, constituted 45% of whole blood — i.e., if the woman's hematocrit ratio is 0.45 — what is her total blood volume?

Problem 2-2

A man weighing 75 kg is given, intravenously, 99.8 g of D_2O (i.e., 100 ml of a 99.8% solution of D_2O) and 100 μCi of radiosulfate (^{35}S-sulfate). Twenty minutes after injection, a blood sample is drawn and treated to obtain a protein-free filtrate of plasma. A second blood sample is drawn 2 hours after the injection and similarly treated. Exactly 1 ml of the first filtrate is found to contain 0.0064 μCi of radiosulfate. The water of the second filtrate is found to contain 0.2 g D_2O per 100 ml of filtrate.

Assume: (a) that 4% of the injected radiosulfate was lost in the urine during the first 20 minutes; (b) that 0.4% of the administered D_2O was lost during the 2 hours; (c) that no other losses of these two substances occurred; and (d) that radiosulfate and D_2O were evenly distributed throughout their compartments after 20 minutes and 2 hours, respectively.

Calculate: (a) total body water, (b) extracellular fluid volume, and (c) intracellular fluid volume.

Problem 2-3

Figure 2-7 is an adaptation of Figure 2-1 in that it combines the plasma and interstitial space into a single extracellular compartment. Given the fact that water moves freely among the body

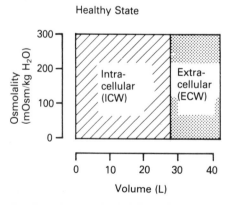

Healthy State

Fig. 2-7 : Volume and osmolality of the major body fluid compartments in an adult human who weighs 70 kg. In this figure, the plasma and the interstitial space have been combined into the single extracellular compartment (ECW). This simplification is often employed in the experimental or clinical analysis of fluid balance. ICW = intracellular compartment.

fluid compartments and that, at equilibrium, the compartments are in osmotic equilibrium, predict the changes in both the volume and osmolality of the intracellular compartment (ICW) and the extracellular compartment (ECW) that would occur with the following perturbations once a new steady state had been established: (a) a loss of isosmotic fluid, as might occur in very severe diarrhea; (b) a loss of "pure" H_2O (i.e., of H_2O without solute), as might occur in a person lost in the desert who is not sweating; (c) a loss of NaCl without a net loss of H_2O, as might occur in a patient with adrenal insufficiency; (d) a gain of isosmotic fluid, as in generalized edema; (e) a gain of NaCl without a net gain of H_2O, as in a person who suddenly goes on a very high salt diet; and (f) a gain of pure H_2O, as in the syndrome of inappropriate ADH secretion (SIADH). (*Hint:* For an approach to this problem, see the analysis of Figure 2-4.)

Selected References

General

Bernard, C. *Leçons sur les Phénomènes de la Vie Communs aux Animaux et aux Végétaux,* vol. 1. Paris: Baillière, 1878.

Boulpaep, E. L. (Guest Ed.). Cellular mechanisms of renal tubular ion transport. *Curr. Top. Membr. Transp.* 13:1, 1980.
The first section of this symposium contains authoritative articles on the ion activity and elemental composition of intraepithelial compartments, as determined by ion selective microelectrodes and electron microprobe analysis.

Conway, E. J. Nature and significance of concentration relations of potassium and sodium ions in skeletal muscle. *Physiol. Rev.* 37:84, 1957.

Dick, D. A. T. *Cell Water.* Washington, D.C.: Butterworth, 1966.

Edelman, I. S., and Leibman, J. Anatomy of body water and electrolytes. *Am. J. Med.* 27:256, 1959.

Edelman, I. S., Liebman, J., O'Meara, M. P., and Birkenfeld, L. W. Interrelations between serum sodium concentration, serum osmolarity and total exchangeable sodium, total exchangeable potassium and total body water. *J. Clin. Invest.* 37:1236, 1958.

Frizzell, R. A. (Chairman). Symposium on probes of cellular composition in epithelia. *Fed. Proc.* 39:2849, 1980.

Gamble, J. L. *Chemical Anatomy, Physiology and Pathology of Extracellular Fluid* (6th ed.). Cambridge: Harvard University Press, 1954.

Hays, R. M. Dynamics of Body Water and Electrolytes. In M. H. Maxwell and C. R. Kleeman (Eds.), *Clinical Disorders of Fluid and Electrolyte Metabolism* (3rd ed.). New York: McGraw-Hill, 1980.

Lechene, C. P. Electron probe microanalysis: Its present, its future. *Am. J. Physiol.* 232 (Renal Fluid Electrolyte Physiol. 1):F391, 1977.

Lockwood, A. P. M. *Animal Body Fluids and Their Regulation.* Cambridge: Harvard University Press, 1966.

Maffly, R. H. The Body Fluids: Volume, Composition, and Physical Chemistry. In B. M. Brenner and F. C. Rector, Jr. (Eds.), *The Kidney* (2nd ed.). Philadelphia: Saunders, 1981.
A very lucid exposition of the principles discussed in this chapter, and at a more detailed level.

Manery, J. F. Water and electrolyte metabolism. *Physiol. Rev.* 34:334, 1954.

Maxwell, M. H., and Kleeman, C. R. (Eds.). *Clinical Disorders of Fluid and Electrolyte Metabolism* (3rd ed.). New York: McGraw-Hill, 1980.

Moore, F. D. *Metabolic Care of the Surgical Patient.* Philadelphia: Saunders, 1959.

Moore, F. D., Oleson, K. H., McMurrey, J. D., Parker, H. V., Ball, M. R., and Boyden, C. M. *The Body Cell Mass and Its Supporting Environment. Body Composition in Health and Disease.* Philadelphia: Saunders, 1963.

Peters, J. P. *Body Water: The Exchange of Fluids in Man.* Springfield, Ill.: Thomas, 1935.

Rose, B. D. *Clinical Physiology of Acid-Base and Electrolyte Disorders.* New York: McGraw-Hill, 1977.

Schmidt-Nielsen, K. *Desert Animals: Physiological Problems of Heat and Water.* London: Oxford University Press, 1964.

Strauss, M. B. *Body Water in Man: The Acquisition and Maintenance of the Body Fluids.* Boston: Little, Brown, 1957.

Walker, J. L., and Brown, H. M. Intracellular ionic activity measurements in nerve and muscle. *Physiol. Rev.* 57:729, 1977.

Welt, L. G. *Clinical Disorders of Hydration and Acid-Base Equilibrium* (2nd ed.). Boston: Little, Brown, 1959.

Widdowson, E. M., and Dickerson, J. W. T. Chemical Composition of the Body. In C. L. Comar and F. Bronner (Eds.), *Mineral Metabolism,* vol. II, part A. New York: Academic, 1964.

Evolution

Macallum, A. B. The paleochemistry of the body fluids and tissues. *Physiol. Rev.* 6:316, 1926.

Maffly, R. H. The Body Fluids: Volume, Composition, and Physical Chemistry. In B. M. Brenner and F. C. Rector, Jr. (Eds.), *The Kidney* (2nd ed.). Philadelphia: Saunders, 1981.

Robertson, J. D. The habitat of the early vertebrates. *Biol. Rev.* 32:156, 1957.

Measurement of
Compartment Size

Brown, E., Hopper, J., Jr., Hodges, J. L., Jr., Bradley, B., Wennesland, R., and Yamauchi, H. Red cell, plasma, and blood volume in healthy women measured by radiochromium cell-labeling and hematocrit. *J. Clin. Invest.* 41:2182, 1962.

Deane, N. Methods of Study of Body Water Compartments. In A. C. Corcoran (Ed.), *Methods in Medical Research,* vol. V. Chicago: Year Book, 1952.

Gaudino, M., and Levitt, M. F. Inulin space as a measure of extracellular fluid. *Am. J. Physiol.* 157:387, 1949.

Moore, F. D., Olesen, K. H., McMurrey, J. D., Parker, H. V., Ball, M. R., and Boyden, C. M. *The Body Cell Mass and Its Supporting Environment. Body Composition in Health and Disease.* Philadelphia: Saunders, 1963.

Schloerb, P. R., Friis-Hansen, B. J., Edelman, I. S., Solomon, A. K., and Moore, F. D. The measurement of total body water in the human subject by deuterium oxide dilution. *J. Clin. Invest.* 29:1296, 1950.

Schultz, A. L., Hammarsten, J. F., Heller, B. I., and Ebert, R. V. A critical comparison of the T-1824 dye and iodinated albumin methods for plasma volume measurement. *J. Clin. Invest.* 32:107, 1953.

Schwartz, I. L., Schachter, D., and Freinkel, N. The measurement of extracellular fluid in man by means of a constant infusion technique. *J. Clin. Invest.* 28:1117, 1949.

Sterling, K., and Gray, S. J. Determination of the circulating red cell volume in man by radioactive chromium. *J. Clin. Invest.* 29:1614, 1950.

Walser, M., Seldin, D. W., and Grollman, A. An evaluation of radiosulfate for the determination of the volume of extracellular fluid in man and dogs. *J. Clin. Invest.* 32:299, 1953.

Zweens, J., Frankena, H., Reichter, A., and Zijlstra, W. G. Infrared-spectrometric determination of D$_2$O in biological fluids. Reappraisal of the method and application to the measurement of total body water and daily water turnover in the dog. *Pflügers Arch. Eur. J. Physiol.* 385:71, 1980.

Regulation of Compartment Size

Ames, A., III, Wright, L., Kowada, M., Thurston, J. M., and Majno, G. Cerebral ischemia: II. The no-reflow phenomenon. *Am. J. Pathol.* 52:437, 1968.

Andreoli, T. E., Grantham, J. J., and Rector, F. C., Jr. (Eds.). *Disturbances in Body Fluid Osmolality.* Bethesda: American Physiological Society, 1977.
Chapters 10 and 11 of this very useful book apply especially to the topics of this chapter.

Appleboom, J. W. T., Brodsky, W. A., Tuttle, W. S., and Diamond, I. The freezing point depression of mammalian tissues after sudden heating in boiling distilled water. *J. Gen. Physiol.* 41:1153, 1958.

Covey, C. M., and Arieff, A. I. Disorders of Sodium and Water Metabolism and Their Effects on the Central Nervous System. In B. M. Brenner and J. H. Stein (Eds.), *Contemporary Issues in Nephrology.* New York: Churchill Livingstone, 1978. Vol. 1, p. 212.

Crone, C., and Christensen, O. Transcapillary transport of small solutes and water. *Int. Rev. Physiol.* 18:149, 1979.

Darrow, D. C., and Yannet, H. The changes in the distribution of body water accompanying increase and decrease in extracellular electrolyte. *J. Clin. Invest.* 14:266, 1935.

Guyton, A. C., Granger, H. J., and Taylor, A. E. Interstitial fluid pressure. *Physiol. Rev.* 51:527, 1971.

Krogh, A. *Osmotic Regulation in Aquatic Animals.* Cambridge: University Press, 1939. (Reprinted unabridged and unaltered by Dover Publications, New York, 1965.)

Landis, E. M. The passage of fluid through the capillary wall. *Harvey Lect.* 32:70, 1936.

Leaf, A., and Macknight, A. D. C. Ischemia and Disturbances in Cell Volume Regulation. In T. E. Andreoli, J. E. Hoffman, and D. D. Fanestil (Eds.), *Physiology of Membrane Disorders.* New York: Plenum, 1978.

Macknight, A. D. C., and Leaf, A. Regulation of cellular volume. *Physiol. Rev.* 57:510, 1977.

Mudge, G. H. Studies on potassium accumulation by rabbit kidney slices: Effect of metabolic activity. *Am. J. Physiol.* 165:113, 1951.

Pappenheimer, J. R. Passage of molecules through capillary walls. *Physiol. Rev.* 33:387, 1953.

Parving, H.-H., Hansen, J. M., Nielsen, S. L., Rossing, N., Munck, O., and Lassen, N. A. Mechanisms of edema formation in myxedema — increased protein extravasation and relatively slow lymphatic drainage. *N. Engl. J. Med.* 301:460, 1979.

Starling, E. H. On the absorption of fluids from the connective tissue spaces. *J. Physiol.* (Lond.) 19:312, 1896.

Starling, E. H. *The Fluids of the Body.* Chicago: Keener, 1909.

Tosteson, D. C., and Hoffman, J. F. Regulation of cell volume by active cation transport in high and low potassium sheep red cells. *J. Gen. Physiol.* 44:169, 1960.

Valtin, H. *Renal Dysfunction: Mechanisms Involved in Fluid and Solute Imbalance.* Boston: Little, Brown, 1979. Chap. 3 on edema.

Zweifach, B. W., and Silberberg, A. The interstitial-lymphatic flow system. *Int. Rev. Physiol.* 18:215, 1979.

3 : Glomerular Filtration

Ultrafiltration

This process occurs at the glomeruli and is filtration under pressure through the permselective glomerular capillary wall. Ultrafiltration separates the plasma water and its nonprotein constituents (often referred to as crystalloids), which enter Bowman's space, from the blood cells and protein macromolecules (the colloids), which stay in the blood. The process is thus qualitatively the same as that occurring in systemic capillaries, although, as we shall see, the two are quantitatively different.

Proof for ultrafiltration by glomeruli was first obtained in 1921 by J. T. Wearn and A. N. Richards, through the technique of micropuncture. They succeeded in collecting fluid from Bowman's space by means of a tiny micropipet having a tip diameter of 7 to 15 μm. The collected fluid contained no protein as measured by methods then available (actually, small amounts of protein are filtered and then reabsorbed), and it had approximately the same composition as plasma in respect to osmolality, electrical conductivity (i.e., total concentration of electrolytes), glucose and other solutes, and pH. Furthermore, the distribution of diffusible electrolytes between glomerular capillary plasma and fluid in Bowman's space conformed to the Gibbs-Donnan relationship. The early results were obtained in amphibians (frog and *Necturus*), and they have since been confirmed in rodents, dogs, primates, and other species.

Forces Involved in Glomerular Ultrafiltration

These are the so-called Starling forces, which were reviewed for systemic capillaries in conjunction with Figure 2-5. Those pertaining to mammalian glomeruli are shown in Figure 3-1. There are several differences. (1) Hydrostatic pressure remains relatively constant in glomerular capillaries, whereas it declines markedly along the length of extrarenal capillaries. (2) Glomerular capillaries are probably less permeable to proteins than systemic capillaries. Hence, the oncotic pressure in Bowman's space is lower than interstitial oncotic pressure. (3) In contrast to the plasma oncotic pressure in systemic capillaries, which stays relatively constant, that in glomerular capillaries rises along the length of the capillary. (4) The hydrostatic pressure in Bowman's space is considerably higher than its systemic analogue, the tis-

44

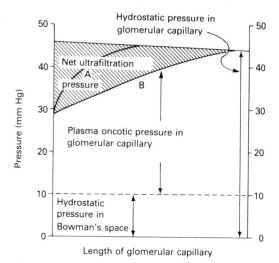

Balance of Mean Values
_____

Hydrostatic pressure in glomerular capillary	45 mm Hg
Hydrostatic pressure in Bowman's space	10
Plasma oncotic pressure in glomerular capillary	27
Oncotic pressure of fluid in Bowman's space	0*
Net ultrafiltration pressure	8 mm Hg

Fig. 3-1 : Starling forces involved in glomerular ultrafiltration in rats (specific values vary with species). As shown, ultrafiltration pressure declines in glomerular capillaries, mainly because plasma oncotic pressure rises. This is in contrast to extrarenal capillaries, in which the decline in ultrafiltration pressure is due mainly to a decrease in intracapillary hydrostatic pressure (see Fig. 2-5). It is not yet known at what point in the capillary the sum of the hydrostatic pressure in Bowman's space and of plasma oncotic pressure exactly balances the hydrostatic pressure in the glomerular capillary. In some species such as dog or man, this point, called *filtration equilibrium,* may not be reached. In those species in which it is attained, the pattern for the rise in plasma oncotic pressure as a function of capillary length is not known precisely, and it can vary. For example, an increase in the rate at which plasma enters the glomerular capillary will lead to a change in the pattern from curve A to curve B, and consequently to a rise in the mean net ultrafiltration pressure. Data from Brenner, B. M., Troy, J. L., and Daugharty, T. M. *J. Clin. Invest.* 50:1776, 1971.

*The concentration of protein in Bowman's space fluid is negligibly small; the estimated oncotic pressure is perhaps 0.3 mm Hg.

sue turgor pressure. Nevertheless, the balance of the forces is such that the mean net ultrafiltration pressure is only slightly higher in glomerular capillaries (Fig. 3-1) than in extrarenal capillaries (Fig. 2-5). In the latter, net ultrafiltration pressure declines because capillary hydrostatic pressure decreases, whereas in glomerular capillaries, net ultrafiltration pressure declines mainly because plasma oncotic pressure increases. Furthermore, in glomerular capillaries, net movement of fluid is primarily or solely out of the capillaries, whereas in systemic capillaries the change in the balance of Starling forces is such that net movement out of the vessels is nearly balanced by net return of fluid into the vessels.

Even though the mean net ultrafiltration pressure (i.e., the balance of the Starling forces) is similar in glomerular and extrarenal capillaries, the transtubular movement of fluid out of glomerular capillaries, the so-called glomerular filtration rate (GFR), far exceeds the analogous flow, $\dot{q}$ of Equation 2-6, in extrarenal capillaries. Hence K_f, the filtration coefficient, must be much larger for glomerular capillaries. As defined in Chapter 2, K_f is a function of total capillary surface area as well as of the permeability per unit of surface area. Both factors are probably involved in raising the K_f of glomerular capillaries. Total glomerular capillary area has been estimated to be from 5,000 to 15,000 cm^2 per 100 g of renal tissue. In contrast, this area is perhaps 7,000 cm^2 per 100 g of skeletal muscle. In addition, per unit of surface area, glomerular capillaries may be at least 100 times more permeable to water and crystalloids than muscle capillaries.

There is one other determinant of glomerular ultrafiltration, at least in some species, and that is the rate at which plasma flows through the capillaries. Other things being equal, the greater the rate at which plasma enters the glomerular capillaries (the so-called initial glomerular plasma-flow rate), the greater will be the rate at which it is filtered into Bowman's space. The reason is that, under these circumstances, the plasma oncotic pressure rises more slowly (as in a shift from curve A to curve B in Figure 3-1), so that the shaded area, which represents the net ultrafiltration pressure, increases. By this means, the net ultrafiltration pressure can vary from 4 mm Hg to 12 mm Hg. Thus, the glomerular plasma-flow rate ultimately exerts its influence through one of the Starling forces, π_p in Equation 2-6, and hence through a change in the mean net ultrafiltration pressure (Fig. 3-1). [The influence of glomerular plasma flow on GFR is most marked when *filtration equilibrium* obtains (see legend to Fig. 3-1); thus, it may not be an important determinant in dog and man. In any case, the Starling forces, not the rate of glomerular plasma flow, are quantitatively the most important determinants of glomerular ultrafiltration in most instances.]

Characteristics of the Glomerular Capillary

The fact that K_f is much greater in glomerular than in systemic capillaries suggests that the glomerular capillary differs from other capillaries, such as those of skeletal muscle. Both glomerular and extrarenal capillaries permit free passage of small molecules such as water (2 Å diameter), urea (3.2 Å diameter), sodium (4 Å diameter), chloride (3.5 Å diameter), and glucose (7 Å diameter); but they do not permit free passage of larger particles such as erythrocytes (80,000 Å diameter) or large plasma

Capillary loops   Bowman's space

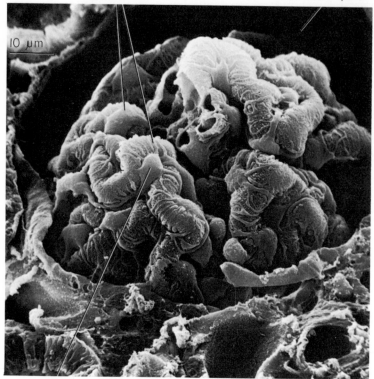

10 μm

Podocyte

A

Fig. 3-2 : Scanning electron micrographs of (A) a glomerulus, magnified about 1,440 times, and (B) a loop of a glomerular capillary, magnified about 7,200 times. An electron micrograph (× 36,000) of a glomerular capillary, viewed in longitudinal section, is shown in (C); the portion on the left indicates the distribution of negative charges in the glomerular capillary wall. Photomicrographs (A) and (B) from Spinelli, F., Wirz, H., and Brücher, C. *Fine Structure of the Kidney Revealed by Scanning Electron-Microscopy.* Basel: Ciba-Geigy, 1972. The electron micrograph (C) was kindly supplied by C. C. Tisher.

proteins. The limits of glomerular capillary permeability are suggested by the fact that hemoglobin (65 Å diameter), as well as smaller plasma proteins such as albumin (36 by 150 Å), are not freely filtered but do get through the membrane in small amounts. In other words, the glomerular capillary behaves as if it were a filtering membrane containing aqueous "pores" with a diameter of 75 to 100 Å.

Given these functional characteristics, anatomists have examined the wall of the glomerular capillary, to see if it contained a structure with fenestrations of the required dimensions. The wall (Fig. 3-2C) consists of three layers: (a) endothelium, (b) basement membrane, and (c) epithelium (podocytes with foot processes).

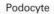

Podocyte

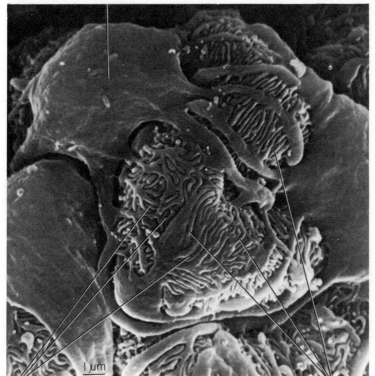

1 μm

Filtration slits

Foot processes

B

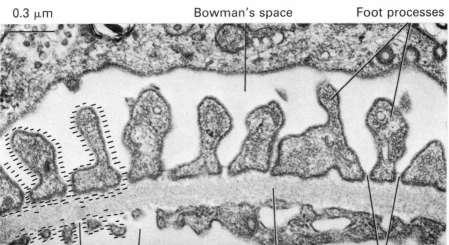

0.3 μm

Bowman's space

Foot processes

Pore in endothelium

Capillary lumen

Basement membrane

Filtration slits

C

The endothelium appears to contain holes with a diameter of 500 to 1,000 Å. Most investigators believe that these apertures, unlike those of other fenestrated capillaries, are not bridged by diaphragms. The glomerular endothelium, therefore, appears to be freely permeable even to large molecules. The basement membrane consists of three filamentous layers (lamina rara interna, lamina densa, and lamina rara externa); the first and third of these layers are fused with the endothelium and epithelium, respectively. Many workers consider the basement membrane to be the restrictive layer, often referred to as the *filtration barrier.* The epithelium consists of highly specialized cells called podocytes, which are attached to the basement membrane by foot processes known as pedicels. Adjacent pedicels are separated by filtration slits measuring about 250 to 600 Å in width, and each gap is bridged by a thin diaphragm. The diaphragms, in turn, contain rectangular "pores" having dimensions of 40 by 140 Å. Thus, the filtration slits with their diaphragms could also constitute the filtration barrier, and some investigators favor this view.

The above deductions are based simply on the size of apertures, which is not the only factor that limits passage of compounds through the glomerular capillary wall. The shape of a molecule (not just its diameter), its flexibility and deformability, and perhaps especially its charge also play important roles. The effect of the last is shown in Fig. 3-3. Dextrans are polysaccharides that can be produced in a range of molecular weights and hence sizes, as well as in an electrically neutral form or with net negative charges (polyanionic dextrans) or net positive charges (poly-

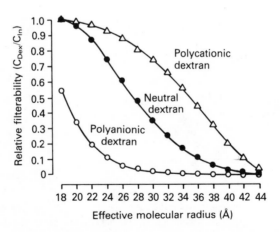

Fig. 3-3 : Influence of electrical charge of a molecule on the filterability of that molecule through the glomerular capillary wall of rats. At any given molecular size, negatively charged dextrans traverse the filtration barrier less readily than do neutral dextrans or, in turn, than do positively charged dextrans. Slightly modified from Bohrer, M. P., et al. *J. Clin. Invest.* 61:72, 1978.

cationic dextrans). At any given effective molecular radius, the dextrans with positive charges pass more readily through the glomerular filter than do neutral dextrans; and negatively charged dextrans encounter even greater hindrance than do neutral dextrans (Fig. 3-3). This selective filterability is explained by the presence of negatively charged glycoproteins (called *glycosialoproteins*) on the surface of all components of the glomerular capillary wall (see left portion of Fig. 3-2C), especially on the endothelium, the lamina rara interna and lamina rara externa of the basement membrane, and the podocytes and foot processes, including the diaphragms in the filtration slits. In other words, the glomerular capillary wall, in addition to discriminating on the basis of size, also acts as an electrostatic barrier.

Although there is not yet consensus on all aspects of the nature of the glomerular filtration barrier, the following is a working model that many workers favor. The endothelium acts as a valve that screens out cells and controls access to the main filter, which is the basement membrane. The epithelium monitors this main filter by phagocytizing macromolecules that have leaked through the filter. There are also mesangial cells, which abut the capillary loops and which are thought to recondition and unclog the filter, and possibly to influence the size and number of fenestrations (and hence K_f) through contractile properties.

Finally, the concept of straight or permanent anatomical pores as such may be naive. The functional characteristics of glomerular capillaries could be accounted for as well if the restrictive barrier were a hydrated gel, with the interstices between glycosialoprotein polymers constituting the channels through which water and crystalloids flow. Whatever the true picture, it does seem clear that the higher transmural filtration rate of glomerular as opposed to extrarenal capillaries is due to a combination of a much greater permeability for water and crystalloids per unit of surface area, a larger capillary surface area per unit of tissue, and a slightly higher mean net ultrafiltration pressure.

Measurement of Glomerular Filtration Rate (GFR)

The quantity of plasma filtered by the glomeruli can be determined by the clearance of inulin, a starch-like polymer of fructose having a molecular weight of about 5,000 (see Table 1-5). It is a foreign substance and must be infused intravenously during the clearance test. Since it is not bound to plasma proteins, has a diameter of about 30 Å, and is not charged, it passes readily through the glomerular capillary membrane. In addition, it is neither reabsorbed nor secreted by renal tubules.

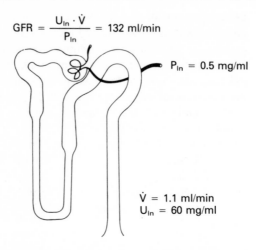

$$GFR = \frac{U_{In} \cdot \dot{V}}{P_{In}} = 132 \text{ ml/min}$$

$P_{In} = 0.5 \text{ mg/ml}$

$\dot{V} = 1.1 \text{ ml/min}$
$U_{In} = 60 \text{ mg/ml}$

Fig. 3-4 : The principle of measuring the glomerular filtration rate (GFR) by means of the inulin clearance. In this figure, the single nephron represents all nephrons from both kidneys of an adult human.

In Figure 3-4, both kidneys of a normal adult human are represented by a single nephron. The principle for measuring GFR by the clearance technique is illustrated by the following steps.

1. Measure the rate of urine flow, $\dot{V}$; $\dot{V}$ = 1.1 ml/min.
2. Measure the concentration of inulin in the urine, U_{In}; U_{In} = 60 mg/ml.
3. Calculate the amount of inulin excreted in the urine per minute.

$$U_{In} \cdot \dot{V} = \frac{60 \text{ mg}}{\text{ml}} \cdot \frac{1.1 \text{ ml}}{\text{min}} = 66 \text{ mg/min}$$

4. If: (a) all inulin reaching the urine got there by filtration, and
   (b) inulin was not reabsorbed from the tubular lumen, and
   (c) inulin was not secreted into the tubular lumen, and
   (d) the plasma concentration of inulin, P_{In}, was 0.5 mg/ml;
   i.e., if each milliliter of plasma contained 0.5 mg of inulin, how many milliliters of plasma must have been filtered in order to excrete 66 mg of inulin?

$$66 \text{ mg} \div \frac{0.5 \text{ mg}}{\text{ml}} = 132 \text{ ml}$$

5. Since 66 mg of inulin was excreted per minute, 132 ml of plasma must have been filtered each minute.

$$\frac{66 \text{ mg}}{\text{min}} \div \frac{0.5 \text{ mg}}{\text{ml}} = \frac{66 \text{ mg}}{\text{min}} \cdot \frac{\text{ml}}{0.5 \text{ mg}} = 132 \text{ ml/min}$$

Thus, during each minute, 132 ml of plasma was separated by ultrafiltration from the blood flowing through the glomerular capillaries. This measurement of the GFR is called the *inulin clearance,* C_{In}, for which the formula is $U_{In} \cdot \dot{V}/P_{In}$. It is defined as the volume of plasma from which, in 1 minute's time, the kidneys remove all inulin.

There is another, intuitive derivation of the formula. The amount of inulin that is filtered into Bowman's space each minute (called the *filtered load of inulin*) is the product of the plasma concentration of inulin and the GFR: $P_{In} \cdot GFR$. The amount of inulin excreted each minute is the product of the urinary concentration of inulin and the urine flow: $U_{In} \cdot \dot{V}$. Since inulin, once deposited in Bowman's space, is neither reabsorbed by the tubules nor secreted by them, the filtered load of inulin is equal to its urinary excretion:

$$P_{In} \cdot GFR = U_{In} \cdot \dot{V}$$

$$\therefore GFR = \frac{U_{In} \cdot \dot{V}}{P_{In}}$$

Several features of this measurement should be noted. (1) The formula for all renal clearances (except the free-water clearance, see Chap. 8) is $U \cdot \dot{V}/P$, where U is the concentration of a given substance in the urine, $\dot{V}$ is the urine flow, and P is the concentration of the same substance in the plasma. *The clearance technique is not confined to the measurement of GFR;* it can be and is applied to many substances besides inulin. (2) *Plasma,* not urine, is being cleared of a given substance, in this case inulin. The units for the inulin clearance refer to the milliliters of *plasma* from which all inulin has been removed. (3) The inulin clearance is independent of the plasma inulin concentration; as P_{In} increases, more inulin will be filtered so that U_{In} will rise in direct proportion to the increase in P_{In} (Fig. 3-4). (4) The inulin clearance is independent of the urine flow; for a given quantity of inulin in the urine, U_{In} will fall proportionately as $\dot{V}$ rises, and vice versa. Points (3) and (4) are illustrated in Problem 3-1, at the end of this chapter.

Concept of Filtration Fraction

Not all the plasma that flows through the glomerular capillaries can be filtered into Bowman's space. This would be an obvious impossibility, for it would require the movement of all plasma out of the capillaries, leaving behind a solid mass of cells and colloids that could not move on into the efferent arterioles. As is shown in Figure 3-1, long before this state is reached, filtration stops because the sum of the hydrostatic pressure in Bowman's space plus the rising plasma oncotic pressure equals the hydrostatic pressure in the glomerular capillaries. Normally, only about one-fifth of the plasma entering the glomerular capillaries is filtered; this is called the *filtration fraction,* the definition and derivation of which are given in Chapter 5.

Inulin: Neither Reabsorbed nor Secreted

Use of the inulin clearance as a measure of GFR is valid only if all the inulin that appears in the urine got there by filtration, i.e., only if inulin is neither reabsorbed nor secreted by the renal tubules. Proof that these conditions are met was obtained through a number of micropuncture experiments, one of which is shown in Figure 3-5. A proximal tubule of a rat was punctured at E from the surface of the kidney, and a column of oil, C, was injected via a micropipet in order to block the tubular lumen. This pipet was then withdrawn, leaving an opening at E through which newly formed glomerular filtrate could escape. A second pipet, A, was then inserted distal to the oil column, and a green dye was injected. This dye traversed the remainder of the proximal tubule and the loop of Henle, and reappeared on the surface of the kidney in the distal tubule belonging to this single nephron. A third pipet, B, was then inserted into the distal segment, and the remainder of the tubule was blocked with a second oil column, D.

A known amount of inulin was now infused into the proximal

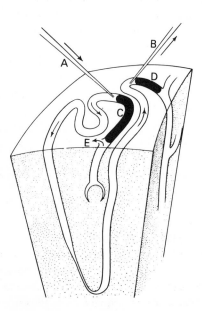

Fig. 3-5 : A micropuncture experiment in a rat kidney. The symbols, as well as the rationale of the experiment, are explained in the text. The arrows indicate the direction of flow of tubular fluid. From Marsh, D., and Frasier, C. *Am. J. Physiol.* 209:283, 1965. Published with permission.

segment through pipet A at the same time that all fluid perfusing that nephron was collected through pipet B. The fact that 99.3% of the injected inulin could be thus recovered strongly suggests that inulin was not reabsorbed. Furthermore, the rate of recovery was the same when the peritubular plasma was loaded with inulin; hence secretion of inulin was also excluded. Finally when oil block D was not present, virtually all the inulin microinjected into the proximal tubule could be recovered in the ureteral urine. Thus, inulin is neither reabsorbed nor secreted in any portion of the nephron.

OTHER SUBSTANCES. There are substances besides inulin that are also freely filtered but neither reabsorbed nor secreted by the renal tubules. Hence such substances, too, can be used to measure GFR; examples include creatinine, vitamin B_{12}, and iothalamate. Some substances meet the criteria in one species but not in others. For example, under physiological conditions, creatinine is neither reabsorbed nor secreted in the dog, and is therefore equal to the inulin clearance. In man, however, the creatinine clearance is slightly higher than the GFR because the renal tubules secrete a small amount of creatinine. The identity of the inulin and creatinine clearances in a dog under physiological conditions is illustrated by the calculations given in Problem 3-2 at the end of this chapter.

Clearance as a General Concept

It was emphasized above that the clearance concept is not restricted to the determination of GFR. One can measure the renal clearance of any substance, and the comparison of that clearance to that of inulin has important functional implications. For example, if, during any given time interval, less plasma is cleared of urea (a small molecule that is freely filterable) than is cleared of inulin, one can deduce that there must have been net reabsorption of urea in its course through the tubular system. (A quantitative example of this deduction is given in the Answers to Problems 4-1 and 8-1 at the end of the text.) Conversely, if, during a given time interval, more plasma is cleared of a substance than is cleared of inulin, that substance must have been added to the urine by an additional process besides glomerular filtration; that process, called tubular secretion, is discussed in Chapter 5.

Finally, it should be stressed that *the clearance concept is by no means restricted to renal function.* One can measure the rates at which the lungs, or the liver, or other organs remove a given substance from plasma; or one can determine the so-called total, or "whole-body," clearance, which represents the sum of the various regional clearances. Such applications of the clearance concept are commonly used in the study of drug or hormone metabolism.

Meaning of TF/P and U/P for Inulin

Not only is inulin freely filtered; it is also a nonelectrolyte and therefore not subject to a Gibbs-Donnan effect. Hence, the concentration of inulin in Bowman's capsule fluid (TF_{In} = inulin concentration in tubular fluid) will be identical to that in plasma, P_{In}. The ratio of the concentration of inulin in Bowman's capsule fluid to that in plasma, referred to as the TF/P inulin, will therefore equal 1. Since inulin is neither reabsorbed from nor secreted into the tubular lumen, its concentration in tubular fluid increases as water is reabsorbed from the various tubular segments; in fact, the concentration of inulin in the tubular fluid will be solely a function of the amount of water reabsorbed up to the point at which the tubule is punctured and a microsample is withdrawn.

For example, if the concentration of inulin in tubular fluid withdrawn from the proximal tubule is twice as great as that in Bowman's space (i.e., twice as great as P_{In}, which is equal to TF_{In} in Bowman's space), it is obvious that 50% of the filtered water must have been reabsorbed. Hence, a TF/P inulin of 2 reflects reabsorption of one-half of the filtered water, and the formula for calculating this fraction is given in Equation 3-1:

$$\text{Fraction of filtered water reabsorbed up to point of micropuncture} = 1 - \frac{1}{\text{TF/P inulin}}$$

$$= 1 - \frac{1}{2} \quad (3\text{-}1)$$

$$= 0.5, \text{ or } 50\%$$

Micropuncture samples withdrawn from the very last segment of a proximal tubule at the surface of the kidney have inulin concentrations that are nearly 3 times greater than the concentration in plasma; that is, TF/P inulin approaches 3, and the fraction of filtered water reabsorbed would be 0.67. This, in fact, constitutes some of the experimental evidence that roughly two-thirds, or 67%, of the filtered fluid is normally reabsorbed in the proximal tubule.

By similar reasoning, the U/P inulin (the ratio of the concentration of inulin in the urine to its concentration in plasma) can be used to calculate the fraction of filtrate reabsorbed in both kidneys, as given in Equation (3-2):

$$\text{Fraction of filtered water reabsorbed by both kidneys} = 1 - \frac{1}{\text{U/P inulin}} \quad (3\text{-}2)$$

In the example given in Figure 3-4, $1 - \frac{1}{120} = 0.992$; i.e., 99.2% of the filtered water was reabsorbed. This point can be verified independently by calculating that the urine flow of 1.1 ml per minute constitutes 0.8% of the amount of fluid filtered, 132 ml per minute. Expressing this point mathematically, and thereby deriving Equation 3-2:

$$\text{Fraction of filtered water excreted} = \frac{\dot{V}}{\text{GFR}}$$

$$= \frac{\dot{V}}{\text{Inulin clearance}}$$

$$= \dot{V} \div \frac{U_{In} \cdot \dot{V}}{P_{In}}$$

$$= \frac{\dot{V}}{1} \cdot \frac{P_{In}}{U_{In} \cdot \dot{V}}$$

$$= \frac{P_{In}}{U_{In}}$$

$$\text{Fraction of filtered water reabsorbed} = 1 - \frac{P_{In}}{U_{In}}$$

$$= 1 - \frac{1}{\text{U/P inulin}} \qquad (3\text{-}2)$$

Note that Equations 3-1 and 3-2 permit one to quantify important aspects about the renal handling of water without actually measuring water flow; all that is needed is the concentration of inulin in tubular fluid and plasma or in urine and plasma, respectively. This fact provides an important advantage, for it obviates the often difficult task of accurately measuring the urine flow or the even more exacting chore of measuring the flow rate of tubular fluid. This simplification can be extended to gauge the renal handling of any other substance through determination of the *clearance ratio.* (For an explanation, see footnote b in Problem 4-1; and for a quantitative example, see Problem 6-1.)

Summary

The initial step in the formation of urine is ultrafiltration of plasma in the glomerular capillaries, which act as permselective filters that discriminate on the basis of molecular size, shape, deformability, and charge. The rate of ultrafiltration is governed by: (a) the balance of Starling forces; (b) the permeability of the glomerular capillary wall to water and small solutes; (c) the total surface area of the capillaries; and (d) the rate at which plasma flows into the glomerular capillaries. The first three factors, especially point (b), are greater in glomerular than in most extrarenal capillaries; hence, the rate of glomerular filtration (GFR) far exceeds analogous movement of fluid across walls of most systemic capillaries.

The GFR can be measured by the inulin clearance, which is defined as the volume of plasma from which, in a minute's time, the kidneys remove all inulin. Normally, about one-fifth of the plasma that flows through the glomerular capillaries is filtered into Bowman's space.

Since inulin, once filtered, is neither reabsorbed from nor secreted into the tubular lumen, the degree to which it is concentrated in tubular fluid will be solely a function of the amount of filtered water that is reabsorbed. Normally, about 70% of the filtered water is reabsorbed in the proximal tubules, and more than 99% is reabsorbed by the entire tubular system of both kidneys.

Problem 3-1 Sample calculations illustrating the independence of the inulin clearance from the plasma concentration of inulin and from the rate of urine flow in a dog. Utilizing the data given, calculate the inulin clearances; indicate the units for clearance.

Urine Flow (ml/min)	Inulin Concentration		Inulin Clearance ( )
	Plasma (mg/ml)	Urine (mg/ml)	
1.2	0.9	45	
1.3	1.4	68	
1.0	2.3	141	
1.4	3.8	168	
1.2	5.7	294	
1.3	0.5	23	
2.1	0.6	17	
3.1	0.4	8	
5.7	0.5	5	
6.6	0.5	4.6	

Modified from Shannon, J. A. *Am. J. Physiol.* 112:405, 1935.

Problem 3-2 Sample calculations illustrating the identity of the inulin and creatinine clearances in a dog under physiological conditions. Utilizing the data given, calculate the inulin and creatinine clearances; supply the units for clearance.

Urine Flow (ml/min)	Inulin			Creatinine		
	Plasma (mg/100 ml)	Urine (mg/100 ml)	Clearance ( )	Plasma (mg/100 ml)	Urine (mg/100 ml)	Clearance ( )
1.0	104	5,076		13.7	673	
1.1	106	4,601		14.7	630	
0.9	108	6,017		16.0	890	
1.0	109	5,137		16.6	792	

Modified from Shannon, J. A. *Am. J. Physiol.* 112:405, 1935.

$$\frac{1 \times 5076}{104}$$

Problem 3-3

In the steady (or equilibrium) state, an organism is in balance, which means that the output of a given substance is equal to the input of that substance. The principle of the steady state is well illustrated in the attainment of balance for inulin as this compound is infused into a subject for the measurement of the GFR. (Although the inulin clearance is seldom used to determine GFR in patients, the principle of balance when applied to urea and endogenous creatinine is so utilized.)

In the study for which data are given in Table 3-1, inulin was infused into the antecubital vein of a healthy human subject whose GFR is 120 ml per minute. The inulin was infused at a steady rate of 72 mg per minute, and periodically blood was withdrawn for determination of the plasma inulin concentration, P_{In}.

1. Fill in the blank column in Table 3-1. *Hint:* Knowing the properties of inulin and how it is handled by the kidneys, you can do the required calculations even though the urinary concentration of inulin and the urine flow are not given.
2. Why does the plasma concentration of inulin increase? At what point will it stop rising?
3. At what point is the steady state reached?
4. Is there a self-contradiction in saying that this person, with a GFR of 120 ml per minute, is healthy when a normal GFR was earlier stated to be 132 ml per minute (Fig. 3-4)?

Table 3-1 : Attainment of a steady state for inulin during a stable intravenous infusion of inulin in a healthy adult human.

Elapsed Time (min)	Rate of Inulin Infusion (mg/min)	GFR (ml/min)	P_{In} (mg/ml)	Urinary Excretion of Inulin (mg/min)
1	72	120	0.005	
5	72	120	0.02	
10	72	120	0.05	
50	72	120	0.24	
100	72	120	0.47	
110	72	120	0.6	
120	72	120	0.6	

Selected References

The Process of Ultrafiltration

Brenner, B. M., Ichikawa, I., and Deen, W. M. Glomerular Filtration. In B. M. Brenner and F. C. Rector, Jr. (Eds.), *The Kidney* (2nd ed.). Philadelphia: Saunders, 1981.

Ichikawa, I., and Brenner, B. M. Of unglazed pottery and glomerular sieving. *Kidney Int.* 10:264, 1976.

Pappenheimer, J. R. Passage of molecules through capillary walls. *Physiol. Rev.* 33:387, 1953.

Pappenheimer, J. R., Renkin, E. M., and Borrero, L. M. Filtration, diffusion and molecular sieving through peripheral capillary membranes: A contribution to the pore theory of capillary permeability. *Am. J. Physiol.* 167:13, 1951.

Physiology Society. Functional and structural determinants of glomerular filtration. A Physiology Society Symposium, chaired by B. M. Brenner. *Fed. Proc.* 36:2599, 1977.
This compilation contains useful articles on the dynamics of glomerular ultrafiltration in rats and dogs and on the structural characteristics of the glomerular filtration barrier.

Richards, A. N. Urine formation in the amphibian kidney. *Harvey Lect.* 30:93, 1935.

Walker, A., Bott, P., Oliver, J., and MacDowell, M. The collection and analysis of fluid from single nephrons of the mammalian kidney. *Am. J. Physiol.* 134:580, 1941.

Wearn, J. T., and Richards, A. N. Observations on the composition of glomerular urine, with particular reference to the problem of reabsorption in the renal tubules. *Am. J. Physiol.* 71:209, 1924.

Forces Determining Glomerular Ultrafiltration

Arendshorst, W. J., and Gottschalk, C. W. Glomerular ultrafiltration dynamics: Euvolemic and plasma volume-expanded rats. *Am. J. Physiol.* 239 (Renal Fluid Electrolyte Physiol. 8):F171, 1980.

Blantz, R. C. The Role of Alterations of the Ultrafiltration Coefficient in the Control of Glomerular Filtrate Formation. In G. H. Giebisch and E. F. Purcell (Eds.), *Renal Function.* New York: Josiah Macy, Jr. Foundation, 1978.

Brenner, B. M., Deen, W. M., and Robertson, C. R. The physiological basis of glomerular ultrafiltration. *Int. Rev. Physiol.* 6:335, 1974.

Brenner, B. M., and Humes, H. D. Mechanics of glomerular ultrafiltration. *N. Engl. J. Med.* 297:148, 1977.

Brenner, B. M., Troy, J. L., Daugharty, T. M., Deen, W. M., and Robertson, C. R. Dynamics of glomerular ultrafiltration in the rat: II. Plasma-flow dependence of GFR. *Am. J. Physiol.* 223:1184, 1972.

Knox, F. G., Marchand, G. R., Osswald, H., Spielman, W. S., and Youngberg, S. P. Regulation of Glomerular Filtration Rate in the Dog. In H. G. Vogel and K. J. Ullrich (Eds.), *New Aspects of Renal Function.* Amsterdam: Excerpta Medica, 1978.

Navar, L. G. The Regulation of Glomerular Filtration Rate in Mammalian Kidneys. In T. E. Andreoli, J. F. Hoffman, and D. D. Fanestil (Eds.), *Physiology of Membrane Disorders.* New York: Plenum, 1978. Chap. 31.

Renkin, E. M., and Gilmore, J. P. Glomerular Filtration. In J. Orloff and R. W. Berliner (Eds.), *Handbook of Physiology,* section 8, Renal Physiology. Washington, D.C.: American Physiological Society, 1973.

Schnermann, J. The Role of the Juxtaglomerular Apparatus in Single Nephron Function. In H. G. Vogel and K. J. Ullrich (Eds.), *New Aspects of Renal Function.* Amsterdam, Excerpta Medica, 1978.
The so-called feedback control of the filtration rate in single glomeruli (sGFR) is discussed in Chapter 6. Other references on this interesting topic, in addition to this article and the review by Wright and Briggs, are cited in Chapter 6.

Wright, F. S., and Briggs, J. P. Feedback control of glomerular blood flow, pressure and filtration rate. *Physiol. Rev.* 59:958, 1979.

Measurement of GFR

Austin, J. H., Stillman, E., and van Slyke, D. D. Factors governing the excretion rate of urea. *J. Biol. Chem.* 46:91, 1921.

Edwards, B. R., and Stern, P. Renal clearances of ^{14}C-inulin and polyfructosan in the rat: Effect of increased ureteral pressure. *Pflügers Arch. Eur. J. Physiol.* 369:281, 1977.

Giebisch, G. (Ed.). Symposium on renal micropuncture techniques. *Yale J. Biol. Med.* 45:187, 1972.
Section I of this symposium, entitled "Micropuncture Collection Techniques and Measurement of Single Nephron GFR," gives definitive discussions of the technical aspects of measuring the glomerular filtration rates of single nephrons.

Gutman, Y., Gottschalk, C. W., and Lassiter, W. E. Micropuncture study of inulin absorption in the rat. *Science* 147:753, 1965.

Jolliffe, N., Shannon, J. A., and Smith, H. W. The excretion of urine in the dog: III. The use of non-metabolized sugars in the measurement of the glomerular filtrate. *Am. J. Physiol.* 100:301, 1932.

Marsh, D., and Frasier, C. Reliability of inulin for measuring volume flow in rat renal cortical tubules. *Am. J. Physiol.* 209:283, 1965.

Mertz, D. P., and Sarre, H. Polyfructosan-S: Eine neue inulin-artige Substanz zur Bestimmung des Glomerulusfiltrates und des physiologisch aktiven extrazellulären Flüssigkeitsvolumens beim Menschen. *Klin. Wochenschr.* 41:868, 1963.

Nelps, W. B., Wagner, H. N., Jr., and Reba, R. C. Renal excretion of vitamin B_{12} and its use in measurement of glomerular filtration rate in man. *J. Lab. Clin. Med.* 63:480, 1964.

O'Connell, J. M. B., Romeo, J. A., and Mudge, G. H. Renal tubular secretion of creatinine in the dog. *Am. J. Physiol.* 203:985, 1962.

Rehberg, P. B. Studies on kidney function: I. The rate of filtration and reabsorption in the human kidney. *Biochem. J.* 20:447, 1926.

Rosenbaum, R. W., Hruska, K. A., Anderson, C., Robson, A. M., Slatopolsky, E., and Klahr, S. Inulin: An inadequate marker of glomerular filtration rate in kidney donors and transplant recipients? *Kidney Int.* 16:179, 1979.

Shannon, J. A. The excretion of inulin by the dog. *Am. J. Physiol.* 112:405, 1935.

Tanner, G. A., and Klose, R. M. Micropuncture study of inulin reabsorption in *Necturus* kidney. *Am. J. Physiol.* 211:1036, 1966.

Clearance Concept

Austin, J. H., Stillman, E., and van Slyke, D. D. Factors governing the excretion rate of urea. *J. Biol. Chem.* 46:91, 1921.

Lauson, H. D. Metabolism of antidiuretic hormones. *Am. J. Med.* 42:713, 1967.

Schwartz, I. L., Breed, E. S., and Maxwell, M. H. Comparison of the volume of distribution, renal and extrarenal clearances of inulin and mannitol in man. *J. Clin. Invest.* 29:517, 1950.

Smith, H. W. *The Kidney: Structure and Function in Health and Disease.* New York: Oxford University Press, 1951.

Characteristics of Glomerular Capillaries

Boylan, J. W., and Van Liew, J. B. (Eds.). Proteinuria. *Kidney Int.* 16:247, 1979.
This very useful symposium considers basic mechanisms of the renal handling of proteins in both health and disease.

Brenner, B. M., Bohrer, M. P., Baylis, C., and Deen, W. M. Determinants of glomerular permselectivity: Insights derived from observations in vivo. *Kidney Int.* 12:229, 1977.

Farquhar, M. G. The primary glomerular filtration barrier — basement membrane or epithelial slits? *Kidney Int.* 8:197, 1975.

Hunsicker, L. G., Shearer, T. P., and Shaffer, S. J. Acute reversible proteinuria induced by infusion of the polycation hexadimethrine. *Kidney Int.* 20:7, 1981.

Karnovsky, M. J. The ultrastructure of glomerular filtration. *Annu. Rev. Med.* 30:213, 1979.

Latta, H. Ultrastructure of the Glomerulus and Juxtaglomerular Apparatus. In J. Orloff and R. W. Berliner (Eds.), *Handbook of Physiology,* section 8, Renal Physiology. Washington, D.C.: American Physiological Society, 1973.

Latta, H., Johnston, W. H., and Stanley, T. M. Sialoglycoproteins and filtration barriers in the glomerular capillary wall. *J. Ultrastruct. Res.* 51:354, 1975.

Rennke, H. G., Cotran, R. S., and Venkatachalam, M. A. Role of molecular charge in glomerular permeability. Tracer studies with cationized ferritins. *J. Cell Biol.* 67:638, 1975.

Rennke, H. G., and Venkatachalam, M. A. Glomerular permeability of macromolecules. Effect of molecular configuration on the fractional clearance of uncharged dextran and neutral horseradish peroxidase in the rat. *J. Clin. Invest.* 63:713, 1979.

Tisher, C. C. Glomerular Morphology and Its Relationship to Glomerular Filtration. In G. H. Giebisch and E. F. Purcell (Eds.), *Renal Function.* New York: Josiah Macy, Jr. Foundation, 1978.

Venkatachalam, M. A., and Rennke, H. G. The structural and molecular basis of glomerular filtration. *Circ. Res.* 43:337, 1978.

Filtration Rate in Single Nephrons (sGFR)

Note: Additional references are cited at the end of Chapter 6, under Autoregulation and Tubuloglomerular Feedback.

de Rouffignac, C., Deiss, S., and Bonvalet, J. P. Détermination du taux individuel de filtration glomérulaire des néphrons accessibles et inaccessibles à la microponction. *Pflügers Arch. Eur. J. Physiol.* 315:273, 1970.

Giebisch, G. (Ed.). Symposium on renal micropuncture techniques. *Yale J. Biol. Med.* 45:187, 1972.
Section I of this symposium is entitled "Micropuncture Collection Techniques and Measurement of Single Nephron GFR."

Hanssen, O. E. The relationship between glomerular filtration and length of the proximal convoluted tubules in mice. *Acta Pathol. Microbiol. Scand.* 53:265, 1961.

Horster, M., and Thurau, K. Micropuncture studies on the filtration rate of single superficial and juxtamedullary glomeruli in the rat kidney. *Pflügers Arch.* 301:162, 1968.

Jamison, R. L. Micropuncture study of superficial and juxtamedullary nephrons in the rat. *Am. J. Physiol.* 218:46, 1970.

Trinh-Trang-Tan, M.-M., Diaz, M., Grünfeld, J.-P., and Bankir, L. ADH-dependent nephron heterogeneity in rats with hereditary hypothalamic diabetes insipidus. *Am. J. Physiol.* 240 (Renal Fluid Electrolyte Physiol. 9):F372, 1981.

4 : Tubular Reabsorption

Water and many solutes are reabsorbed from the tubular lumen into the peritubular interstitial fluid and thence into the blood. Since the activities of water and small molecules in interstitial fluid are virtually identical to those in plasma, we often speak of reabsorption directly into the blood. The term *reabsorption* refers to the *direction* of transport, i.e., out of the tubular lumen; it may be applied to all modes of transport in that direction, be they active or passive.

Generally speaking, tubular reabsorption facilitates the conservation of substances that are essential to normal function — e.g., water, glucose and other sugars, amino acids, and electrolytes. Many of these substances, such as glucose and amino acids, are reabsorbed primarily or exclusively by the proximal tubules, whereas others, such as water and sodium, are also reabsorbed at more distal sites in the nephron.

Qualitative Evidence for Reabsorption

The most obvious examples are water, and Na^+ with its main accompanying anions, Cl^- and HCO_3^-. For these substances, which are considered in subsequent chapters, more than 99% of the loads that are filtered are reabsorbed (see Table 1-1). In this chapter, however, we shall concentrate on the reabsorption of solutes other than sodium and its attendant anions. Glucose is a simple case in point. This sugar, having a molecular diameter of about 7 Å and not being bound to plasma proteins, is freely filtered through the glomerular capillary wall and appears in Bowman's space fluid at the same concentration as in plasma. The fact that normally almost no glucose appears in the urine (Table 1-1) therefore shows that the sugar must be reabsorbed. Micropuncture studies have shown that more than 98% of the filtered glucose is reabsorbed in the proximal tubule, nearly all of this in the first half of the proximal tubule. Furthermore, since the plasma concentration of glucose is much higher than that in urine, glucose must be reabsorbed against a concentration gradient; i.e., its reabsorption must be at least in part active.

Reabsorption of glucose can be blocked by a glucoside, phlorizin. When this compound is given to an animal, glucose appears in the urine, and the U/P ratio for glucose (i.e., the ratio of the concentration of glucose in urine to that in plasma) is identical to the U/P ratio for inulin. As reviewed in Chapter 3, the U/P ratio for inulin is a function solely of water reabsorption. Hence, the identity of the two ratios during administration of phlorizin must mean that all glucose reabsorption was blocked so that urinary glucose was concentrated by water reabsorption, to the same extent as inulin. (See footnote b to Problem 4-1 for amplification of this point.)

Quantifying Reabsorption

Net reabsorption for all nephrons combined can be measured using the following formula:

$$\text{Quantity excreted} = \text{Quantity filtered} - \text{Quantity reabsorbed} \quad (4\text{-}1)$$

For inorganic phosphate, an electrolyte that is actively reabsorbed — i.e., reabsorbed against an electrochemical potential gradient at the expense of energy derived from metabolism:

$$\text{Quantity excreted} = U_{Phos} \cdot \dot{V}$$

$$\text{Quantity filtered} = P_{Phos} \cdot GFR$$

where U_{Phos} = the concentration of inorganic phosphate in urine

$\dot{V}$ = the rate of urine flow

P_{Phos} = the concentration of inorganic phosphate in plasma

GFR = the glomerular filtration rate.

If GFR is determined by the clearance of inulin, substituting and rearranging Equation 4-1:

$$\text{Phosphate reabsorbed} = \left(\frac{U_{In} \cdot \dot{V}}{P_{In}} \cdot P_{Phos} \right) - (U_{Phos} \cdot \dot{V}) \quad (4\text{-}2)$$

A precise determination of the filtered quantity — often referred to as the *filtered load* — of a solute must correct for: (a) the effect of the Donnan equilibrium, which of course applies only to electrolytes, and (b) possible binding of the solute to plasma proteins, since the bound portion cannot be filtered. For many substances, these correction factors are small or nonexistent. Hence, the corrections have been ignored throughout this book. Nevertheless, it should be noted that most substances in the body are probably bound to plasma proteins; by and large, however, this is not true of the compounds considered in this text.

Problem 4-1 and its solution in the Answers section list raw data from an experiment that tested the characteristics of inorganic phosphate transport in dogs. A few of the derived values, converted from milligrams of phosphorus to millimoles of phosphate (see footnote to Problem 4-1), are shown in Table 4-1, and they have been plotted in Figure 4-1.

Transport Maximum (Tm)

Note that at low plasma concentrations all phosphate that is filtered is reabsorbed. Then the amount that is reabsorbed reaches a maximal value that does not vary even though more and more phosphate is filtered into Bowman's space. This constant value of reabsorbed phosphate, expressed as amount per minute, is known as the *transport maximum (Tm)*. Many other substances that are reabsorbed by the kidneys have a Tm. Examples include glucose and other sugars, sulfate, many amino acids, uric acid, and probably albumin.

Normally the plasma phosphate concentration is at a level where slightly more phosphate is filtered than the tubules can reabsorb. In other words, normally Tm for inorganic phosphate is exceeded, so that small amounts of phosphate are excreted. This fact enables the kidneys to help regulate phosphate balance: If intake of inorganic phosphate increases and its plasma concentration rises, the surcharge is excreted (Fig. 4-1); conversely, if intake decreases and the plasma concentration falls even slightly, virtually all of the filtered phosphate is conserved. Such fine adjustments are not possible for compounds such as glucose, where Tm is reached only at abnormally high plasma concentrations (see Fig. 4-3). In other words, the kidney is an important regulator of phosphate balance but not of glucose balance (see legend to Fig. 4-1).

Characteristics of Active Transport

Active transport may be defined as the net movement of a particle against an electrochemical potential gradient, at the expense

Table 4-1 : Renal handling of inorganic phosphate as a function of plasma phosphate concentration.

Plasma Phosphate Concentration (mM/L)	Filtered Load of Phosphate (mM/min)	Phosphate	
		Reabsorbed (mM/min)	Excreted (mM/min)
0.404	0.035	0.035	0
0.329	0.027	0.027	0
1.195	0.098	0.088	0.010
3.015	0.248	0.099	0.149
4.197	0.352	0.098	0.254
10.234	0.775	0.103	0.672

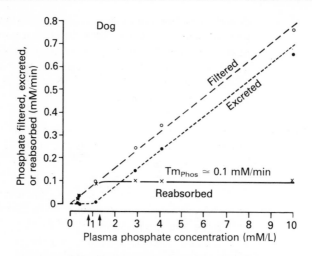

Fig. 4-1 : Renal filtration, reabsorption, and excretion of inorganic phosphate in dogs, plotted as a function of plasma phosphate concentration. The arrows span the range of normal plasma inorganic phosphate concentration; plasma phosphate exists mainly in two forms: HPO_4^{2-} and $H_2PO_4^-$ (see Table 1-2 and Fig. 9-5). Normally, small amounts of phosphate are excreted. Note that Tm_{Phos} refers to the maximal amount of phosphate that the tubules can transport per unit time. This amount varies under different physiological conditions; for example, Tm_{Phos} is decreased in the presence of high plasma concentrations of parathyroid hormone. Slightly modified from Pitts, R. F., and Alexander, R. S. *Am. J. Physiol.* **142**:648, 1944.

of metabolic energy. (An uncharged particle, which is not influenced directly by electrical forces, will be subject only to the chemical potential gradient.) The net movement of an electrolyte may be down its chemical concentration gradient and still require energy if it has to move against a relatively higher electrical potential gradient; the converse, net movement down an electrical potential gradient but against a relatively greater chemical concentration gradient, would also require energy and would therefore be called active.

METABOLIC INHIBITION. It follows from the above definition that if a system is deprived of metabolic energy, the net flux of an actively transported substance against its electrochemical potential gradient should be diminished or abolished. Such inhibition of transport is commonly seen if a system is cooled, or deprived of oxygen, or exposed to specific metabolic inhibitors such as dinitrophenol (DNP), which prevents the formation of high-energy phosphate bonds (see Fig. 2-6).

TM. The nonlinear relationship shown in Figure 4-1, between the plasma concentration of a given substance and its rate of transport, is another characteristic feature of many substances that are transported actively. The Tm phenomenon is apparently not due to exhaustion of the energy supply, but possibly to saturation of a hypothetical "carrier." For this reason, the term *saturation kinetics* is often used to describe the Tm phenomenon.

One possible scheme for visualizing active transport is depicted in Figure 4-2. Although the figure refers to a renal tubular cell, the diagram presumably applies to many other cells as well. A substance, S, is thought to combine with a carrier, C, having a high affinity for S and being located within the cellular membrane; in the case of many substances, the carrier also combines with Na$^+$, possibly even prior to the attachment of S (see Cotransport, below). After traversing the membrane, the so-called ternary complex, S $\cdot$ C $\cdot$ Na, dissociates, and S and Na$^+$ move through the cytoplasm and peritubular membrane into the peritubular fluid and blood. In the process of dissociation, the carrier acquires a new form, C', which probably has a diminished affinity for S and Na$^+$. One energy-requiring step in active transport may occur either in the transformation of C to C' or in the reconversion of C' to C. Another such step involves the direct input of energy to the pump that carries Na$^+$ across the peritubular membrane (see Cotransport, below; also Fig. 7-2).

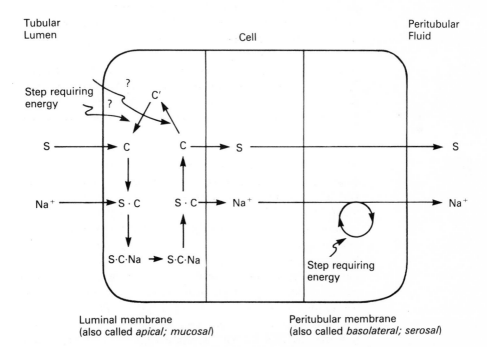

Fig. 4-2 : One hypothetical scheme for a carrier-mediated active transport system. Description and definition of symbols are given in the text. It is possible that Na$^+$ attaches to the carrier before S combines with it. Adapted from Scriver, C. R. and Rosenberg, L. E. *Amino Acid Metabolism and Its Disorders.* Philadephia: Saunders, 1973.

Although the scheme depicted in Figure 4-2 is still hypothetical, many parts of it are now being defined. It is likely that the carrier is a membrane protein whose chemical structure is specific for the substance that it transports. Also, the scheme varies in detail, depending on the substance in question. For example, S may first move passively through the luminal membrane and cytoplasm, and the energy-requiring step involving the complex may occur at the peritubular membrane; or, for some substances, as for glucose, there may be a carrier — albeit of different specifications — in each membrane; etc.

COMPETITIVE INHIBITION. This is the process by which some substances can diminish the rate of transport of certain other substances, presumably by competing for attachment to the same carrier. For example, an intravenous infusion of fructose will diminish or abolish the tubular reabsorption of glucose. Similarly, many amino acids can compete against one another for what appears to be a common carrier system. The inhibitory effect of phlorizin on renal glucose reabsorption, referred to earlier, is probably a competitive phenomenon.

It must be emphasized that substances that are actively transported do not necessarily manifest all these characteristics. For example, in Chapter 7 we present the experimental evidence that Na^+ can be transported against an electrochemical potential gradient, not only by renal tubular cells but also by most other cells. Although this process requires energy (see Figs. 2-6 and 4-2), a Tm for Na^+ has not been demonstrated. Furthermore, the carrier concept and saturation kinetics are not limited to active transport, for in some instances passive transport processes may also be carrier-mediated.

Cotransport

The epithelial transport of a number of compounds — e.g., glucose, uric acid, amino acids, and phosphate — is enhanced by Na^+ or can occur only in the presence of Na^+; the reverse — the enhancement of Na^+ transport by some of the organic compounds — is also true (see Fig. 7-3C). The explanation for this phenomenon, called *cotransport,* is not fully known. It appears likely that the affinity of a carrier for a certain compound (say, glucose) is somehow enhanced by the attachment of Na^+ to that carrier, or that the mobility of the ternary complex, $S \cdot C \cdot Na$, across the membrane may be augmented by Na^+, or both (Fig. 4-2). The latter effect might arise because the electrochemical potential gradient for Na^+ across the luminal membrane supplies the driving force for the reabsorption of Na^+ which, being attached to the same carrier, thereby transports with it, so to speak, glucose, or phosphate, or amino acids, or some other compounds. Note from Figure 4-2 that Na^+ is carried across the peritubular membrane by a metabolic pump that derives energy directly from adenosine triphosphate (ATP) (discussed in Chap. 7). Since this primary active transport lowers the intracellular concentration of Na^+, it increases the electrochemical potential gradient for Na^+ across the luminal membrane and thereby secondarily enhances the reabsorption of the substance that is co-transported; hence, the term *secondary active transport.* The phenomenon of cotransport is not restricted to reabsorption but applies as well to some instances of tubular secretion (Chap. 5).

Glucose Titration Curve

The glucose titration curve is constructed by determining the amount of glucose that is reabsorbed at increasing plasma glucose concentrations. If the GFR stays constant, increasing the plasma concentration of glucose will lead to a progressive rise in the filtered load of glucose ($GFR \cdot P_{Gluc}$), i.e., in the amount of glucose presented to the proximal tubules for reabsorption. In this way, the system is titrated to determine the plasma concentration at which the carrier for glucose becomes saturated and glucose is spilled in the urine. The plasma concentration of glucose at which the sugar first appears in the urine is known as the *renal threshold* for glucose.

A typical glucose titration curve in man is presented in Figure 4-3. It is apparent that the curve has the form that is characteristic of a Tm-limited active transport system; in fact, it was the first renal Tm-limited system to be described. At first, virtually all the filtered glucose is reabsorbed and 0.1% or less of that which was filtered is excreted (see Table 1-1). This is the case at normal plasma glucose concentrations, as denoted by the arrows on the abscissa. Then, as the maximal capacity of the tubules for reabsorbing glucose is reached, much more glucose is excreted in the urine. (In the experiment shown in Figure 4-3, the amount filtered, and hence that which was excreted, fell off slightly at higher plasma concentrations because the GFR decreased slightly.)

As discussed earlier in this chapter [under Transport Maximum (Tm)], the fact that normally the plasma glucose concentration is far below the value needed to saturate the reabsorptive mechanism means that the kidney is not a major regulator of glucose balance; that is, within a wide margin, virtually all of the filtered glucose will be reabsorbed whether the plasma glucose concentration falls or rises (Fig. 4-3).

Splay

Note that Tm for glucose is approached somewhat gradually, along a curve, rather than abruptly with a sharp deflection. The curve is known as the *splay,* and it probably has at least two explanations. The first involves the kinetics of the chemical reac-

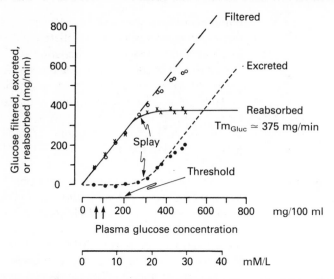

Fig. 4-3 : Renal handling of glucose as a function of increasing plasma glucose concentrations. The curve for reabsorption is known as the glucose titration curve because it determines the plasma concentration at which the carrier for glucose becomes saturated. Tm_{Gluc} refers to the maximal amount of glucose that can be transported per unit time. The range of normal plasma glucose concentration (70 to 100 mg/100 ml; see Table 1-2) is spanned by the arrows on the abscissa; note that normally virtually all the filtered glucose is reabsorbed. The significance of the splay is explained in the text. In the clinical laboratory, plasma glucose concentrations are ordinarily expressed as milligrams per 100 ml of plasma; corresponding concentrations, in millimoles per liter, are given on the second abscissa. Data from Smith, H. W. *Principles of Renal Physiology.* New York: Oxford University Press, 1956.

tion between glucose and the postulated carrier. To the extent that the carrier has a finite affinity for glucose, a "supersaturating" concentration of glucose in the tubular fluid will be needed to saturate the carrier. Hence, glucose will be spilled in the urine before Tm is reached, and some splay will result.

The second explanation involves the concept of morphological glomerulotubular imbalance. It has been shown that there is considerable variation in the anatomical dimensions of glomeruli and renal tubules. In any one person, for example, there may be an eightfold difference in the glomerular surface area available for filtration, and a twofold to threefold variation in the volume of the proximal tubule. Unless the glucose reabsorptive capacity of each proximal tubule is tailored precisely to the glucose-filtering capacity of its own glomerulus, some nephrons will excrete glucose before Tm_{Gluc} for most nephrons is reached, and other nephrons will continue to reabsorb glucose after Tm_{Gluc} has been exceeded in most nephrons. Thus, the degree of splay in the glucose titration curve partly reflects the extent of anatomical glomerulotubular balance. The fact that this splay is small means that the balance is remarkably precise, so that despite the great variation in anatomical dimensions the balance between filtering and reabsorptive capacity in the majority of individual nephrons is similar to this balance for the kidney as a whole.

The concept of glomerulotubular balance is not limited to glucose but may be applied to all substances that are filtered and reabsorbed. Furthermore, the term *glomerulotubular* balance is used in two contexts: (a) when comparing the amount of a substance filtered with the *maximal* capacity of the tubular system to reabsorb that substance, as in the case of glucose; and (b) when comparing the amount of a substance filtered with the *fraction* of the filtered load that the tubules reabsorb. The latter meaning (usually referred to as G-T balance) has special significance for Na^+ balance and it is discussed in detail in Chapter 7.

Passive Reabsorption: Urea

The influence of acute changes in the rate of urine flow on the urinary excretion of urea is shown in Figure 4-4A. The rate of excretion increases markedly with increments in urine flow up to about 2 ml per minute, and thereafter it increases at a lesser rate. The increased excretion could be due to an increase in the amount of urea filtered $(GFR \cdot P_{Urea})$ or to decreased reabsorption of urea, or to a combination of the two. Since the plasma concentration of urea and the GFR stayed relatively constant in the experiment depicted in Figure 4-4, the filtered load of urea did not change; hence the increased excretion with rising urine flows must have been due to decreased tubular reabsorption, as depicted in Figure 4-4B.

The relationship between the rate of urine flow and the reabsorptive rate for urea is characteristic of a substance that undergoes passive tubular reabsorption. The increase in urine flow shown in Figure 4-4 was due to decreased reabsorption of water from the distal tubules and collecting ducts; that is, there was increased flow of tubular fluid, mainly water, in the distal convolutions and collecting ducts. Consequently, the concentration of urea in these tubular structures, and hence the difference in urea concentration between tubular and interstitial fluid, declined. Since passive transport of a nonelectrolyte depends largely on its chemical concentration gradient, the reabsorption of urea decreased. The decline in the reabsorptive rate is much steeper at low than at high urine flows because the concentration gradient, i.e., the driving force for passive reabsorption, decreases more per linear unit rise in urine flow at low flow rates than it does at high flow rates.

Having emphasized the importance of urea as a solute that is passively reabsorbed, we must now admit that a small portion of

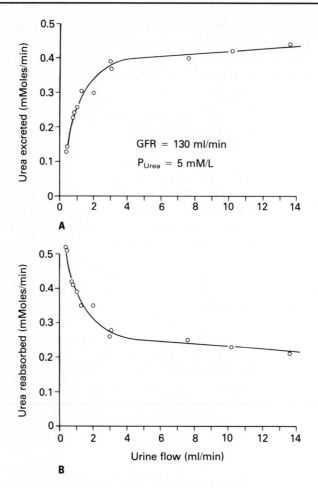

GFR = 130 ml/min

P_{Urea} = 5 mM/L

A

B

Urine flow (ml/min)

Fig. 4-4 : A. An experiment in man showing the influence of the rate of urine flow on urea excretion. The points represent values in a single individual in whom urine flow was decreased by withdrawing drinking water, and subsequently increased by having him ingest large amounts of water. Since the filtered load of urea (GFR · P_{Urea}) did not change with increasing urine flow, the increased excretion must have been due to decreased reabsorption (Eq. 4-1); this fact is shown in (B). Data adapted from Austin, J. H., Stillman, E., and Van Slyke, D. D. J. Biol. Chem. 46:91, 1921.

that which is filtered *may* be actively reabsorbed by the mammalian nephron. Under most physiological conditions, however, the majority probably is reabsorbed passively. To compound the confusion, urea is actively secreted by some amphibians and, as discussed below, is passively secreted into the loops of Henle of mammals.

Bidirectional Transport

Equation 4-1 can give a measure only of *net* reabsorption. When we describe the renal handling of a substance as involving filtration and reabsorption, we mean filtration followed by net flux from tubular lumen to blood. The statement does not exclude the possibility that the substance is simultaneously secreted, i.e., moved from blood into tubular fluid. In fact, for many or most substances, net tubular reabsorption or net secretion is the algebraic sum of fluxes in both directions; and the mode of transport in any one direction may be passive or active, or a combination of the two. For example, Na^+ undergoes net reabsorption, but it moves across the tubular wall in two directions, being actively reabsorbed and passively secreted.

Some substances undergo net transport in one direction in one part of the nephron, and net movement in the opposite direction in another part. Thus, K^+ (Chap. 11) is usually reabsorbed in proximal tubules and loops of Henle, secreted in distal tubules and cortical collecting ducts, and reabsorbed in medullary collecting ducts. For the entire kidney, there may be net reabsorption or net secretion of K^+, depending on the conditions. Certain weak acids and bases, including many drugs such as the antimalarials and salicylate (a metabolic product of aspirin), undergo active secretion in the proximal tubule and passive reabsorption predominantly in the distal tubule.

There are also a number of compounds that undergo either net reabsorption or net secretion through carrier-mediated processes in the same tubular segment. For example, uric acid is thought to be both reabsorbed and secreted in this manner in the proximal tubule, the net movement in one direction or the other depending on a variety of experimental conditions.

In the preceding section, we stressed the reabsorption of urea from the collecting ducts. Actually the renal handling of urea is much more complicated. The scheme shown in Figure 4-5 is based on micropuncture studies, mainly in rats, at normal rates of urine flow. The numbers within the lumen denote the percentage of the filtered load of urea that flows at the various sites. About 50% of the filtered urea is reabsorbed in the proximal tubules. Yet, 100% or more of the filtered amount of urea is found at the beginning of the distal tubules; therefore, urea must diffuse into the intermediate segments, i.e., the loops of Henle (which, in some classifications, include the late proximal tubules; see legend to Fig. 1-2A). At normal rates of urine flow, urea is then again reabsorbed from the collecting ducts, so that about 40% of the filtered load of urea is excreted. Thus, urea also exhibits bidirectional transport. It undergoes net reabsorption from the proximal tubules and collecting ducts, and net secretion into the loops of Henle, possibly including the pars recta of the proximal tubules. The possible advantage of this seemingly complicated handling of urea, for the process of urinary concentration, is

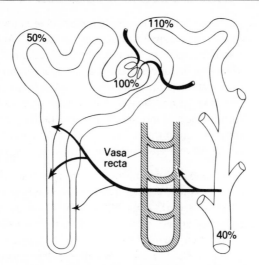

Fig. 4-5 : Renal handling of urea at normal rates of urine flow. The numbers within the lumen denote the percentage of the filtered amount of urea that flows at the various sites. The urea that is reabsorbed from the collecting ducts flows partly into the vasa recta and partly into the tubular segments that lie between the late proximal and early distal convolutions. This process, called "medullary recycling of urea," may occur predominantly in short (as opposed to long) loops of Henle. Data adapted from Lassiter, W. E., Gottschalk, C. W., and Mylle, M. *Am. J. Physiol.* 200:1139, 1961.

considered in Chapter 8 (see Role of Urea in the Countercurrent System).

Summary

The term *tubular reabsorption* refers to the direction of tubular transport, from tubular lumen, through peritubular interstitium, into blood. This definition applies to all modes of transport in the reabsorptive direction. Many of the compounds that undergo net tubular reabsorption are essential to homeostasis, e.g., Na^+, HCO_3^-, H_2O, glucose, and amino acids.

When we speak of a compound as being handled by filtration and reabsorption, we usually mean filtration followed by *net* reabsorption; such net transport can be deduced from Equation 4-1 as the difference between the amount filtered and that which is excreted in the urine.

Many substances, such as Na^+, inorganic phosphate, and glucose, are actively reabsorbed, i.e., against an electrochemical potential gradient at the expense of metabolic energy. Many such compounds exhibit the characteristic features of active transport: metabolic inhibition, transport maximum (Tm), and competitive inhibition. Na^+, however, exhibits no Tm even though it is actively reabsorbed. Several compounds — notably glucose, amino acids, and phosphate — undergo cotransport, in which the presence of Na^+ enables or accelerates their reabsorption; or vice versa, in which the reabsorption of the compounds enhances the transport of Na^+. The degree of splay in a curve showing Tm (e.g., the glucose titration curve) is probably a function of two phenomena: (a) affinity of the carrier for the transported substance and (b) anatomical glomerulotubular imbalance.

The rate of tubular reabsorption of urea, which in mammals is mainly by passive diffusion, varies as a function of the rate of urine flow. Like many other compounds, urea exhibits bidirectional transport; it undergoes net reabsorption in the proximal tubules and collecting ducts, and net secretion into the loops of Henle and possibly the partes rectae.

Problem 4-1 Renal handling of inorganic phosphate in dogs. Utilizing the data given, complete the blank columns.

Urine Flow (ml/min)	Phosphate Phosphorus[a]			Creatinine			Phosphate Phosphorus[a]			Clearance Ratio: Phosphate Clearance/Creatinine Clearance[b]
	Plasma (mg/100 ml)	Urine (mg/100 ml)	Clearance (ml/min)	Plasma (mg/100 ml)	Urine (mg/100 ml)	Clearance (ml/min)	Filtered (mg/min)	Excreted (mg/min)	Reabsorbed (mg/min)	
6.8	1.25	0.07		33.9	427					
9.2	2.75	0.46		31.2	283					
9.7	3.70	2.95		32.5	274					
8.7	4.64	9.10		33.3	321					
6.7	9.34	69.0		34.5	423					
8.2	13.0	95.7		34.5	352					
10.0	31.7	208		38.7	293					

[a]The values were measured as phosphate phosphorus (see Table 1-2); they have been converted from milligrams to millimoles of inorganic phosphate in Table 4-1 and Figure 4-1.

[b]The so-called clearance ratio is the ratio of the clearance of any substance to the clearance of inulin or of creatinine, i.e., to the GFR. In the case of phosphate, the clearance ratio has the following formula: $U_{Phos} \cdot \dot{V}/P_{Phos} \div U_{In} \cdot \dot{V}/P_{In}$. The $\dot{V}$s cancel out, and the formula is reduced to $U_{Phos}/P_{Phos} \div U_{In}/P_{In}$, which has the great advantage that the clearance ratio — and the important information that it yields — can be determined without having to measure urine flow. The ratio can be applied to any substance; when the clearance ratio is <1.0, the substance in question undergoes net reabsorption; when the ratio is >1.0, the substance is secreted; and when the ratio is 1.0, the substance is, in the net, neither reabsorbed nor secreted. Numerical examples of the use of clearance ratios are given in the Answers to Problem 4-1, to Problem 4-1, to Problem 4-2 (footnote), and to Problem 8-1 (*How to compute the fraction of a filtered substance that is reabsorbed*). Examples of how the clearance ratio is applied to micropuncture samples — and hence to quantifying the handling of a given substance by various tubular segments — are presented in Problem 6-1 (parts 2 and 3) and in Figure 11-1. Slightly modified from Pitts, R. F., and Alexander, R. S. *Am. J. Physiol.* 142:648, 1944. Used with permission of the American Physiological Society.

Problem 4-2 Handling of urea by the kidneys of an adult human at varying rates of urine flow. Utilizing the data given, complete the blank columns.

V̇ (ml/min)	Urine Concentration Inulin (mg/ml)	Urine Concentration Urea (mM/L)	Plasma Concentration Inulin (mg/ml)	Plasma Concentration Urea (mM/L)	GFR (ml/min)	Urea Filtered (mM/min)	Urea Excreted (mM/min)	Urea Reabsorbed (mM/min)	Urea Excreted (% of filtered load)	Urea Reabsorbed (% of filtered load)
0.4	144	300	0.5	5						
0.8	75	263	0.5	5						
1.0	60	240	0.5	5						
3.1	20	119	0.5	5						
10.2	5.8	37	0.5	5						

**Selected
References**

General

Forster, R. P. Renal transport mechanisms. *Fed. Proc.* 26:1008, 1967.

Lotspeich, W. D. *Metabolic Aspects of Renal Function.* Springfield, Ill.: Thomas, 1959.

Kinne, R. Membrane-molecular aspects of tubular transport. *Int. Rev. Physiol.* 11:169, 1976.

Kinne, R. Metabolic Correlates of Tubular Transport. In G. Giebisch (Ed.), *Transport Organs,* vol. IVB. New York: Springer-Verlag, 1979.

Mudge, G. H., Berndt, W. O., and Valtin, H. Tubular Transport of Urea, Glucose, Phosphate, Uric Acid, Sulfate, and Thiosulfate. In J. Orloff and R. W. Berliner (Eds.), *Handbook of Physiology,* section 8, Renal Physiology. Washington, D.C.: American Physiological Society, 1973.

Pitts, R. F. *Physiology of the Kidney and Body Fluids* (3rd ed.). Chicago: Year Book, 1974. Chap. 6.

Smith, H. W. *The Kidney: Structure and Function in Health and Disease.* New York: Oxford University Press, 1951.

Stein, W. D. *The Movement of Molecules Across Cell Membranes.* New York: Academic, 1967.

Torretti, J., and Weiner, I. M. The Renal Excretion of Drugs. In M. Martinez-Maldonado (Ed.), *Methods in Pharmacology,* vol. 4A, *Renal Pharmacology.* New York: Plenum, 1976.

Ullrich, K. J. Renal Transport of Organic Solutes. In G. Giebisch (Ed.), *Transport Organs,* vol. IVA. New York: Springer-Verlag, 1979.

Vogel, H. G., and Ullrich, K. J. (Eds.). *New Aspects of Renal Function.* Amsterdam: Excerpta Medica, 1978.
Contains many useful, up-to-date summaries.

Wearn, J. T., and Richards, A. N. Observations on the composition of glomerular urine with particular reference to the problem of reabsorption in the renal tubules. *Am. J. Physiol.* 71:209, 1924.

Glucose

Bradley, S. E., Laragh, J. H., Wheeler, H. O., MacDowell, M., and Oliver, J. Correlation of structure and function in the handling of glucose by nephrons of the canine kidney. *J. Clin. Invest.* 40:1113, 1961.

Davison, J. M., and Cheyne, G. A. Renal reabsorption of glucose. *Lancet* 1:787, 1972.

Frohnert, P. P., Höhmann, B., Zwiebel, R., and Baumann, K. Free flow micropuncture studies of glucose transport in the rat nephron. *Pflügers Arch. Eur. J. Physiol.* 315:66, 1970.

Kinne, R. Properties of the glucose transport system in the renal brush border membrane. *Curr. Top. Membr. Transp.* 8:209, 1976.

Kinne, R., Keljo, D., Gmaj, P., and Murer, H. The Energy Source of Glucose and Calcium Transport in the Renal Proximal Tubule. In H. G. Vogel and K. J. Ullrich (Eds.), *New Aspects of Renal Function.* Amsterdam: Excerpta Medica, 1978.

Lotspeich, W. D. Phlorizin and the cellular transport of glucose. *Harvey Lect.* 56:63, 1961.

Oliver, J., and MacDowell, M. The structural and functional aspects of the handling of glucose by the nephrons and the kidney and their correlation by means of structural-functional equivalents. *J. Clin. Invest.* 40:1093, 1961.

Rohde, R., and Deetjen, P. Die Glucoseresorption in der Ratenniere. Mikropunktionsanalysen der tubulären Glucosekonzentration bei freiem Fluss. *Pflügers Arch. Ges. Physiol.* 302:219, 1968.

Shannon, J. A., and Fisher, S. The renal tubular reabsorption of glucose in the normal dog. *Am. J. Physiol.* 122:765, 1938.

Smith, H., Goldring, W., Chasis, H., Ranges, H. A., and Bradley, S. E. The application of saturation methods to the study of glomerular and tubular function in the human kidney. *Mt. Sinai J. Med.* (N.Y.) 10:59, 1943.

van Liew, J. B., Deetjen, P., and Boylan, J. W. Glucose reabsorption in the rat kidney: Dependence on glomerular filtration. *Pflügers Arch. Ges. Physiol.* 295:232, 1967.

Cotransport

Aronson, P. S., Hayslett, J. P., and Kashgarian, M. Dissociation of proximal tubular glucose and Na^+ reabsorption by amphotericin B. *Am. J. Physiol.* 236 (Renal Fluid Electrolyte Physiol. 5):F392, 1979.

Aronson, P. S., and Sacktor, B. The Na^+ gradient-dependent transport of D-glucose in renal brush border membranes. *J. Biol. Chem.* 250:6032, 1975.

Costanzo, L. S., Windhager, E. E., and Taylor, A. Sodium-Calcium Interaction in the Distal Tubule. In H. G. Vogel and K. J. Ullrich (Eds.), *New Aspects of Renal Function.* Amsterdam: Excerpta Medica, 1978.

Crane, R. K. The gradient hypothesis and other models of carrier-mediated active transport. *Rev. Physiol. Biochem. Pharmacol.* 78:101, 1977.

Fairclough, P. D., Malathi, P., Preiser, H., and Crane, R. K. Glucose Transport in Renal Brush Border Membranes and Reconstituted Liposomes. *Proceedings VII International Congress of Nephrology.* Basel: Karger, 1978, p. 161.

Frömter, E. Primary and Secondary Active Transport Mechanisms in Rat Renal Proximal Tubule. In H. G. Vogel and K. J. Ullrich (Eds.), *New Aspects of Renal Function.* Amsterdam: Excerpta Medica, 1978.

Kinne, R., and Murer, H. Recent Advances in the Understanding of Renal Amino Acid and Sugar Transport. *Proceedings VII International Congress of Nephrology.* Basel: Karger, 1978, p. 601.

Murer, H., and Kinne, R. Sidedness and Coupling of Transport Processes in Small Intestinal and Renal Epithelia. In G. Semenza and E. Carafoli (Eds.), *Biochemistry of Membrane Transport.* Berlin: Springer, 1977.

Sacktor, B. Transport in membrane vesicles isolated from the mammalian kidney and intestine. *Curr. Top. Bioeng.* 6:39, 1977.

Schultz, S. G. Sodium-coupled solute transport by small intestine: A status report. *Am. J. Physiol.* 233 (Endocrinol. Metab. Gastrointest. Physiol. 2):E249, 1977.

Schultz, S. G., and Curran, P. F. Coupled transport of sodium and organic solutes. *Physiol. Rev.* 50:637, 1970.

Ullrich, K. J. Sugar, amino acid, and Na$^+$ cotransport in the proximal tubule. *Annu. Rev. Physiol.* 41:181, 1979.

Urea and
Uric Acid

Note: Further references on urea can be found at the end of Chapter 8.

Clapp, J. Renal tubular reabsorption of urea in normal and protein-depleted rats. *Am. J. Physiol.* 210:1304, 1966.

Fanelli, G. M., Jr. Drugs Affecting the Renal Handling of Uric Acid. In M. Martinez-Maldonado (Ed.), *Methods in Pharmacology,* vol. 4A, *Renal Pharmacology.* New York: Plenum, 1976.

Forster, R. P. Active cellular transport of urea by frog renal tubules. *Am. J. Physiol.* 179:372, 1954.

Goldberg, M., Wojtczak, A. M., and Ramirez, M. A. Uphill transport of urea in the dog kidney: Effects of certain inhibitors. *J. Clin. Invest.* 46:388, 1967.

Hays, R. M. Familial azotemia. *N. Engl. J. Med.* 298:160, 1978.

Hsu, C. H., Kurtz, R. W., Massari, P. U., Ponze, S. A., and Chang, B. S. Familial azotemia. Impaired urea excretion despite normal renal function. *N. Engl. J. Med.* 298:117, 1978.

Irish, J. M., III, and Grantham, J. J. Renal Handling of Organic Anions and Cations. In B. M. Brenner and F. C. Rector, Jr. (Eds.), *The Kidney* (2nd ed.). Philadelphia: Saunders, 1981.

Kawamura, S., and Kokko, J. P. Urea secretion by the straight segment of the proximal tubule. *J. Clin. Invest.* 58:604, 1976.

Lassiter, W. E. Uric Acid and the Kidney. In L. E. Earley and C. W. Gottschalk (Eds.), *Strauss and Welt's Diseases of the Kidney* (3rd ed.). Boston: Little, Brown, 1979. Chap. 34.

Lassiter, W. E., Gottschalk, C. W., and Mylle, M. Micropuncture study of net transtubular movement of water and urea in nondiuretic mammalian kidney. *Am. J. Physiol.* 200:1139, 1961.

Lassiter, W. E., Mylle, M., and Gottschalk, C. W. Net transtubular movement of water and urea in saline diuresis. *Am. J. Physiol.* 206:669, 1964.

Lassiter, W. E., Mylle, M., and Gottschalk, C. W. Micropuncture study of urea transport in rat renal medulla. *Am. J. Physiol.* 210:965, 1966.

May, D. G., and Weiner, I. M. The renal mechanisms for the excretion of m-hydroxybenzoic acids in *Cebus* monkeys: Relationship to urate transport. *J. Pharmacol. Exp. Ther.* 176:407, 1971.

Mudge, G. H., Berndt, W. O., and Valtin, H. Tubular Transport of Urea, Glucose, Phosphate, Uric Acid, Sulfate, and Thiosulfate. In J. Orloff and R. W. Berliner (Eds.), *Handbook of Physiology,* section 8, Renal Physiology. Washington, D.C.: American Physiological Society, 1973.

Roch-Ramel, F., and Peters, G. Urinary Excretion of Uric Acid in Nonhuman Mammalian Species. In W. N. Kelley and I. M. Weiner (Eds.), *Handbook of Experimental Pharmacology,* vol. 51, *Uric Acid.* Berlin: Springer-Verlag, 1978.

Roch-Ramel, F., and Weiner, I. M. Renal excretion of urate: Factors determining the actions of drugs. *Kidney Int.* 18:665, 1980.

Schmidt-Nielsen, B. Urea excretion in mammals. *Physiol. Rev.* 38:139, 1958.

Schmidt-Nielsen, B. (Ed.). *Urea and the Kidney.* Amsterdam: Excerpta Medica, 1970.
A most useful source for authoritative information on numerous aspects of urea metabolism and excretion.

Shannon, J. A. Urea excretion in the normal dog during forced diuresis. *Am. J. Physiol.* 122:782, 1938.

Stewart, J. Urea handling by the renal countercurrent system: Insights from computer simulation. *Pflügers Arch. Eur. J. Physiol.* 356:133, 1975.

Ullrich, K. J., Rumrich, G., and Baldamus, C. A. Mode of Urea Transport Across the Mammalian Nephron. In B. Schmidt-Nielsen (Ed.), *Urea and the Kidney.* Amsterdam: Excerpta Medica, 1970.

Phosphate and Calcium

Agus, Z. S., Chiu, P. J. S., and Goldberg, M. Regulation of urinary calcium excretion in the rat. *Am. J. Physiol.* 232 (Renal Fluid Electrolyte Physiol. 1):F545, 1977.

Costanzo, L. S., and Windhager, E. E. Calcium and sodium transport by the distal convoluted tubule of the rat. *Am. J. Physiol.* 235 (Renal Fluid Electrolyte Physiol. 4):F492, 1978.

DeFronzo, R. A., Goldberg, M., and Agus, Z. S. The effects of glucose and insulin on renal electrolyte transport. *J. Clin. Invest.* 58:83, 1976.

Dennis, V. M., Stead, W. W., and Myers, J. L. Renal handling of phosphate and calcium. *Annu. Rev. Physiol.* 41:257, 1979.

Edwards, B. R., Baer, P. G., Sutton, R. A. L., and Dirks, J. H. Micropuncture study of diuretic effects on sodium and calcium reabsorption in the dog nephron. *J. Clin. Invest.* 52:2418, 1973.

Goldberg, M., Agus, Z. S., and Goldfarb, S. Renal handling of calcium and phosphate. *Int. Rev. Physiol.* 11:211, 1976.

Hamburger, R. J., Lawson, N. L., and Schwartz, J. H. Response to parathyroid hormone in defined segments of proximal tubule. *Am. J. Physiol.* 230:286, 1976.

Hellman, D., Baird, H. R., and Bartter, F. C. Relationship of maximal tubular phosphate reabsorption to filtration rate in the dog. *Am. J. Physiol.* 207:89, 1964.

Kempson, S. A., Colon-Otero, G., Ou, S.-Y. L., Turner, S. T., and Dousa, T. P. Possible role of nicotinamide adenine dinucleotide as an intracellular regulator of renal transport of phosphate in the rat. *J. Clin. Invest.* 67:1347, 1981.

Knox, F. G., Osswald, H., Marchand, G. R., Spielman, W. S., Haas, J. A., Berndt, T., and Youngberg, S. P. Phosphate transport along the nephron. *Am. J. Physiol.* 233 (Renal Fluid Electrolyte Physiol. 2):F261, 1977.

Lang, F. Renal handling of calcium and phosphate. *Klin. Wochenschr.* 58:985, 1980.

Lassiter, W. E., Gottschalk, C. W., and Mylle, M. Micropuncture study of renal tubular reabsorption of calcium in normal rodents. *Am. J. Physiol.* 204:771, 1963.

Lemann, J., Adams, N. D., and Gray, R. W. Urinary calcium excretion in human beings. *N. Engl. J. Med.* 201:535, 1979.

Massry, S. G. (Ed.). *Renal Handling of Phosphate.* New York: Plenum, 1980.

Mudge, G. H., Berndt, W. O., and Valtin, H. Tubular Transport of Urea, Glucose, Phosphate, Uric Acid, Sulfate, and Thiosulfate. In J. Orloff and R. W. Berliner (Eds.), *Handbook of Physiology,* section 8, Renal Physiology. Washington, D.C.: American Physiological Society, 1973.

Pastoriza-Muñoz, E., Colindres, R. E., Lassiter, W. E., and Lechene, C. Effect of parathyroid hormone on phosphate reabsorption in rat distal convolution. *Am. J. Physiol.* 235 (Renal Fluid Electrolyte Physiol. 4):F321, 1978.

Physiology Society. Renal handling of calcium. A Physiology Society Symposium, chaired by J. H. Dirks and reported on by R. A. L. Sutton, and J. H. Dirks. *Fed. Proc.* 37:2112, 1978.

Pitts, R. F., and Alexander, R. S. The renal reabsorptive mechanism for inorganic phosphate in normal and acidotic dogs. *Am. J. Physiol.* 142:648, 1944.

Shareghi, G. R., and Stoner, L. C. Calcium transport across segments of the rabbit distal nephron in vitro. *Am. J. Physiol.* 235 (Renal Fluid Electrolyte Physiol. 4):F367, 1978.

Staum, B. B., Hamburger, R. J., and Goldberg, M. Tracer microinjection study of renal tubular phosphate reabsorption in the rat. *J. Clin. Invest.* 51:2271, 1972.

Strickler, J. C., Thompson, D. D., Klose, R. M., and Giebisch, G. Micropuncture study of inorganic phosphate excretion in the rat. *J. Clin. Invest.* 43:1596, 1964.

Sutton, R. A. L., Quamme, G. A., and Dirks, J. H. Transport of Calcium, Magnesium and Inorganic Phosphate in the Kidney. In G. Giebisch (Ed.), *Transport Organs,* vol. IVA. New York: Springer-Verlag, 1979.

Walser, M. Calcium-Sodium Interdependence in Renal Transport. In J. W. Fisher (Ed.), *Renal Pharmacology.* New York: Appleton-Century-Crofts, 1971.

Sulfate

Lotspeich, W. D. Renal tubular reabsorption of inorganic sulfate in the normal dog. *Am. J. Physiol.* 151:311, 1947.

Mudge, G. H., Berndt, W. O., and Valtin, H. Tubular Transport of Urea, Glucose, Phosphate, Uric Acid, Sulfate, and Thiosulfate. In J. Orloff and R. W. Berliner (Eds.), *Handbook of Physiology,* section 8, Renal Physiology. Washington, D.C.: American Physiological Society, 1973.

Amino Acids
and Proteins

Beyer, K. H., Wright, L. D., Skeggs, H. R., Russo, H. F., and Shaner, G. A. Renal clearance of essential amino acids: Their competition for reabsorption by the renal tubules. *Am. J. Physiol.* 151:202, 1947.

Brown, J. L., Samiy, A. H., and Pitts, R. F. Localization of amino-nitrogen reabsorption in the nephron of the dog. *Am. J. Physiol.* 200:370, 1961.

Cortney, M. A., Sawin, L. L., and Weiss, D. D. Renal tubular protein absorption in the rat. *J. Clin. Invest.* 49:1, 1970.

Cusworth, D. C., and Dent, C. E. Renal clearances of amino acids in normal adults and in patients with aminoaciduria. *Biochem. J.* 74:550, 1960.

Kamin, H., and Handler, P. Effect of infusion of single amino acids upon excretion of other amino acids. *Am. J. Physiol.* 164:654, 1951.

Leber, P. D., and Marsh, D. J. Micropuncture study of concentration and fate of albumin in rat nephron. *Am. J. Physiol.* 219:358, 1970.

Maunsbach, A. B. Absorption of I^{125}-labeled homologous albumin by rat kidney proximal tubule cells: A study of microperfused single proximal tubules by electron microscopic autoradiography and histochemistry. *J. Ultrastruct. Res.* 15:197, 1966.

Maunsbach, A. B. Cellular mechanisms of tubular protein transport. *Int. Rev. Physiol.* 11:145, 1976.

Oken, D. E., Cotes, S. C., and Mende, C. W. Micropuncture study of tubular transport of albumin in rats with aminonucleoside nephrosis. *Kidney Int.* 1:3, 1972.

Oken, D. E., and Weise, M. Micropuncture studies of the transport of individual amino acids by the *Necturus* proximal tubule. *Kidney Int.* 13:445, 1978.

Robson, E. B., and Rose, G. A. The effect of intravenous lysine on the renal clearances of cystine, arginine and ornithine in normal subjects, in patients with cystinuria and Fanconi syndrome and in their relatives. *Clin. Sci. Mol. Med.* 16:75, 1957.

Rosenberg, L. E., Downing, S. J., and Segal, S. Competitive inhibition of dibasic amino acid transport in rat kidney. *J. Biol. Chem.* 237:2265, 1962.

Scriver, C. R., and Bergeron, M. Amino Acid Transport in Kidney. The Use of Mutation to Dissect Membrane and Transepithelial Transport. In W. L. Nyhan (Ed.), *Heritable Disorders of Amino Acid Metabolism: Patterns of Clinical Expression and Genetic Variation.* New York: Wiley, 1974.

Scriver, C. R., and Rosenberg, L. E. *Amino Acid Metabolism and Its Disorders.* Philadelphia: Saunders, 1973.

Segal, S., and Thier, S. O. The Renal Handling of Amino Acids. In J. Orloff and R. W. Berliner (Eds.), *Handbook of Physiology,* section 8, Renal Physiology. Washington, D.C.: American Physiological Society, 1973.

Silbernagl, S. Renal transport of amino acids. *Klin. Wochenschr.* 57:1009, 1979.

Silbernagl, S., Foulkes, E. C., and Deetjen, P. Renal transport of amino acids. *Rev. Physiol. Biochem. Pharmacol.* 74:105, 1975.

Ullrich, K. J. Renal tubular mechanisms of organic solute transport. *Kidney Int.* 9:134, 1976.

Webber, W. A., Brown, J. L., and Pitts, R. F. Interactions of amino acids in renal tubular transport. *Am. J. Physiol.* 200:380, 1961.

5 : Tubular Secretion

The term *secretion* refers to the *direction* of movement, from peritubular blood, or interstitium, or tubular cell into the tubular lumen, regardless of whether the transport is passive or active. The term excludes entry of substances into the tubular lumen via glomerular filtration.

Many of the substances that are secreted by renal tubules are either weak acids or weak bases, and many fall into one or more of the following categories. (1) They are foreign to the body. Drugs, such as penicillin, certain diuretics, and salicylate (a breakdown product of aspirin), are examples; H^+ and NH_3 are notable exceptions. (2) They are not metabolized, but are excreted unchanged in the urine, e.g., para-aminohippuric acid (PAH). (3) They are metabolized slowly, incompletely, and with difficulty, e.g., thiamine (vitamin B_1). Thus, tubular secretion may be viewed as a supplement to glomerular filtration, to help in the elimination of compounds that cannot be disposed of by metabolism alone. It may also serve as a means of getting some drugs (e.g., diuretics) from the blood into the tubular fluid and thence to their sites of action in the luminal membrane (Fig. 4-2) of the cell.

The fact that secreted substances are mainly compounds that are foreign to the body has often raised the question whether the tubular secretory mechanism normally plays any essential physiological role. Julius Cohen and his associates have suggested that one such role may be the acquisition, by renal cells, of essential metabolic substrates. For example, α-ketoglutarate is selectively taken up by the kidneys and the liver, and it is actively transported across the basolateral membrane (see Fig. 4-2), from the blood into renal and hepatic cells. Another role, in analogy with that cited above for diuretics, may be to transport certain endogenous compounds, such as prostaglandins, from their sites of synthesis within the kidney, via the tubular fluid, to their sites of action on tubular cells. It may be a mere concomitant resulting from structural similarity that foreign organic compounds such as PAH can utilize the same carrier mechanisms and thus be efficiently excreted by the kidney.

Qualitative Evidence for Secretion

The possibility that some substances might be secreted was vehemently rejected for a long time. As mentioned in Chapter 1, Cushny considered the process of tubular secretion so vitalistic as to be inconceivable. (In an introductory letter to the monograph, in which Cushny presented his view, he stated: "If it [the monograph] serves as an advanced post from which others may issue against the remaining ramparts of vitalism, its purpose will be served." It is an ironic twist that Cushny entitled the monograph *The Secretion of the Urine;* the definition of secretion that is given above was introduced after the appearance of Cushny's book.)

The first convincing evidence for tubular secretion appeared in 1923, when E. K. Marshall, Jr., and J. L. Vickers showed that as much as 70% of an injected dye, phenolsulfonphthalein (PSP), could appear in the urine in a single circulation through the kidneys. Since about 75% of PSP is bound to plasma proteins, only 25% was available for filtration, and only about one-fifth of that portion could be filtered (see Concept of Filtration Fraction, Chap. 3, and Filtration Fraction, below.) Hence, only 5% of the injected PSP could have reached the urine by filtration, and 65% therefore must have been secreted. Those who objected to the concept of tubular secretion, however, pointed out that PSP is a foreign substance and that Marshall's demonstration therefore might have little physiological meaning. Five years later, Marshall and A. L. Grafflin showed that endogenous compounds such as creatine and creatinine were excreted in the urine of the goosefish, *Lophius,* which has virtually no glomeruli. Nevertheless, this report was purportedly met by some obstinate skeptics with the comment that ". . . at last Marshall has found an animal that fits in with his theory."

Tubular secretion was subsequently demonstrated in numerous animals and preparations. For example, it was shown by direct visualization that PSP could be concentrated several thousand-fold within the lumina of separated tubules without glomeruli, and that this accumulation could be prevented by the metabolic poison, dinitrophenol (DNP), or by depriving the preparation of oxygen. Thus, the secretion of at least some substances must be an active transport process. The reality of tubular secretion became fully accepted with the development of the inulin clearance as a means of quantifying the rate of glomerular filtration. With this tool, as is shown in Equation 5-1, it could be clearly shown in vivo that the rate of urinary excretion of many substances far exceeded the rate at which they are filtered (see footnote b to Problem 4-1).

**Quantifying
Secretion**

The calculation is based on the following equation:

Quantity excreted = Quantity filtered + Quantity secreted   (5-1)

For PAH:

Quantity excreted = $U_{PAH} \cdot \dot{V}$

Quantity filtered   = $P_{PAH} \cdot C_{In}$

where U_{PAH} = the concentration of PAH in the urine (mg/ml)
$\dot{V}$ = the rate of urine flow (ml/min)
P_{PAH} = the concentration of PAH in the plasma (mg/ml).
(As discussed in conjunction with Eq. 4-2, this
concentration should be corrected for several
factors, including the binding of PAH to plasma
proteins. Since only about 10% of PAH is thus
bound, however, this correction will be ignored.
For an example of when the correction cannot be
ignored, see discussion of PSP, above.)
C_{In} = the clearance of inulin, i.e., GFR (ml/min).

Substituting, and rearranging Equation 5-1:

$$\text{Quantity of PAH secreted} = (U_{PAH} \cdot \dot{V}) - \left(P_{PAH} \cdot \frac{U_{In} \cdot \dot{V}}{P_{In}} \right) \quad (5\text{-}2)$$

PAH is actively secreted by the proximal tubules, from the
peritubular blood into the tubular lumen. We might therefore
anticipate a secretory transport maximum, Tm, for PAH. The
existence of this maximum is shown in Figure 5-1, which depicts
the handling of PAH by the kidneys of a normal adult human as
the plasma concentration of PAH is raised progressively by intravenous infusion. Note that, at plasma concentrations above 20
mg per 100 ml, PAH secretion becomes constant because Tm_{PAH}
has been reached. In a normal adult person, the maximal amount
of PAH that can be transported by all proximal tubular cells
combined is approximately 80 mg per minute.

**Measurement of
Renal Plasma Flow**

In Chapter 3 we stressed that only about one-fifth of the plasma
that enters the glomerular capillaries can be filtered into Bowman's space. Inulin can get into the tubular system only by
filtration, i.e., as a solute dissolved in plasma. It follows, therefore, that only about one-fifth of the inulin can be removed from
the plasma as blood courses through the kidneys at any one
time. However, a substance like PAH, which besides being

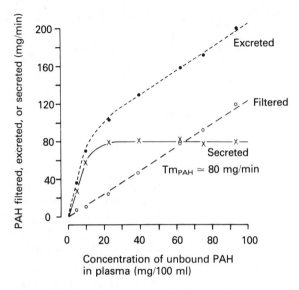

Fig. 5-1 : Rates of filtration, excretion, and secretion of para-aminohippuric acid (PAH) in an adult human, at increasing plasma concentrations of PAH. The plasma concentrations refer to that portion of the PAH that is not bound to plasma proteins (approximately 90%) and that is therefore freely filterable. Slightly modified from Pitts, R. F. *Physiology of the Kidney and Body Fluids* **(3rd ed.). Chicago: Year Book, 1974.**

filtered also undergoes active tubular secretion, can be almost "completely" removed. This has been proved by simultaneously sampling arterial and renal venous blood; as the blood enters the kidney, it has a finite concentration of PAH, and as the blood leaves the kidney, the concentration is virtually zero. "Complete" removal is possible because the substance does not need to be dissolved in plasma in order to be transported by the "carrier" into the tubular fluid.

Obviously, "complete" removal in a single circuit of the blood through the kidneys is possible only if the secretory Tm for PAH has not been reached. Consequently, the procedure for *estimating* renal plasma flow with PAH is as follows:

1. Infuse PAH intravenously at a rate that will result in a steady, low plasma concentration, which will not saturate the secretory transport mechanism, i.e., which will maintain the rate of secretion well below Tm.
2. Measure the concentration of PAH in the urine; U_{PAH} = 25.5 mg/ml.
3. Measure the rate of urine flow; $\dot{V}$ = 1.1 ml/min.
4. Calculate the rate of urinary excretion of PAH; $U_{PAH} \cdot \dot{V}$ = 28 mg/min.

5. Measure the concentration of PAH in arterial plasma; P_{PAH} = 0.05 mg/ml.
6. If each milliliter of plasma flowing through the glomeruli and peritubular vessels contributed 0.05 mg of PAH to the urine (which must be so if the renal venous concentration of PAH is zero), how many milliliters of plasma must have passed through the kidneys in order to have excreted 28 mg of PAH?

$$28 \text{ mg} \div \frac{0.05 \text{ mg}}{\text{ml}} = \frac{28 \text{ mg}}{1} \cdot \frac{\text{ml}}{0.05 \text{ mg}} = 560 \text{ ml}$$

Since 28 mg was excreted in one minute, 560 ml of plasma must have passed through the kidneys during this 1 minute. Note that, when we express the value in milliliters per minute, we have calculated the clearance of PAH, $U_{PAH} \cdot \dot{V}/P_{PAH}$.

Effective Renal Plasma Flow (ERPF)

In the above description, the word *complete* has been in quotation marks because actually the concentration of PAH in renal venous blood is not zero but rather about one-tenth of its concentration in renal arterial blood. This is probably so because some blood flows through renal tissue that does not remove PAH, e.g., the renal capsule, the renal pelvis, the perirenal fat, and possibly the inner medulla and parts of the outer medulla. Since the procedure described above measures the flow that traverses tissue that *effectively* removes PAH from the plasma, the rate of flow thus determined is called the *effective renal plasma flow* (ERPF). Hence, at low plasma concentration of PAH, the clearance of PAH is a measure of ERPF.

$$C_{PAH} = \frac{U_{PAH} \cdot \dot{V}}{P_{PAH}} = \text{ERPF (ml/min)} \qquad (5\text{-}3)$$

Exact Renal Plasma Flow (RPF). Extraction of PAH

By simultaneously measuring the concentration of PAH in renal arterial and renal venous plasma, one can determine exactly how much PAH was extracted from each milliliter of plasma flowing through the kidneys. In this way one can precisely measure the renal plasma flow (RPF), as opposed to the ERPF. In fact, whenever an exact determination of RPF is needed, the extraction of PAH is measured. This is necessary not only because under control conditions only 85 to 90% is extracted, but also because the rate of extraction can vary by 20% or more during various physiological and experimental conditions. This fact and sample calculations of RPF using the extraction of PAH are given in Problem 5-1 and in the corresponding Answer.

Moreover, one can measure RPF precisely by determining the extraction of any one of a number of substances. This point can be illustrated for inulin. If the urinary concentration of inulin is 150 mg per milliliter, and the urine flow is 1.1 ml per minute, the urinary excretion of inulin is 165 mg per minute. If, while this excretion rate was measured, the concentration of inulin in renal arterial plasma was 1.25 mg per milliliter, and that in renal venous plasma was 1.00 mg per milliliter, each milliliter of plasma traversing the kidneys must have contributed 0.25 mg to the 165 mg that was excreted. Hence the RPF must have been

$$\frac{165 \text{ mg}}{\text{min}} \div \frac{0.25 \text{ mg}}{\text{ml}} = \frac{165 \text{ mg}}{\text{min}} \cdot \frac{\text{ml}}{0.25 \text{ mg}} = 660 \text{ ml/min} = \text{RPF}$$

It will be apparent that this method of measuring RPF is an application of the Fick principle (see Eq. 6-2). The urinary excretion of inulin is in a sense the renal consumption of inulin and thus analogous to the $\dot{V}_{O_2}$ of Equation 6-2; and the concentration of 0.25 mg per milliliter is the difference between the renal arterial and renal venous concentrations of inulin and is thus analogous to the a-v oxygen difference of Equation 6-2. Thus, the formula for measuring RPF by substance X (be it PAH, or inulin, or some other substance) is:

$$\text{RPF} = \frac{U_X \cdot \dot{V}}{Pa_X - Pv_X} \tag{5-4}$$

where Pa_X = the concentration of substance X in renal arterial plasma

Pv_X = the concentration of X in renal venous plasma.

The reason PAH, rather than inulin, is ordinarily used for this purpose is that the a-v difference is greater for PAH, so that errors due to measurement influence the results less with PAH than with inulin.

Another way of deriving Equation 5-4 is through the principle of balance. The input of substance X to the kidney is equal to the product of the concentration of X in renal arterial plasma, Pa_X, and the plasma flow rate in the renal artery, RPF_a (Fig. 5-2). The output of X by the kidney is equal to the urinary output of X ($U_X \cdot \dot{V}$) plus the flow of X in the renal vein ($Pv_X \cdot RPF_v$). (The small difference between RPF in the renal artery and that in the renal vein, which is due to urine flow, may be ignored in this example.) In the steady state, input equals output, and solving the balance equation in Figure 5-2 leads to Equation 5-4.

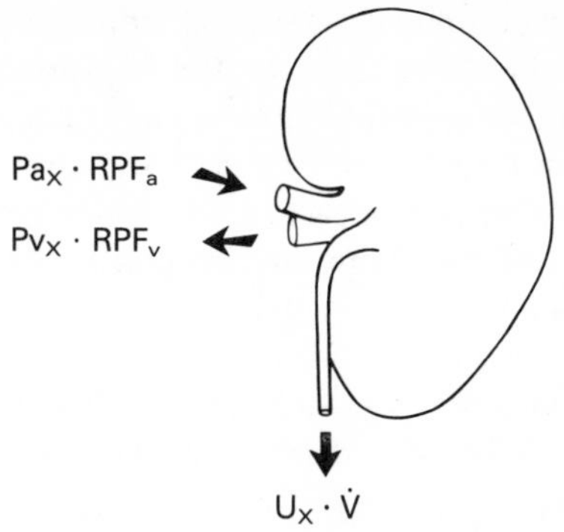

$$Input = Output$$

$$\overline{(Pa_X \cdot RPF_a) = (U_X \cdot \dot{V}) + (Pv_X \cdot RPF_v)}$$

$$(Pa_X \cdot RPF_a) - (Pv_X \cdot RPF_v) = (U_X \cdot \dot{V})$$

$$RPF (Pa_X - Pv_X) = U_X \cdot \dot{V}$$

$$RPF = \frac{U_X \cdot \dot{V}}{Pa_X - Pv_X} \qquad \text{(Eq. 5-4)}$$

Fig. 5-2 : Application of the principle of balance to the derivation of Equation 5-4. Symbols are explained in the text.

EXTRACTION RATIO (E). This ratio yields the fraction of a given substance that is removed from the plasma in a single passage through the kidneys. It is calculated by the following equation:

$$E_X = \frac{Pa_X - Pv_X}{Pa_X} \qquad (5\text{-}5)$$

The ratio can be calculated for any substance. For PAH at low plasma concentrations, Pv_{PAH} approaches zero, and E is about 0.85 to 0.90; for glucose, which is normally almost completely reabsorbed, E will be virtually 0.

From Equation 5-5, $E_X \cdot Pa_X = Pa_X - Pv_X$; substituting in Equation 5-4:

$$RPF = \frac{U_X \cdot \dot{V}}{Pa_X \cdot E_X} \qquad (5\text{-}6)$$

Catheterization of the renal artery and vein is a fairly routine, safe procedure that is frequently done, even in unanesthetized human patients. The procedure is usually carried out for diagnostic purposes other than the determination of RPF, however. In most studies on humans, renal plasma flow is either measured by some method other than the Fick principle (see Chap. 6) or ap-proximated as ERPF (Eq. 5-3). But in experimental work on ani-mals, the Fick principle and Equation 5-6 are commonly em-ployed. For a substance such as PAH, which is not metabolized by any organ, and not excreted by any organ other than the kidneys, a sample from any peripheral vessel can be used to determine Pa_X.

Calculation of Renal Blood Flow (RBF)

If the hematocrit (Hct) — i.e., the fraction of whole blood that is cells — is 0.45 or 45%, the fraction of whole blood that is plasma is 0.55. Hence,

$$\frac{RPF}{0.55} = \frac{RBF}{1.00}, \text{ and}$$

$$RBF = \frac{RPF}{0.55} = \frac{RPF}{1.00 - Hct} \tag{5-7}$$

Substituting 660 ml per minute for RPF,

$$RBF = \frac{660}{1.00 - 0.45} = \frac{660}{0.55} = 1,200 \text{ ml/min}$$

Filtration Fraction (FF)

The filtration fraction, alluded to in Chapter 3, is that fraction of the plasma flowing through the kidneys that is filtered into Bow-man's space. It is calculated by the following formula:

$$FF = \frac{GFR}{RPF}$$

Substituting 132 ml per minute for GFR (see Fig. 3-4) and 660 ml per minute for RPF (above)

$$FF = \frac{132}{660} = 0.20$$

This is simply restating that normally about one-fifth, or 20%, of the plasma entering the glomerular capillaries is filtered. Changes in this value can alter the oncotic pressure in peritubu-lar capillaries and thereby the reabsorption of tubular fluid (see Fig. 7-9).

Summary

Tubular secretion refers to the transport of substances into the tubular lumen by means other than glomerular filtration. Se-cretion defines the direction of transport, not the mode. When we speak of a substance as being filtered and secreted, we usually mean *net* secretion; this net transport can be quantified by means of Equation 5-1.

The process of secretion may be viewed as helping the body to get rid of potentially harmful compounds, especially when they are bound to plasma proteins and therefore cannot be filtered in large amounts. Secretion may also serve as a means to get metabolic substrates into tubular cells, and to bring certain drugs and certain endogenous compounds that act at the luminal membrane of tubular cells to these sites.

At low plasma concentrations — i.e., below Tm_{PAH} — 85 to 90% of the PAH is removed from the plasma in a single circuit through the kidneys. Hence, at low plasma concentrations of PAH, the clearance of PAH, C_{PAH}, yields a fairly close approximation of the renal plasma flow; this approximation is known as the effective renal plasma flow (ERPF). The exact renal plasma flow (RPF) can be determined through application of the Fick principle, and this is often done by measuring the renal extraction of PAH.

The rate of renal blood flow (RBF) can be calculated by means of a simple proportionality if the fraction of whole blood that is made up of cells (the hematocrit) is known.

The filtration fraction (FF) is normally about 0.20; that is, normally about 20% of the plasma that traverses the kidneys is filtered into Bowman's space.

Problem 5-1 Determination of renal plasma flow (RPF), renal blood flow (RBF), and filtration fraction (FF), using PAH and inulin in dogs. The extraction ratio of PAH (E_{PAH}) changes during the postnatal period, when these data were obtained. Utilizing the data given, fill in the blank columns.

Age (days)	Urine Flow (μl per min per g of kidney)[c]	U_{PAH} (mg/100 ml)	Pa_{PAH}[a] (mg/100 ml)	Pv_{PAH}[a] (mg/100 ml)	E_{PAH}	RPF (μl per min per g of kidney)[c]	RBF[b] (μl per min per g of kidney)[c]	C_{In} (μl per min per g of kidney)[c]	FF
2	3.8	104	2.60	2.16				130	
21	2.7	283	1.70	1.08				270	
40	5.2	664	3.00	1.23				630	
60	3.2	672	1.20	0.34				790	
74	2.3	3,516	3.10	0.52				1,200	

[a]Pa_{PAH} and Pv_{PAH} = concentration of PAH in arterial and renal venous plasma, respectively.
[b]Assume that the hematocrit = 0.45.
[c]Values have been expressed per gram of kidney in order to correct for any changes that might be due to growth of the kidney during the postnatal period.
Abstracted from Horster, M., and Valtin, H. *J. Clin. Invest.* 50:779, 1971.

**Selected
References**

*The Process of
Secretion*

Bayliss, L. E. The Process of Secretion. In F. R. Winton (Ed.), *Modern Views on the Secretion of Urine.* London: Churchill, 1956.

Chambers, R., and Kempton, R. T. Indications of function of the chick mesonephros in tissue culture with phenol red. *J. Cell. Comp. Physiol.* 3:131, 1933.

Cross, R. J., and Taggart, J. V. Renal tubular transport: Accumulation of p-aminohippurate by rabbit kidney slices. *Am. J. Physiol.* 161:181, 1950.

Cushny, A. R. *The Secretion of the Urine.* London: Longmans, Green, 1917.

Dantzler, W. H., and Bentley, S. K. Effects of inhibitors in lumen on PAH and urate transport by isolated renal tubules. *Am. J. Physiol.* 236 (Renal Fluid Electrolyte Physiol. 5):F379, 1979.

Forster, R. P. Active cellular transport of urea by the frog renal tubules. *Am. J. Physiol.* 179:372, 1954.

Forster, R. P. Urea and the Early History of Renal Clearance Studies. In B. Schmidt-Nielsen (Ed.), *Urea and the Kidney.* Amsterdam: Excerpta Medica, 1970.

Grantham, J. J. Fluid secretion in the nephron: Relation to renal failure. *Physiol. Rev.* 56:248, 1976.

Marshall, E. K., Jr., and Crane, M. The secretory function of the renal tubules. *Am. J. Physiol.* 70:465, 1924.

Marshall, E. K., Jr., and Grafflin, A. L. The structure and function of the kidney of *Lophius piscatorius. Bull. Johns Hopkins Hosp.* 43:205, 1928.

Marshall, E. K., Jr., and Vickers, J. L. The mechanism of the elimination of phenolsulphonphthalein by the kidney: A proof of secretion by the convoluted tubules. *Bull. Johns Hopkins Hosp.* 34:1, 1923.

Mudge, G. H., and Taggart, J. V. Effect of acetate on the renal excretion of p-aminohippurate in the dog. *Am. J. Physiol.* 161:191, 1950.

Pitts, R. F. *Physiology of the Kidney and Body Fluids* (3rd ed.). Chicago: Year Book, 1974.

Shannon, J. A. The renal excretion of phenol red by the aglomerular fishes, *Opsanus tau* and *Lophius piscatorius. J. Cell. Comp. Physiol.* 11:315, 1938.

Shannon, J. A. Renal tubular excretion. *Physiol. Rev.* 19:63, 1939.

Smith, H. W. Newer Methods of Study of Renal Function in Man. In *Lectures on the Kidney.* Lawrence: University of Kansas Press, 1943. Pp. 25–46.

Smith, H. W. *The Kidney: Structure and Function in Health and Disease.* New York: Oxford University Press, 1951.

*Organic Acids
and Bases*

Berndt, W. O., and Grote, D. The accumulation of C^{14}-dinitrophenol by slices of rabbit kidney cortex. *J. Pharmacol. Exp. Ther.* 164:223, 1968.

Berner, W., and Kinne, R. Transport of p-aminohippuric acid by plasma membrane vesicles isolated from rat kidney cortex. *Pflügers Arch. Eur. J. Physiol.* 361:269, 1976.

Beyer, K. H., Peters, L., Woodward, R., and Verwey, W. F. The enhancement of the physiological economy of penicillin in dogs by the simultaneous administration of para-aminohippuric acid. *J. Pharmacol. Exp. Ther.* 82:310, 1944.

Beyer, K. H., Russo, H. F., Tilson, E. K., Miller, A. K., Verwey, W. F., and Gass, S. R. Benemid, p-(di-n-propylsulfamyl)-benzoic acid: Its renal affinity and its elimination. *Am. J. Physiol.* 166:625, 1951.

Cohen, J. J., Chesney, R. W., Brand, P. H., Neville, H. F., and Blanchard, C. F. α-Ketoglutarate metabolism and K^+ uptake by dog kidney slices. *Am. J. Physiol.* 217:161, 1969.

Cohen, J. J., and Wittmann, E. Renal utilization and excretion of α-ketoglutarate in dog: Effect of alkalosis. *Am. J. Physiol.* 204:795, 1963.

Dantzler, W. H. Urate and p-aminohippurate transport by isolated, perfused reptilian renal tubules. *Physiologist* 21 (No. 5):5, 1978.

Forster, R. P., and Copenhaver, J. H., Jr. Intracellular accumulation as an active process in a mammalian renal transport system *in vitro:* Energy dependence and competitive phenomena. *Am. J. Physiol.* 186:167, 1956.

Grantham, J. J., and Irish, J. M., III. Organic Acid Transport and Fluid Secretion in the Pars Recta (PST) of the Proximal Tubule. In H. G. Vogel and K. J. Ullrich (Eds.), *New Aspects of Renal Function.* Amsterdam: Excerpta Medica, 1978.

Greger, R., Lang, F., and Deetjen, P. Renal excretion of purine metabolites, urate and allantoin, by the mammalian kidney. *Int. Rev. Physiol.* 11:257, 1976.

Hong, S. K., and Forster, R. P. Further observations on the separate steps involved in the active transport of chlorphenol red by isolated renal tubules of the flounder in vitro. *J. Cell. Comp. Physiol.* 54:237, 1959.

Mudge, G. H., and Taggart, J. V. Effect of 2,4-dinitrophenol on renal transport mechanisms in the dog. *Am. J. Physiol.* 161:173, 1950.

Rennick, B. R. Proximal Tubular Transport and Renal Metabolism of Organic Cations and Catechol. In M. Martinez-Maldonado (Ed.), *Methods in Pharmacology,* vol. 4A, *Renal Pharmacology.* New York: Plenum, 1976.

Selleck, B. H., and Cohen, J. J. Specific localization of α-ketoglutarate uptake to dog kidney and liver *in vivo. Am. J. Physiol.* 208:24, 1965.

Sperber, I. Secretion of organic anions in the formation of urine and bile. *Pharmacol. Rev.* 11:109, 1959.

Taggart, J. V., and Forster, R. P. Renal tubular transport: Effect of 2,4-dinitrophenol and related compounds on phenol red transport in the isolated tubules of the flounder. *Am. J. Physiol.* 161:167, 1950.

Torretti, J., and Weiner, I. M. The Renal Excretion of Drugs. In M. Martinez-Maldonado (Ed.), *Methods in Pharmacology,* vol. 4A, *Renal Pharmacology.* New York: Plenum, 1976.

Weiner, I. M. Transport of Weak Acids and Bases. In J. Orloff and R. W. Berliner (Eds.), *Handbook of Physiology,* section 8, Renal Physiology. Washington, D.C.: American Physiological Society, 1973.

Weiner, I. M., and Mudge, G. H. Renal tubular mechanisms for excretion of organic acids and bases. *Am. J. Med.* 36:743, 1964.

Woodhall, P. B., Tisher, C. C., Simonton, C. A., and Robinson, R. R. Relationship between para-aminohippurate secretion and cellular morphology in rabbit proximal tubules. *J. Clin. Invest.* 61:1320, 1978.

Renal Plasma Flow,
Renal Blood Flow,
Extraction

Note: For further references on these topics, see Selected References at the end of Chapter 6.

Horster, M., and Lewy, J. E. Filtration fraction and extraction of PAH during the neonatal period in the rat. *Am. J. Physiol.* 219:1061, 1970.

Horster, M., and Valtin, H. Postnatal development of renal function: Micropuncture and clearance studies in the dog. *J. Clin. Invest.* 50:779, 1971.

Pilkington, L. A., Binder, R., deHaas, J. C. M., and Pitts, R. F. Intrarenal distribution of blood flow. *Am. J. Physiol.* 208:1107, 1965.

Reubi, F. Objections à la théorie de la séparation intrarénale des hématies et du plasma (Pappenheimer). *Helv. Med. Acta* 25:516, 1958.

Smith, H. W. The Renal Blood Flow in Normal Subjects. In *Lectures on the Kidney.* Lawrence: University of Kansas Press, 1943. Pp. 47–62.

Smith, H. W. *The Kidney: Structure and Function in Health and Disease.* New York: Oxford University Press, 1951.

6 : Renal Hemodynamics and Oxygen Consumption

The two kidneys of an adult human together weigh about 300 g, and thus constitute less than 0.5% of the body weight. Yet, they are perfused by an amount of blood that is equal to 20 to 25% of the cardiac output, i.e., in excess of 1,000 ml per minute. The reason for this very high rate of perfusion is probably related to the evolutionary development of an organ with a high filtering capacity, as discussed in Chapter 1.

In addition to the high rate of flow, the renal circulation has a number of other characteristic features, some of which are unique. This chapter will concentrate on these features.

Hydrostatic Pressures and Resistances in the Renal Vascular Tree

Hydrostatic pressures in the major renal vessels are shown in Figure 6-1. The data are from rats; although absolute values in humans and other species might be slightly different, the profile is almost certainly similar. Of particular importance are the large decreases in pressure that occur in the afferent and efferent arterioles, identifying these two vessels as the major sites of vascular resistance. Changes in the resistance within either of these

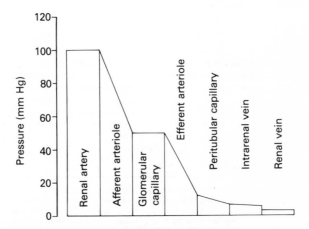

Fig. 6-1 : **Hydrostatic pressure profile in the renal vascular tree of the rat. Data from Brenner, B. M., Troy, J. L., and Daugharty, T. M.** J. Clin. Invest. **50:1776, 1971; and** Proceedings of the XXV International Congress of Physiological Sciences, **Abstract No. 229.**

vessels will alter the renal blood flow (RBF); but it is the differential changes in the resistances within both vessels that will determine the hydrostatic pressure within the glomerular capillaries, and hence the rate of glomerular ultrafiltration (see Fig. 3-1).

It is possible that the afferent and efferent arterioles of outer cortical nephrons have properties different from those of the corresponding vessels of juxtamedullary nephrons. Such differences, which might involve types of nerve supply or responses to humoral agents, could partly account for the differential behavior of the renal circulation in different regions of the kidney, which are described below.

Intrarenal Differences in Glomerular Filtration

Two types of nephron, the outer cortical and the juxtamedullary, were described in Chapter 1. Besides having anatomical distinctions, these nephrons also differ functionally. As shown in Table 6-1, under control conditions the so-called *single nephron* glomerular filtration rate (sGFR, as distinct from GFR, which refers to the glomerular filtration rate of the entire kidney) of a juxtamedullary nephron is greater than that of a nephron lying in more superficial parts of the cortex. Furthermore, differential changes in these filtration rates occur during various conditions. Water diuresis (defined in Chap. 7) is accompanied by a reduction in the sGFR of juxtamedullary nephrons but no change in that of outer cortical nephrons. An increase in sodium intake, on the other hand, may be associated with an increase in the sGFR of outer cortical nephrons.

The functional significance of these changes is not yet clear; it is possible that they involve the regulation of sodium and water balance (Chaps. 7 and 8). Nor have the mechanisms responsible for these changes been identified. The fact that the sGFR of juxtamedullary nephrons is higher in the control state than during

Table 6-1 : Intrarenal differences in the glomerular filtration rates of single nephrons (sGFR) of rats, under varying conditions.

Condition	Outer Cortical Nephron (nl/min)[b]	Juxtamedullary Nephron (nl/min)[b]
Control (ADH present)[a]	30	50
Water diuresis (ADH absent)	30	35
High sodium intake	40	50

[a]ADH = antidiuretic hormone (see Chap. 8).
[b]Note units: nanoliters per minute.
Note: All values are approximations that have been rounded off. They have been taken from the following: Horster, M., and Thurau, K. *Pflügers Arch. Ges. Physiol.* 301:162, 1968; Jamison, R. L. *Am. J. Physiol.* 218:46, 1969; de Rouffignac, C., Deiss, S., and Bonvalet, J. P. *Pflügers Arch. Eur. J. Physiol.* 315:273, 1970; Davis, J. M., and Schnermann, J. *Pflügers Arch. Eur. J. Physiol.* 330:323, 1971; Daugharty, T. M., Troy, J. L., and Brenner, B. M. *Proceedings of the XXV International Congress of Physiological Sciences,* Abstract No. 383.

water diuresis probably reflects a relative increase in the resistance of the efferent as opposed to the afferent arteriole in the presence of antidiuretic hormone (ADH) (see Fig. 6-2); the mechanism for this change in resistance is not yet known (see p. 104).

Intrarenal Differences in Blood Flow

Control

The total renal blood flow can be measured by relatively direct techniques, as with an electromagnetic flow meter attached to the renal artery, or indirectly through application of the Fick principle (see Chap. 5, Exact Renal Plasma Flow [RPF]. Extraction of PAH). Other methods, however, must be used to detect differences in blood flow to the major regions of the kidney. Such methods are based, variously, on the fractional tissue uptake of dyes or radioactive markers, on filling of the renal vasculature with a silicone rubber compound, on dye dilution curves recorded by tiny detectors inserted into the renal tissue, or on the rate of washout of certain markers from the tissue. Results obtained in dogs by the last two techniques are summarized in Table 6-2; the situation is similar in humans. More than 90% of the total renal blood flow perfuses the cortical region. Considering that about one-quarter of the cardiac output goes to the kidneys, this amounts to a perfusion rate per unit of cortical tissue that is more than 100 times higher than that of resting muscle. Only a very small portion of the total renal blood flow enters the outer medulla, and only about 1% perfuses the inner medulla. Again, however, since total renal blood flow is so great, the absolute flow per unit even of inner medullary tissue is still approximately the same as that of resting muscle.

The high cortical perfusion rate is almost certainly related to the evolutionary development of the kidney as a filtering organ and not to its oxygen requirements. The relatively low medullary

Table 6-2 : Distribution of total renal blood flow (RBF) in dogs under control conditions.

Region	RBF (ml/100 g of kidney · min)	Proportion of Total Renal Blood Flow (%)
Cortex	340	93
Outer medulla	21	6
Inner medulla	2.5	0.7

Note: All values are averages taken from the work of: Kramer, K., et al. *Pflügers Arch. Ges. Physiol.* 270:251, 1960; Deetjen, P., et al. *Pflügers Arch. Ges. Physiol.* 279:281, 1964; and Thorburn, G. D., et al. *Circ. Res.* 13:290, 1963.

perfusion, in turn, is crucial to the important function of the kidneys to conserve water; this is considered in detail in Chapter 8 (under Countercurrent Exchange in Vasa Recta).

The mechanisms that so strikingly decrease the medullary blood flow as compared to cortical flow have not been entirely identified. It seems clear, however, that they do not involve a decrease in the vascular volume per unit of renal tissue, which is roughly the same — 20% — in the cortex, outer medulla, and inner medulla. There is, rather, an increased resistance to flow; this resistance lies mainly in the descending vasa recta, and it may be related to their length; to the smooth muscles in their efferent arterioles and their innervation; to other factors, such as increased viscosity of medullary blood; or to all of these.

Hemorrhage

The renal circulation is exquisitely sensitive to blood loss. Even relatively small hemorrhages, which do not decrease the systemic blood pressure, can result in striking decreases in the renal blood flow. The reduction affects primarily the superficial cortex. In contrast to the control situation, when there is uniform filling of the vessels throughout the cortex (see Fig. 1-1B), after hemorrhage there is a selective reduction in the blood flow to the superficial cortex and increased filling in the juxtamedullary and outer medullary regions. A similar change in the distribution of renal blood is seen in other conditions, such as heart or liver failure. The fact that this pattern is also seen when the renal sympathetic nerves are stimulated may be a clue to at least one of the mechanisms that may cause the change in distribution.

Antidiuretic Hormone (ADH)

Normally, this hormone is present in the blood; its effect on the renal blood flow has been tested by first removing ADH from the circulation and then restoring it, usually in the same animal. In the absence of ADH, i.e., in water diuresis, blood flow to the superficial cortex is increased over the control situation, flow in the juxtamedullary region and outer medulla is decreased, and that in the inner medulla is increased. These changes in the distribution of renal blood flow can be returned to that of the control state by administering ADH. These results have been interpreted to reflect a vasoconstrictor action of ADH.

Mechanisms Causing Changes in GFR and RBF

The examples cited above are only a few of many influences that can alter the GFR and the RBF. It is important to realize at this point not only that these two functions can change, but also that each may simultaneously undergo different alterations in various regions of the kidney, and that there may be divergent shifts in the filtration rate and blood flow. These points are illustrated in

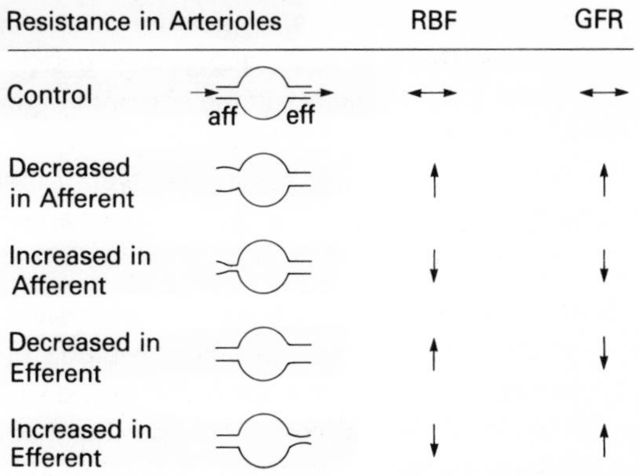

Resistance in Arterioles		RBF	GFR
Control	aff — eff	↔	↔
Decreased in Afferent		↑	↑
Increased in Afferent		↓	↓
Decreased in Efferent		↑	↓
Increased in Efferent		↓	↑

Fig. 6-2 : Changes in renal blood flow (RBF) and glomerular filtration rate (GFR) that will occur when resistance is altered in either the afferent or the efferent arterioles, provided that renal perfusion pressure does not change. Details are discussed in the text.

Figure 6-2. We assume that the hydrostatic pressure in the renal artery (the so-called renal perfusion pressure) does not change in the following examples.

If resistance decreases in the afferent arterioles, then there will be an increase in RBF; this conclusion follows from the relationship

$$\dot{Q} = \frac{\Delta P}{R} \tag{6-1}$$

where $\dot{Q}$ = the rate of blood flow (i.e., RBF)

ΔP = the difference in hydrostatic pressure between two points in the axial circuit (i.e., between the renal artery and the renal vein)

R = the vascular resistance (i.e., the total renal resistance).

Inasmuch as the decrease in afferent resistance will raise the hydrostatic pressure within the glomerular capillaries (P_c of Equation 2-6; *note* that this equation must be used to assess changes in GFR, not Equation 6-1), there will also be an increase in GFR. Exactly the opposite reasoning applies when resistance in the afferent arterioles is increased: By the formula $\dot{Q} = \Delta P/R$, RBF will diminish, and because P_c in Equation 2-6 falls, GFR will also decline.

Changes in resistance within efferent arterioles, on the other hand, will lead to divergent alterations in RBF and GFR. Thus, if there is a decrease in efferent resistance, then (by Eq. 6-1) RBF will rise and (by Eq. 2-6) P_c, and therefore GFR, will fall. And the opposite changes occur when efferent resistance increases.

Note, then, that when resistance is altered in the afferent arterioles, RBF and GFR change in the same direction, whereas alteration of resistance in the efferent arterioles will cause movements of RBF and GFR in opposite directions. Finally, the schema depicted in Figure 6-2 will hold even if there are simultaneous changes of resistance in both afferent and efferent arterioles, so long as the net change in any instance is that shown in the figure.

With so many variables simultaneously influencing both the glomerular filtration rate and the blood flow, not only for the entire kidney but also for each nephron and depending on its location, it is perhaps not surprising that the mechanisms of control are not yet clear. Although normal renal function may be maintained after complete denervation, there is nevertheless evidence that the autonomic innervation of the kidneys has a functional role under some circumstances. There are also data that show the influence of humoral agents, such as the catecholamines, angiotensin, the prostaglandins, the kinins, ADH, and the adrenal steroids. What is not yet clear, however, is on which vessel(s) some of these factors exert their influence, in which region of the kidney, and under what circumstances.

Autoregulation of RBF and GFR

The phenomenon of autoregulation is illustrated in Figure 6-3, which portrays the RBF and the GFR measured simultaneously in dogs as their renal arterial pressure is varied. Note that over a range of pressure from about 80 to 180 mm Hg, a 100% increase in perfusion pressure causes an increase in RBF of less than 10%. This, by the formula $\dot{Q} = \Delta P/R$, must mean that somehow an increase in perfusion pressure is accompanied by a nearly equivalent increase in vascular resistance. By the deductions referred to in relation to Figure 6-2, the simultaneous "constancy" of GFR and RBF (shown in Fig. 6-3) indicates that the predominant change in resistance must have occurred in the afferent arterioles.

Autoregulation persists even after complete renal denervation, after adrenal demedullation, and in a completely isolated kidney perfused with plasma in vitro. Hence, as the term is meant to indicate, autoregulation must be due to a change exclusively within the kidney, and brought about when the arterial perfusion pressure is altered.

The mechanism of autoregulation has not been fully identified. It seems likely that it involves varying tone of smooth muscle in afferent arterioles, which may be governed in part through a mechanism described by W. M. Bayliss many years ago. That mechanism is an intrinsic property of arterial smooth muscle whereby that muscle contracts when it is stretched and relaxes

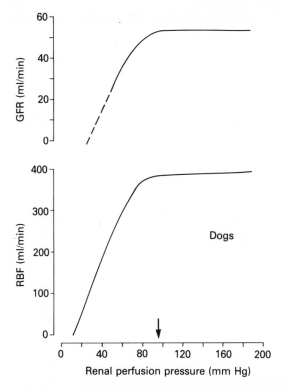

Fig. 6-3 : **Autoregulation of the renal blood flow (RBF) and glomerular filtration rate (GFR) in dogs as the renal perfusion pressure is varied. The arrow indicates the approximate normal mean pressure in the renal arteries. The fact that RBF and GFR are simultaneously kept constant must mean that the net change in resistance occurs in the afferent arterioles. Note that within the so-called autoregulatory range of approximately 80 to 180 mm Hg (and assuming a hematocrit of 45% — Eq. 5-7), the filtration fraction in this example is 0.25, or 25%. Adapted from Navar, L. G.** *Am. J. Physiol.* **234 (Renal Fluid Electrolyte Physiol. 3):F357, 1978.**

when it is shortened. Additionally, or alternatively, autoregulation may be attributable to a phenomenon known as *tubuloglomerular feedback.*

Tubuloglomerular Feedback

This mechanism, as the name implies, involves a feedback loop in which the flow rate of tubular fluid, or some derivative thereof, is sensed at the macula densa of the juxtaglomerular apparatus (JGA) and in turn governs the filtration rate of the single glomerulus (sGFR) to which that JGA is apposed (see Chap. 1, under The Juxtaglomerular Apparatus). It has been shown, for example, that when a single loop of Henle is microperfused at an abnormally high rate (thus simulating an increased rate of filtration), the sGFR in that particular nephron is reduced, mainly because of a decreased hydrostatic pressure in glomerular capillaries (P_c of Eq. 2-6, and Fig. 6-1). The opposite also holds, although to a lesser degree: When tubular flow rate through the loop of Henle is decreased, P_c and sGFR are increased.

The major unknowns about tubuloglomerular feedback concern the variable(s) that is sensed at the JGA as well as the effector substance(s) that alters the tone of the arteriolar smooth muscle — probably of the afferent arteriole. It is possible that the specialized macula densa cells of the distal tubule (see Fig. 1-3) monitor the NaCl within the tubular fluid at this point; but it is not known whether the variable that is sensed is the concentration of Cl^-, or the amount of Cl^- that is reabsorbed, or some other correlate of the tubular flow rate — or whether indeed it is Cl^- at all rather than Na^+ or Ca^{2+} or osmolality. Nor is it settled whether the effector mechanism involves mainly renin-angiotensin or possibly some other vasoactive substances, such as the prostaglandins, the catecholamines, the kinins, or other substances.

Tubuloglomerular feedback and autoregulation may have evolved to subserve the critical function of salt balance (see Chap. 7, under Renal Regulation of Na^+ Balance). That is, as sGFR increases and therefore an abnormally large amount of NaCl is filtered, this fact might be quickly sensed at the JGA and corrected through a negative feedback loop that decreases the sGFR. The concomitant autoregulation of RBF (Fig. 6-3) could be a mere by-product of one mechanism by which the kidneys maintain salt balance; or, since the rate of plasma flow through glomerular capillaries can in part determine the rate of glomerular filtration (see Chap. 3, Forces Involved in Glomerular Ultrafiltration), autoregulation of RBF might be an integral part of autoregulation of GFR.

Renal Oxygen Consumption

According to the Fick principle, the oxygen consumption of an organ, $\dot{V}_{O_2}$, is related directly to the rate of blood flow to that organ, $\dot{Q}$, and to the difference in oxygen content between the artery, Ca_{O_2}, and vein, Cv_{O_2}, of that organ.

$$\dot{V}_{O_2} = \dot{Q}(Ca_{O_2} - Cv_{O_2}) \tag{6-2}$$

In most organs, such as skeletal muscle, the resting oxygen consumption remains constant as the blood flow to that organ is reduced. Consequently, the arteriovenous (a-v) oxygen content difference rises in proportion to the decrease in flow (Eq. 6-2). The heart is an exception, since even at rest the coronary a-v oxygen difference is very high, about 11 vol%. Therefore, when coronary blood flow decreases, the oxygen supply to the myocardium is deficient. For this reason, the heart is known as a flow-limited organ.

There are two seeming paradoxes in renal oxygen consumption. (1) Even though this consumption per weight of renal tissue is greater than that of any other organ save the heart, the renal a-v oxygen difference is only about 1.7 vol%, probably the lowest of any organ. (2) Despite the very low a-v oxygen difference, the kidneys behave like flow-limited organs. The solution to these paradoxes is illustrated in Figure 6-4; it involves the fact that the main renal requirement for oxidative energy is the tubular reabsorption of sodium.

As is shown in Figure 6-4A, the relationship among renal blood flow, renal oxygen consumption, and renal a-v oxygen difference goes through three phases as the blood flow is decreased. At first, down to a blood flow of approximately 150 ml per 100 g of kidney per minute, the oxygen consumption decreases proportionally, so that the a-v oxygen difference does not change; that is, from about 700 to 150 ml of blood flow, the kidneys act like flow-limited organs. As blood flow decreases further, the kidneys behave like most other organs, i.e., they extract more oxygen from each unit of blood flowing through them, thereby meeting basal needs to keep renal cells alive and functioning. At extremely low levels of renal blood flow (below approximately 75 ml per 100 g of kidney per minute), no more oxygen can be extracted even as the flow decreases; consequently, at this point the renal cells will undergo ischemic damage and they may die.

These relationships puzzled renal physiologists until it became clear that the true independent variable is not the renal blood flow but rather the glomerular filtration rate and hence the amount of sodium that is filtered ($P_{Na} \cdot$ GFR). There is a direct correlation between the filtration rate and the oxygen consumption (Fig. 6-4B). With a stable plasma sodium concentration (P_{Na}), the amount of sodium filtered into the tubular system varies in direct proportion to the GFR. And since virtually all the filtered sodium is reabsorbed (Table 1-1), the true independent variable that determines renal oxygen consumption is the amount of sodium that must be reabsorbed. This fact is illustrated in Figure 6-4C, which is based on experiments that showed a linear correlation between renal oxygen consumption and sodium reabsorption as the latter was varied by a number of maneuvers.

When GFR, and hence sodium reabsorption, ceases (Fig. 6-4B and C), the remaining oxygen consumption reflects the basal requirements of the renal tissue, amounting to about one-third of the total oxygen consumption of the normally functioning kidney. Interestingly, this basal consumption of a little less than 100 μMoles per 100 g of kidney per minute is about the same as that

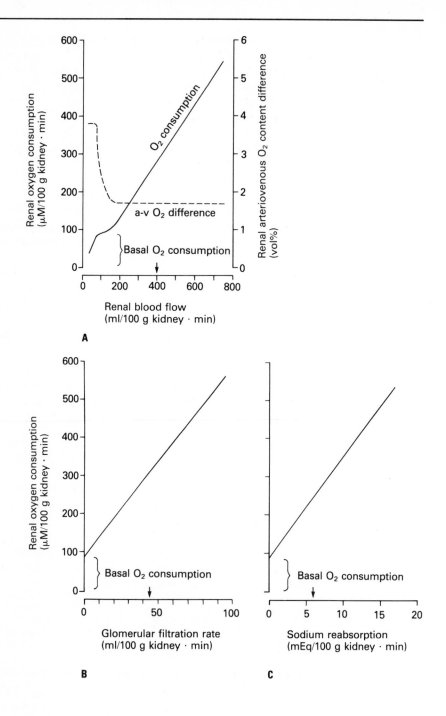

A

B

C

of other epithelial tissues. It is only in this range of oxygen requirements that the kidneys act like many other organs, i.e., by extracting more oxygen when the rate of flow is insufficient to meet the minimal needs.

Sodium reabsorption is an active process (see Chap. 7) which, according to the direct correlation shown in Figure 6-4C, depends largely on energy derived from oxidative metabolism. This deduction fits well with the fact that most of the filtered sodium is reabsorbed in the proximal and distal tubules (see Fig. 7-7), i.e., in the renal cortex, which has a very high rate of aerobic metabolism; in contrast, renal medullary structures derive much energy from anaerobic as well as from aerobic metabolism. The cost of reabsorbing filtered sodium is about 1 μMole of oxygen for every 28 μEq of sodium reabsorbed.

Summary

The mammalian renal circulation has a number of unique features. Per unit of tissue weight, the kidneys are perfused by more blood and they consume more oxygen than does almost any other organ. Yet, the renal arteriovenous (a-v) oxygen content difference is lower than that of other organs. The rate of renal blood flow (RBF) and the filtration rate of individual glomeruli (sGFR) vary not only under different conditions but also in different regions of the kidney. Ordinarily, both variables are

---

Fig. 6-4 : Experiments in dogs, which solved the puzzle that even though oxygen consumption is very high per unit of renal tissue, the renal arteriovenous (a-v) oxygen content difference is very low; and that despite the low a-v oxygen content difference, the kidneys act like flow-limited organs over a wide range of renal blood flow. The arrows indicate approximate normal values for renal blood flow, glomerular filtration rate, and sodium reabsorption.

A. As renal blood flow decreases to about 150 ml per 100 g of kidney per minute, renal oxygen consumption decreases proportionally, so that the a-v oxygen content difference does not change (Eq. 6-2). In these experiments, the changes in renal blood flow were either spontaneous or induced by altering renal perfusion pressure after autoregulation had been abolished.

B. In these experiments, the glomerular filtration rate (GFR) varied directly as the renal blood flow. The relationship between the filtration rate and renal oxygen consumption was linear over the entire range of GFR. Since plasma sodium concentration did not change, the rate at which sodium was filtered ($P_{Na} \cdot$ GFR) must have varied in direct proportion to the GFR, suggesting that the oxidative energy required to reabsorb sodium might be the true independent variable that determines the rate of renal oxygen consumption.

C. This suggestion was confirmed by varying the rate of renal sodium reabsorption by means other than, and in addition to, changes in GFR. The experimental maneuvers included constriction of the renal vein, and intravenous infusions of Na^+ salts. No matter how sodium reabsorption was varied, oxygen consumption changed proportionately.

These graphs are based on data from the following references: Kramer, K., and Deetjen, P. *Pflügers Arch. Ges. Physiol.* 271:782, 1960; Lassen, N. A., Munck, O., and Thaysen, J. H. *Acta Physiol. Scand.* 51:371, 1961; Deetjen, P., and Kramer, K. *Pflügers Arch. Ges. Physiol.* 273:636, 1961.

autoregulated in most nephrons — in part through an intrinsic mechanism of arteriolar smooth muscle described by W. M. Bayliss, and partly by tubuloglomerular feedback.

These unique features are best understood in the context of salt and water balance. Probably through evolutionary forces, the kidney became an organ of high filtering capacity. As a necessary concomitant, the RBF is far in excess of the basal oxygen requirements, so that the a-v oxygen content difference is very low. In most terrestrial mammals, the potential liability of high filtration is counteracted by virtually complete reabsorption of the filtered water and sodium. The latter requires energy (see Chap. 7) and is, in fact, the process that accounts for the high rate of renal oxygen consumption (which amounts to about 10% of the total body oxygen uptake). But since an increased rate of filtration is ordinarily accompanied by an increase in the RBF, the greater need for oxygen is "automatically" met so that an increase in oxygen extraction is not required. The *raison d'être* for autoregulation of the GFR may well be the regulation of sodium balance. Simultaneous autoregulation of the blood flow might be a mere coincidental event or it might be an integral part of the mechanism by which GFR is attuned. Finally, the intrarenal distribution of the blood flow and filtration rate may also be governed primarily by the need for the conservation of sodium and water.

Problem 6-1

This problem has been adapted from two reports: Horster, M., and Thurau, K. *Pflügers Arch. Ges. Physiol.* 301:162, 1968; Jamison, R. L. *Am. J. Physiol.* 218:46, 1969.

An anesthetized rat, which weighed 140 g, was prepared for renal micropuncture. The animal was given inulin by intravenous infusion to attain a steady plasma concentration for this compound. A late segment of a proximal tubule was punctured at the surface of the kidney, and a droplet of oil was instilled into the tubular lumen through the micropipet. (To visualize this procedure, see Fig. 3-5.) All of the tubular fluid flowing just proximal to the oil droplet was then collected for a period of 3 minutes, during which time a sample of blood was obtained from a femoral artery. This procedure was repeated three times in other proximal tubules.

Next, the papilla was exposed by incision of the renal pelvis (see Fig. 1-1; rats have only a single papilla), the bend of a loop of Henle was punctured, and tubular fluid was collected quantitatively, as described above for a proximal tubule. Again, samples of arterial blood were obtained during each collection of tubular fluid. This procedure was applied to two other bends of loops of Henle.

Table 6-3 : Results obtained on micropuncture samples.

Flow Rate of Tubular Fluid (v̇) (nl/min)	Concentrations in Tubular Fluid (TF)		Concentrations in Arterial Plasma (P)	
	Na⁺ (mEq/L)	Inulin (mg/100 ml)	Na⁺ (mEq/L)	Inulin (mg/100 ml)
Micropunctures of proximal tubules				
11.21	140	209	137	98
Micropunctures of bends of loops of Henle				
9.14	283	583	138	93

Each sample of tubular fluid was analyzed for its total volume and its concentration of inulin and of Na^+. Each sample of arterial blood was centrifuged, and the plasma was analyzed for its concentration of inulin and Na^+. Average values for the two types of collection are given in Table 6-3.

1. What was the glomerular filtration rate of single nephrons (sGFR) at the surface of the kidney? What was the sGFR of nephrons arising deep in the cortex? Explain the difference.
2. What fraction of the glomerular filtrate was reabsorbed by the end of the proximal tubule at the surface of the kidney? What fraction had been reabsorbed up to the bend of the loop of Henle?
3. What fraction of the filtered Na^+ was reabsorbed up to the end of the proximal tubule at the surface of the kidney? What fraction of the filtered Na^+ had been reabsorbed up to the bend of the loop of Henle?

Selected References

General

Andreoli, T. E. (Section Editor). Renal physiology. *Annu. Rev. Physiol.* 42:529, 1980.
The entire section is devoted to the renal circulation, and it offers six authoritative articles on various aspects of the subject.

Aukland, K. Renal blood flow. *Int. Rev. Physiol.* 11:23, 1976.

Barger, A. C., and Herd, J. A. Renal Vascular Anatomy and Distribution of Blood Flow. In J. Orloff and R. W. Berliner (Eds.), *Handbook of Physiology,* section 8, Renal Physiology. Washington D.C.: American Physiological Society, 1973.

Beeuwkes, R., III, Ichikawa, I., and Brenner, B. M. The Renal Circulation. In B. M. Brenner and F. C. Rector, Jr. (Eds.), *The Kidney* (2nd ed.). Philadelphia: Saunders, 1981.

Fourman, J., and Moffat, D. B. *The Blood Vessels of the Kidney.* Oxford: Blackwell, 1971.

Kiil, F. Blood Flow and Oxygen Utilization by the Kidney. In J. W. Fisher (Ed.), *Kidney Hormones.* New York: Academic, 1971.

Sherwood, T., and Lavender, J. P. Renal medullary perfusion: Direct observations by fine detail angiography in the dog. *Nephron* 8:317, 1971.

Thurau, K., and Levine, D. Z. The Renal Circulation. In C. Rouiller and A. F. Muller (Eds.), *The Kidney,* vol. III. New York: Academic, 1971.

Trueta, J., Barclay, A. E., Daniel, P. M., Franklin, K. J., and Prichard, M. M. C. *Studies of the Renal Circulation.* Oxford: Blackwell, 1948.

Winton, F. R. Present concepts of the renal circulation. *Arch. Intern. Med.* 103:495, 1959.

Methods

Bankir, L., Trinh Trang Tan, M.-M., and Grünfeld, J.-P. Measurement of glomerular blood flow in rabbits and rats: Erroneous findings with 15-µm microspheres. *Kidney Int.* 15:126, 1979.

Davis, J. M., and Schnermann, J. The effect of antidiuretic hormone on the distribution of nephron filtration rates in rats with hereditary diabetes insipidus. *Pflügers Arch. Eur. J. Physiol.* 330:323, 1971.

de Rouffignac, C., Deiss, S., and Bonvalet, J. P. Détermination du taux individuel de filtration glomérulaire des néphrons accessibles et inaccessibles à la microponction. *Pflügers Arch. Eur. J. Physiol.* 315:273, 1970.

Fourman, J., and Moffat, D. B. *The Blood Vessels of the Kidney.* Oxford: Blackwell, 1971.

Giebisch, G. H. (Ed.). Symposium on renal micropuncture techniques. *Yale J. Biol. Med.* 45:187, 1972.
Section I of this symposium considers pitfalls and techniques for measuring filtration rates in single nephrons.

Hanssen, O. D. The relationship between glomerular filtration and length of the proximal convoluted tubules in mice. *Acta Pathol. Microbiol. Scand.* 53:265, 1961.

Horster, M., and Thurau, K. Micropuncture studies on the filtration rate of single superficial and juxtamedullary glomeruli in the rat kidney. *Pflügers Arch. Ges. Physiol.* 301:162, 1968.

Jamison, R. L. Micropuncture study of superficial and juxtamedullary nephrons in the rat. *Am. J. Physiol.* 218:46, 1970.

Kramer, K., Thurau, K., and Deetjen, P. Hämodynamik des Nierenmarks: I. Mitteilung. Capilläre Passagezeit, Blutvolumen, Durchblutung, Gewebshämatokrit und O_2-Verbrauch des Nierenmarks in situ. *Pflügers Arch. Ges. Physiol.* 270:251, 1960.

Smith, H. W. *The Kidney: Structure and Function in Health and Disease.* New York: Oxford University Press, 1951.

Thorburn, G. D., Kopald, H. H., Herd, J. A., Hollenberg, M., O'Morchoe, C. C. C., and Barger, A. C. Intrarenal distribution of nutrient blood flow determined with Krypton 85 in the unanesthetized dog. *Circ. Res.* 13:290, 1963.

Thurau, K. Renal hemodynamics. *Am. J. Med.* 36:698, 1964.

Wright, F. S., and Giebisch, G. Glomerular filtration in single nephrons. *Kidney Int.* 1:201, 1972.

Intrarenal Distribution of Blood Flow and Glomerular Filtration

Birtch, A. G., Zakheim, R. M., Jones, L. G., and Barger, A. C. Redistribution of renal blood flow produced by furosemide and ethacrynic acid. *Circ. Res.* 21:869, 1967.

Carriere, S., Thorburn, G. D., O'Morchoe, C. C. C., and Barger, A. C. Intrarenal distribution of blood flow in dogs during haemorrhagic hypotension. *Circ. Res.* 19:167, 1966.

Davis, J. M., Brechtelsbauer, H., Prucksunand, P., Weigl, J., Schnermann, J., and Kramer, K. Relationship between salt loading and distribution of nephron filtration rates in the dog. *Pflügers Arch. Eur. J. Physiol.* 350:259, 1974.

Davis, J. M., and Schnermann, J. The effect of antidiuretic hormone on the distribution of nephron filtration rates in rats with hereditary diabetes insipidus. *Pflügers Arch. Eur. J. Physiol.* 330:323, 1971.

Davis, J. M., Schütz, W., and Schnermann, J. The effect of experimental alterations in urine concentration on nephron filtration rate. *Pflügers Arch. Eur. J. Physiol.* 344:69, 1973.

Fisher, R. D., Grünfeld, J.-P., and Barger, A. C. Intrarenal distribution of blood flow in diabetes insipidus: Role of ADH. *Am. J. Physiol.* 219:1348, 1970.

Horster, M., and Thurau, K. Micropuncture studies on the filtration rate of single superficial and juxtamedullary glomeruli in the rat kidney. *Pflügers Arch. Ges. Physiol.* 301:162, 1968.

Jamison, R. L. Micropuncture study of superficial and juxtamedullary nephrons in the rat. *Am. J. Physiol.* 218:46, 1970.

Johnson, M. D., Park, C. S., and Malvin, R. Antidiuretic hormone and distribution of renal cortical blood flow. *Am. J. Physiol.* 232 (Renal Fluid Electrolyte Physiol. 1):F111, 1977.

Kew, M. C., Varma, R. R., Williams, H. S., Brunt, P. W., Hourigan, K. J., and Sherlock, S. Renal and intrarenal blood-flow in cirrhosis of the liver. *Lancet* 2:504, 1971.

Ladefoged, J., and Munck, O. Distribution of Blood Flow in the Kidney. In J. W. Fisher (Ed.), *Kidney Hormones.* New York: Academic, 1971.

Levinsky, N. G. The renal kallikrein-kinin system. *Circ. Res.* 44:441, 1979.

Pomeranz, B. H., Birtch, A. G., and Barger, A. C. Neural control of intrarenal blood flow. *Am. J. Physiol.* 215:1067, 1968.

Schmid-Schönbein, H., Wells, R. E., and Goldstone, J. Effect of ultrafiltration and plasma osmolarity upon the flow properties of blood: A possible mechanism for control of blood flow in the renal medullary vasa recta. *Pflügers Arch. Eur. J. Physiol.* 338:93, 1973.

Autoregulation and Tubuloglomerular Feedback

Anderson, R. J., Taher, M. S., Cronin, R. E., McDonald, K. M., and Schrier, R. W. Effect of β-adrenergic blockade and inhibitors of angiotensin II and prostaglandins on renal autoregulation. *Am. J. Physiol.* 229:731, 1975.

Arendshorst, W. J., Finn, W. F., and Gottschalk, C. W. Autoregulation of blood flow in the rat kidney. *Am. J. Physiol.* 228:127, 1975.

Assaykeen, T. A. (Ed.). *Control of Renin Secretion. Advances in Experimental Medicine and Biology,* vol. XVII. New York: Plenum, 1972.

Bayliss, W. M. On the local reactions of the arterial wall to changes of internal pressure. *J. Physiol.* (Lond.) 28:220, 1902.

Bell, P. D., Thomas, C., Williams, R. H., and Navar, L. G. Filtration rate and stop-flow pressure feedback responses to nephron perfusion in the dog. *Am. J. Physiol.* 234 (Renal Fluid Electrolyte Physiol. 3):F154, 1978.

Cook, W. F. Cellular Localization of Renin. In J. W. Fisher (Ed.), *Kidney Hormones.* New York: Academic, 1971.

Davis, J. O. (Ed.). Symposium on advances in our knowledge of the renin-angiotensin system. *Fed. Proc.* 36:1753, 1977.

Forster, R. P., and Maes, J. P. Effects of experimental neurogenic hypertension on renal blood flow and glomerular filtration rates in intact denervated kidneys of unanesthetized rabbits with adrenal glands demedullated. *Am. J. Physiol.* 150:534, 1947.

Frega, N. S., Davalos, M., and Leaf, A. Effect of endogenous angiotensin on the efferent glomerular arteriole of rat kidney. *Kidney Int.* 18:323, 1980.

Goormaghtigh, N. Existence of an endocrine gland in the media of the renal arterioles. *Proc. Soc. Exp. Biol. Med.* 42:688, 1939.

Gorgas, K. Struktur und Innervation des juxtaglomerulären Apparates in der Ratte. *Adv. Anat. Embryol. Cell Biol.* 54 (Fasc. 2):1, 1978.

Hall, J. E., Guyton, A. C., and Cowley, A. W., Jr. Dissociation of renal blood flow and filtration rate autoregulation by renin depletion. *Am. J. Physiol.* 232 (Renal Fluid Electrolyte Physiol. 1):F215, 1977.

Johnson, P. C. (Ed.). Autoregulation of blood flow. *Circ. Res.* 15:I-1, 1964. *Section 4 of this symposium presents the various theories for the mechanism of autoregulation of the renal blood flow and glomerular filtration rate.*

Moore, L. C., Schnermann, J., and Yarimizu, S. Feedback mediation of SNGFR autoregulation in hydropenic and DOCA- and salt-loaded rats. *Am. J. Physiol.* 237 (Renal Fluid Electrolyte Physiol. 6):F63, 1979.

Navar, L. G. Renal autoregulation: Perspectives from whole kidney and single nephron studies. *Am. J. Physiol.* 234 (Renal Fluid Electrolyte Physiol. 3):F357, 1978.

Navar, L. G., Burke, T. J., Robinson, R. R., and Clapp, J. R. Distal tubular feedback in the autoregulation of single nephron glomerular filtration rate. *J. Clin. Invest.* 53:516, 1974.

Schnermann, J. The Role of the Juxtaglomerular Apparatus in Single Nephron Function. In H. G. Vogel and K. J. Ullrich (Eds.), *New Aspects of Renal Function.* Amsterdam: Excerpta Medica, 1978.

Schnermann, J., Persson, A. E. G., and Ågerup, B. Tubuloglomerular feedback: Nonlinear relation between glomerular hydrostatic pressure and loop of Henle perfusion rate. *J. Clin. Invest.* 52:862, 1973.

Schnermann, J. Schubert, G., Hermle, M., Herbst, R., Stowe, N. T., Yarimizu, S., and Weber, P. C. The effect of inhibition of prostaglandin synthesis on tubuloglomerular feedback in the rat kidney. *Pflügers Arch. Eur. J. Physiol.* 379:269, 1979.

Stowe, N., Schnermann, J., and Hermle, M. Feedback regulation of neph-ron filtration rate during pharmacologic interference with the renin-angiotensin and adrenergic systems in rats. *Kidney Int.* 15:473, 1979.

Thurau, K., and Mason, J. The intrarenal function of the juxtaglomerular apparatus. *Int. Rev. Physiol.* 6:357, 1974.

Thurau, K., Schnermann, J., Nagel, W., Horster, M., and Wahl, M. Com-position of tubular fluid in the macula densa segment as a factor regulat-ing the function of the juxtaglomerular apparatus. *Circ. Res.* 21 (Suppl. 2):79, 1967.

Tobian, L. Physiology of the juxtaglomerular cells. *Ann. Intern. Med.* 52:395, 1960.

Tucker, B. J., Steiner, R. W., Gushwa, L. C., and Blantz, R. C. Studies on the tubulo-glomerular feedback system in the rat. The mechanism of reduction in filtration rate with benzolamide. *J. Clin. Invest.* 62:993, 1978.

Vander, A. J. Control of renin release. *Physiol. Rev.* 47:359, 1967.

Wright, F. S., and Briggs, J. P. Feedback control of glomerular blood flow, pressure, and filtration rate. *Physiol. Rev.* 59:958, 1979.

Renal Metabolism

Bernanke, D., and Epstein, F. H. Metabolism of the renal medulla. *Am. J. Physiol.* 208:541, 1965.

Cohen, J. J. Is the function of the renal papilla coupled exclusively to an anaerobic pattern of metabolism? *Am. J. Physiol.* 236 (Renal Fluid Elec-trolyte Physiol. 5):F423, 1979.

Cohen, J. J., and Barac-Nieto, M. Renal Metabolism of Substrates in Relation to Renal Function. In J. Orloff and R. W. Berliner (Eds.), *Hand-book of Physiology,* section 8, Renal Physiology. Washington, D.C.: American Physiological Society, 1973.

Cohen, J. J., and Kamm, D. E. Renal Metabolism: Relation to Renal Func-tion. In B. M. Brenner and F. C. Rector, Jr. (Eds.), *The Kidney* (2nd ed.). Philadelphia: Saunders, 1981.

Deetjen, P. Normal and Critical Oxygen Supply of the Kidney. In D. W. Lubbers, U. C. Luft, G. Thews, and E. Witzleb (Eds.), *Oxygen Transport in Blood and Tissue.* Stuttgart: Thieme, 1968.

Deetjen, P., and Kramer, K. Die Abhängigkeit des O_2-Verbrauchs der Niere von der Na-Rückresorption. *Pflügers Arch. Ges. Physiol.* 273:636, 1961.

Friedman, P. A., and Torretti, J. Regional glucose metabolism in the cat kidney in vivo. *Am. J. Physiol.* 234 (Renal Fluid Electrolyte Physiol. 3):F415, 1978.

Kiil, F., Aukland, K., and Refsum, H. E. Renal sodium transport and oxy-gen consumption. *Am. J. Physiol.* 201:511, 1961.

Krebs, H. A. Renal Carbohydrate and Fatty Acid Metabolism. In K. Thurau and H. Jahrmärker (Eds.), *Renal Transport and Diuretics.* New York: Springer-Verlag, 1969.

Lassen, N. A., Munck, O., and Thaysen, J. H. Oxygen consumption and sodium reabsorption in the kidney. *Acta Physiol. Scand.* 51:371, 1961.

Lee, J. B., and Peter, H. M. Effect of oxygen tension on glucose metabolism in rabbit kidney cortex and medulla. *Am. J. Physiol.* 217:1464, 1969.

Lymph Flow

Bell, R. D., Keyl, M. J., Shrader, F. R., Jones, E. W., and Henry, L. P. Renal lymphatics: The internal distribution. *Nephron* 5:454, 1968.

Kriz, W., and Dieterich, H. J. Das Lymphgefäss-system der Niere bei einigen Säugetieren. Licht- und elektronenmikroskopische Untersuchungen. *Z. Anat. Entwicklungsgesch.* 131:111, 1970.

LeBrie, S. J. Renal lymph and osmotic diuresis. *Am. J. Physiol.* 215:116, 1968.

LeBrie, S. J., and Mayerson, H. S. Influence of elevated venous pressure on flow and composition of renal lymph. *Am. J. Physiol.* 198:1037, 1960.

Mayerson, H. S. The Physiologic Importance of Lymph. In W. F. Hamilton and P. Dow (Eds.), *Handbook of Physiology,* section 2, Circulation, vol. II. Washington, D.C.: American Physiological Society, 1963.

Yoffey, J. M., and Courtice, F. C. *Lymphatics, Lymph and the Lymphomyeloid Complex.* New York: Academic, 1970. Chap. 4.

7 : Na^+ and H_2O Transport. Na^+ Balance

Definitions

The following definitions conform to the common usage of the terms in renal physiology.

Na^+ balance: the balance between the total input of Na^+ into the body and the total output of that ion, usually during a 24-hour period. When the input exceeds the output, the body is in positive balance for Na^+; when the output exceeds the input, the balance is negative; and when input equals output during the same period of time, the balance is zero and the organism is said to be in balance for Na^+.

Frequently (but not necessarily), when we speak of Na^+ balance we mean balance for NaCl, or salt. This extended meaning arises from the fact that Na^+ and Cl^-, being the most abundant solute particles in extracellular fluid (Fig. 2-2), together determine the volume of that fluid (Eq. 2-1), and the further fact that when Na^+ is transported, an anion must accompany it or a cation must be transported in the opposite direction so that electroneutrality of the fluid compartments is maintained. Usually, Na^+ and Cl^- are transported together, but there are important exceptions, as in the early proximal tubule (Fig. 7-3C) or in disturbances of H^+ balance (Fig. 11-5B). (See also the introductory paragraph under Renal Regulation of Na^+ Balance, this chapter.)

Diuresis: urine flow that is greater than normal, i.e., in excess of about 1 ml per minute in an adult human being.

Osmotic diuresis: increased urine flow that is due to extra amount of nonreabsorbed solute within the tubular lumen. A common example is mannitol diuresis (see p. 172).

Water diuresis: increased urine flow that is due to decreased reabsorption of "free" (i.e., solute-free) water. This type of diuresis is seen in persons who have drunk large amounts of dilute fluid (see Problem 8-1 and the corresponding Answer) and in patients with diabetes insipidus, who have some abnormality of the antidiuretic hormone (ADH or vasopressin).

Antidiuresis: urine flow that is less than normal, usually below about 0.5 ml per minute in an adult human. The term is also frequently used to connote the excretion of urine that is hyperosmotic to plasma.

Osmolality: the concentration of discrete — i.e., osmotically active — particles in solution. Osmolality is a function of the number of particles in solution, regardless of their mass, charge, or size. The common units in biological fluids are milliosmoles per kilogram of H_2O (mOsm/kg H_2O). The term *osmolality* is commonly used interchangeably with the term *osmolarity*, which has a slightly but negligibly different value, being the number of discrete particles per liter of total solution.

Isosmotic: equal to the osmolality of plasma, which normally is about 290 mOsm/kg H_2O (see Table 1-2). Because it is a round figure that is easy to remember, 300 mOsm/kg H_2O is frequently used for plasma.

The term is also used to connote equality with the osmolality of any other solution, be that more or less concentrated than plasma; e.g., isosmotic absorption by the gallbladder refers to the reabsorbate having the same osmolality as the luminal fluid. This additional meaning is sometimes also applied to "hyperosmotic" and "hyposmotic."

Hyperosmotic: greater than the osmolality of plasma. Maximally concentrated human urine has an osmolality of about 1,200 mOsm/kg H_2O at the same time that plasma osmolality remains around 295 mOsm/kg H_2O.

Hyposmotic: less than the osmolality of plasma. Maximally dilute human urine has an osmolality of about 50 mOsm/kg H_2O at the same time that plasma osmolality remains around 285 mOsm/kg H_2O.

Correlation of Na$^+$ and H_2O Transport

The balance of Na$^+$ and H_2O depends critically on these substances being avidly reabsorbed by the renal tubules (see Table 1-1). Water reabsorption by renal tubules (and in fact by all epithelia) is a passive process that depends upon osmotic gradients between the tubular fluid and the peritubular interstitial fluid and plasma. Hence, water diffuses passively in response to an osmotic gradient set up mainly by NaCl, $NaHCO_3$ and, to a lesser extent, organic solutes that are transported with Na$^+$ (see Chap. 4, Cotransport).

Na$^+$, Cl$^-$, and H_2O Reabsorption in Proximal Tubules

Early micropuncture experiments suggested that fluid reabsorbed from the proximal tubule was isosmotic; that is, even after two-thirds of the fluid that was filtered had been reabsorbed, the fluid remaining within the proximal tubular lumen appeared to have the same osmolality as plasma (Fig. 7-4). The concentration of Na$^+$ in this tubular fluid was also identical with that in plasma. These findings could be interpreted as reflecting reabsorption of water as the initial event, followed secondarily by reabsorption of Na$^+$ and Cl$^-$, whose concentrations had been raised by the withdrawal of water; conversely, the primary event could have been reabsorption of Na$^+$ and Cl$^-$, setting up a slight osmotic gradient for the reabsorption of water. The experiment illustrated in Figure 7-1 showed that the latter alternative is correct.

Na$^+$ Reabsorption Is Primary and Active

The experiment was performed on the proximal tubule of *Necturus;* the important results have been confirmed in proximal and distal tubules of mammalian species, only some specific numerical values being different. The rationale of the experiment was that if the primary reabsorption of water initiated the reabsorption of NaCl, net flux of water should be independent of the intratubular concentration of NaCl; but if the converse were the case — i.e., if water reabsorption followed the osmotic gradient set up by the reabsorption of NaCl — there should be a correlation between the intratubular concentration of NaCl and the net flux of water, especially if the reabsorption of NaCl depended in part on its concentration in tubular fluid.

Figure 7-1A illustrates the technique of stop-flow microperfusion. In step 1, the early part of the proximal tubule is filled with oil. By means of a micropipet inserted into the middle of the oil column, the tubular lumen is then filled with solution, thereby splitting the column of oil (step 2). The solution, which has different concentrations of NaCl (50, 62.5, 75, and 100 mMoles/liter), is left within the tubular lumen until a steady concentration of NaCl has been attained. The time interval required to reach a steady concentration is 20 minutes in *Necturus* and about 30 seconds in rats. The fluid is then withdrawn (step 3). In addition to NaCl at varying concentrations, the injected fluid column (step 2) contains trace amounts of inulin, and enough mannitol to render the fluid isosmotic with plasma.

The results of such an experiment in the proximal tubule of *Necturus* are shown in Figure 7-1B. Net flux of water could be calculated from the inulin concentration of the fluid that was withdrawn in step 3 (see Chap. 3, Meaning of TF/P and U/P for Inulin). At NaCl concentrations above 66 mMoles/liter, water was reabsorbed from the tubule, but at concentrations below this value, water entered the tubule. Clearly, then, the net flux of water is correlated with the intratubular concentration of NaCl, strongly arguing, by the rationale of the experiment, that movement of NaCl is the primary event.

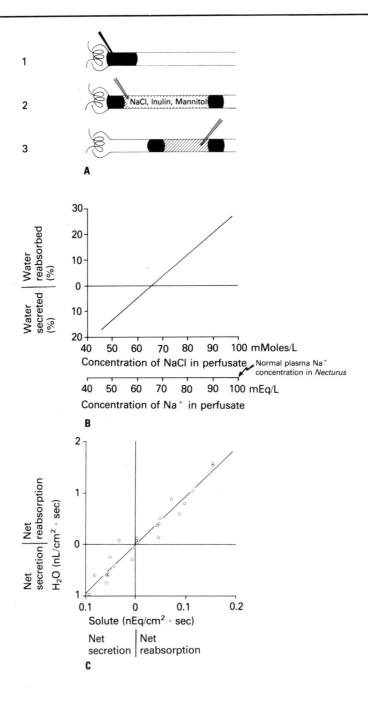

1

2

NaCl, Inulin, Mannitol

3

A

30

20

10

Water reabsorbed (%)

0

10

Water secreted (%)

20

40 50 60 70 80 90 100 mMoles/L

Concentration of NaCl in perfusate

Normal plasma Na$^+$
concentration in *Necturus*

40 50 60 70 80 90 100 mEq/L

Concentration of Na$^+$ in perfusate

B

2

1

Net reabsorption

0

1

Net secretion

H$_2$O (nL/cm^2 · sec)

0.1 0 0.1 0.2

Solute (nEq/cm^2 · sec)

Net secretion | Net reabsorption

C

This conclusion is supported by a further argument. Active transport of water by the kidney had been rejected earlier on the basis of thermodynamic arguments. Calculations suggested that the rate of expenditure of free energy that would be required to maintain observed differences in osmolality between plasma and hyperosmotic urine through the active transport of water was about 1,000 times greater than the maximal rate for living cells. In fact, to date, active water transport has not been demonstrated in any biological system. Thus, the movement of water shown in Figure 7-1B was presumably passive, and since the experiment was so designed, through the addition of mannitol, that no osmotic gradients existed between tubular fluid and interstitium when the fluid was first instilled, water movement could not have been primary.

Na$^+$ TRANSPORT AGAINST A CHEMICAL GRADIENT. In the lower abscissa of Figure 7-1B, the intratubular concentration of NaCl has been expressed as milliequivalents of Na$^+$ per liter. The Na$^+$ concentration in plasma of *Necturus* is about 100 mEq/liter. Hence, in that portion of the experiment in which water moved out of the tubule (reflecting primary movement of NaCl), Na$^+$ must have been reabsorbed against a concentration gradient. At Na$^+$ concentrations below 66 mEq/liter, Na$^+$ (and hence water) moved into the tubule. These findings have been interpreted to mean that the proximal tubular epithelium of *Necturus* cannot transport Na$^+$ against a concentration difference exceeding about 34 mEq/liter (the "limiting" concentration difference). When this maximal difference is surpassed, there is net movement of Na$^+$ (and Cl$^-$) into the lumen, and water follows. The concentration of 66 mEq/liter is called the limiting steady-state Na$^+$ concentration. In the proximal tubule of rats, this concentration has a value of about 107 mEq/liter. Since the plasma Na$^+$ concentration of rats is about 140 mEq/liter, the limiting concen-

---

Fig. 7-1

A. Illustration of the technique of stop-flow microperfusion.

B. Results of stop-flow microperfusion experiments in the proximal tubule of *Necturus*. Inasmuch as the net flux of NaCl in and out of the tubule depends in part on the intratubular concentration of NaCl, the direct relationship shown here strongly suggests that solute flux is primary and water follows passively. This point is further illustrated in (C).

C. Direct and linear correlation between net flux of solute and net flux of water in the same experiment. Since water moves passively in all biological systems that have been examined, and there were no initial osmotic gradients (step 2), water must have moved secondarily in response to movement of solute.

Modified from Shipp, J. C., et al. *Am. J. Physiol.* 195:563, 1958; and Windhager, E. E., et al. *Am. J. Physiol.* 197:313, 1959.

tration difference against which their proximal tubules can transport Na^+ is also in the range of 35 mEq/liter.

That NaCl did in fact move out of the tubule when water was reabsorbed, and into the tubule when water was secreted, is shown in Figure 7-1C. In the same type of experiment that is shown in Figure 7-1A and B, net flux was calculated not only for water but also for solute, and the results demonstrate a direct and linear correlation between these two variables.

Na^+ TRANSPORT AGAINST AN ELECTRICAL POTENTIAL GRADIENT. The experiment depicted in Figure 7-1 shows that movement of NaCl is the initial event, and that Na^+ is reabsorbed against a chemical concentration gradient. In order to determine whether the transport of Na^+ is active, one must in addition know the electrical potential differences (P.D.'s) across the proximal tubular cells. These are shown, for a mammalian kidney, in Figure 7-2. Electrical P.D.'s were measured by inserting microelectrodes into the tubular lumen and into the cell, taking peritubular fluid

Proximal Tubule

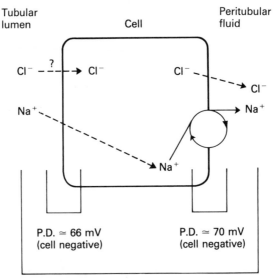

Fig. 7-2 : Electrical potential profile and transport of Na^+ and Cl^- across a mammalian proximal tubular cell. The transepithelial electrical potential difference (P.D.) is directed lumen negative in the early proximal tubule and it becomes lumen positive in the intermediate and late portions of the proximal tubule (Fig. 7-3C); for the sake of simplicity, it is shown here as 4 mV, lumen negative.

as a zero reference. In proximal tubules of mammals, the trans-epithelial P.D. (i.e., the P.D. between peritubular fluid and tubular lumen) is at first approximately 3 to 8 millivolts (mV) with the lumen being negative in respect to peritubular fluid, and it then becomes lumen positive in later portions of the proximal tubule (Fig. 7-3C); in *Necturus* it is approximately 15 mV (lumen negative). For the sake of clarity, the value of 4 mV (lumen negative) has been used in Figure 7-2. The P.D. between cell interior and peritubular fluid has a value of about 70 mV, the interior of the cell being negative to the peritubular fluid. The P.D. across the luminal membrane is then about 66 mV, the cell interior being negative in relation to the luminal fluid.

Since the intracellular Na$^+$ concentration is relatively low as compared to that of plasma (Fig. 2-2) and hence to that of prox-imal tubular fluid, Na$^+$ movement from lumen into cell need not be active, but could proceed passively down an electrochemical potential gradient. This fact is expressed by the broken down-ward arrow. In its movement from cell interior to peritubular fluid and blood, however, Na$^+$ must be transported against an electrochemical potential gradient. Hence, this movement is indi-cated by a solid upward arrow involving an energy-consuming pump at the peritubular cell membrane.

A similar analysis of the electrochemical gradient for the nega-tively charged Cl ion yields the conclusion that there would have to be a small active component for the entry of this ion from the lumen into the cell. This possibility is indicated by the question mark over the broken arrow in Figure 7-2. Once in the cell, Cl$^-$ can diffuse passively into the peritubular fluid, even against its chemical concentration gradient, since the electrical potential gradient favors its movement out of the cell. However, it appears likely that most chloride is transported across the luminal mem-brane as the electrically neutral NaCl salt, and hence passively. In addition, Cl$^-$ could move down an electrochemical gradient by a route to be described in conjunction with Figure 7-3C, i.e., be-tween cells via lateral intercellular spaces. In both instances, pas-sive transport is aided by elevation of the Cl$^-$ concentration within luminal fluid in later portions of the proximal tubules, brought about by preferential reabsorption of NaHCO$_3$, and hence of water, in the early proximal tubules (see discussion of Fig. 7-3C and Isosmotic Fluid Reabsorption).

Thus, the combined chemical and electrical analysis of the prox-imal tubule indicates that Na$^+$ is transported actively, and Cl$^-$ possibly entirely passively; H$_2$O is reabsorbed passively as a consequence of the movement of NaCl.

Reabsorptive Events
Along Proximal
Tubules

Although the foregoing description illustrates the type of analysis by which transport across epithelia is defined, the actual situation is considerably more complicated than the events depicted in Figure 7-2. Not only is Na$^+$ reabsorbed in combination with different solutes in the early, as opposed to the later, portions of the proximal tubule, but the route for solute and water flow includes a paracellular pathway (i.e., alongside or between cells). These points are shown in Figure 7-3C. The description will be limited to reabsorption and to certain major substances; other transport processes in the proximal tubule, such as secretion of organic acids and H$^+$ or reabsorption of K$^+$, are considered elsewhere (e.g., Chaps. 5, 10, 11).

EARLY PROXIMAL TUBULE. By "early" we mean approximately the first half of the proximal convolutions (Fig. 1-2A). In this portion, Na$^+$ is reabsorbed preferentially in association with HCO$_3^-$ rather than with Cl$^-$, and Na$^+$ is also reabsorbed in cotransport with glucose, amino acids, lactate, inorganic phosphate, and other substances (see Chap. 4, Cotransport). The reabsorption of all these solutes in association with Na$^+$ is accompanied by the reabsorption of water in amounts that leave the osmolality of luminal fluid and peritubular fluid equal, i.e., isosmotic (at least as gauged by the methods with which we usually measure osmolality; see below, under Isosmotic Fluid Reabsorption).

The mode of transport varies with the substance in question: Na$^+$ is transported much as shown in Figure 7-2 except that the active step which requires a direct input of energy from adenosine triphosphate (ATP) (denoted by the circular pump) is not confined to the peritubular membrane but is located all along the basolateral membrane, including the membranes that line the lateral intercellular spaces (Fig. 7-3C); glucose is probably transported by carriers (not requiring ATP) that are located in both the luminal and peritubular membranes, with only the former being linked with Na$^+$; and transport of amino acids involves a carrier in cotransport with Na$^+$ in the luminal membrane, as shown in Figure 4-2. More variations could be cited, but these examples suffice to make the point that only the net and predominant movements are shown in Figure 7-3C, and that many details have been omitted.

The large open arrows in Figure 7-3C are not meant to imply that the movement of solutes and water is necessarily through cells. The several possible routes are indicated in the figure. Of the four paths shown, two are probably much more common than the others: A, B, E, i.e., tubular lumen, into cell, into lateral intercellular space, and thence across the basement membrane into the peritubular fluid; and D, E, i.e., across the tight junction into the lateral intercellular space and into peritubular fluid. The proximal epithelium has a high permeability for water and major solutes and a high electrical conductance, and it is the so-called intercellular or paracellular shunt pathway (i.e., the tight junction, the lateral intercellular space, and the basement membrane) that is thought to constitute the route of low resistance (see Fig. 7-3B for the extensive arborization of lateral intercellular spaces). Solute and water transport along this route — i.e., D, E in Figure 7-3C, and in some instances A, B, E as well — does not entail active processes, and as much as one-third (or even more) of reabsorption in the entire proximal tubule may occur by passive means. The double arrows within the lateral intercellular spaces mark these channels as the major route for back-leak of Na$^+$ or NaCl and water. In Chapter 4 (under Bidirectional Transport) we mentioned that net reabsorption of Na$^+$ and water is the algebraic sum of reabsorption and passive secretion; under some circumstances, during net secretion in Figures 7-1B and C, the passive back-leak can exceed the reabsorptive rate for solute and water.

LATE PROXIMAL TUBULE. By "late" is meant approximately the second half of the proximal convolution and the pars recta (see Fig. 1-2A). The events in the early proximal tubule — namely, isosmotic reabsorption of water resulting from transport of Na$^+$ that is coupled to HCO$_3^-$ and organic solutes in preference to Cl$^-$ — lead to an increase in the tubular fluid concentration of Cl$^-$ (TF$_{Cl^-}$) in the later portions of the proximal tubule. The resulting concentration difference for Cl$^-$ between tubular and peritubular fluid (higher in lumen) provides the driving force for passive reabsorption of Cl$^-$; and the change in P.D. with lumen positive (which can be related to the difference in tubular fluid composition between early and late portions) provides a driving force for reabsorption of Na$^+$. Thus, the predominant species being reabsorbed in the late proximal tubule is NaCl, and as much as 40% of this transport may be passive. Again, water follows in roughly isosmotic proportions (for mechanisms, see Isosmotic Fluid Reabsorption, below). The remaining events, such as routes of solute and water flow and active transport of Na$^+$ into the lateral intercellular spaces, are probably similar in early and late segments of the proximal tubule.

HETEROGENEITY. The differences in function between the early and late proximal tubule are due to intrinsic differences between these segments, which are reflected as well in morphological dissimilarities. The early part, for example, has more extensive microvilli, more lateral intercellular spaces, and more mitochondria than does the later portion. Such structural and functional

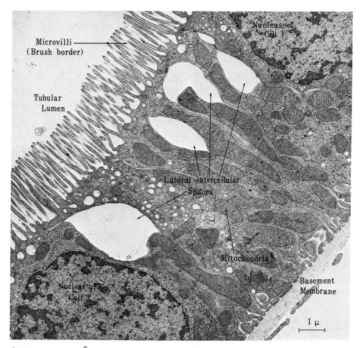

A

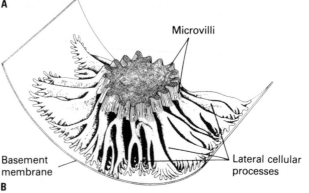

B

Fig. 7-3 : Anatomical and functional characteristics of the proximal tubule.

A. Electron micrograph of early proximal tubular epithelium from a rat. The lateral intercellular spaces follow a serpentine course, so it is seldom possible to portray a single channel extending from the apex to the base of the cell. Micrograph kindly supplied by C. C. Tisher.

B. Three-dimensional model of an early proximal tubular cell, constructed by morphometric techniques. Scanning electron micrographs have proved this model to be remarkably correct (see Welling, D. J., and Welling, L. W. *Fed. Proc.* 38:121, 1979). The lateral cellular processes of one cell interdigitate with corresponding processes of adjacent cells to produce an extensive and complicated network of lateral intercellular channels. The configuration of late proximal tubular cells is similar but less complex. From Welling, L. W., and Welling, D. J. *Kidney Int.* 9:385, 1976. Published with permission.

C. Reabsorptive processes in the early and late proximal tubules; "early" constitutes approximately the first half of the proximal convolutions, and "late" is the remainder, including the pars recta. TF = tubular fluid. For detailed description, see text.

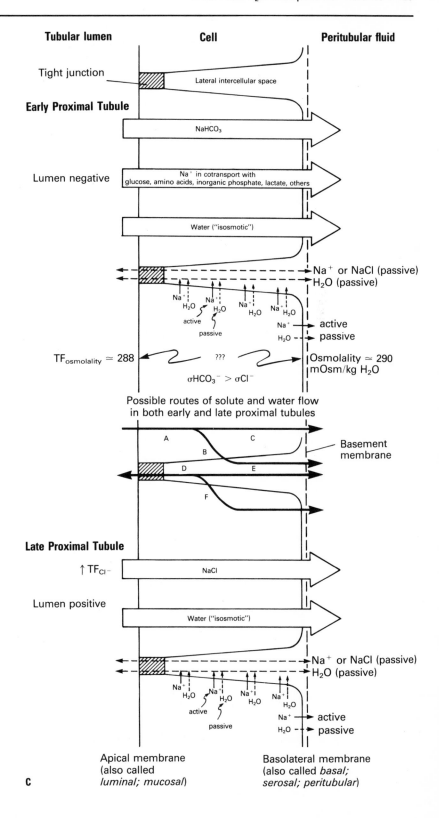

Possible routes of solute and water flow
in both early and late proximal tubules

differences, known as *heterogeneity,* almost certainly play important roles in major renal functions, such as balance for salt and water. Over the years, the concept of heterogeneity has progressed from recognition of two populations of nephrons, the outer cortical and juxtamedullary (see Fig. 1-2), to differences between analogous segments of these two types of nephron (e.g., the pars recta of an outer cortical nephron vs. the pars recta of a juxtamedullary nephron), to identification of differences within major components of the same nephron, as within the proximal tubule (Fig. 7-3C), the distal tubule, or the collecting duct.

Isosmotic Fluid Reabsorption

It has already been mentioned that the fluid that is reabsorbed from the proximal tubules is "isosmotic" with plasma. This fact, which is illustrated in Figure 7-4, is characteristic of Na^+ and water transport in many epithelial membranes, including, among others: the gallbladder; the ileum; and the secretion of gastric juice, pancreatic juice, and cerebrospinal fluid. The word *isosmotic* has been put in quotation marks because, if we had more sensitive means for measuring osmolality, we might detect a very small difference. In fact, it is the inability to measure osmolality precisely that epitomizes the problem of identifying the mechanism by which isosmotic reabsorption occurs. Passive, bulk flow of water takes place in response to a difference in osmotic pressure between two points. Knowing the very high water permeability (more specifically, the hydraulic conductivity) of the proximal tubular epithelium, one can calculate that a difference in osmolality of as little as 2 mOsm/kg H_2O might suffice to account for the rate at which water is reabsorbed from this part of the nephron. Since such a small difference cannot be established with confidence by current techniques, it is possible that an undetectable osmotic gradient (as shown in Fig. 7-3C) supplies the driving force for "isosmotic" reabsorption.

An alternative or additional mechanism involves the reflection coefficient, σ, which gives a measure of the relative effectiveness of a solute as an osmotic force. For the proximal epithelium, HCO_3^- has a higher reflection coefficient than does Cl^-, which means that once absorbed from the tubular lumen into the peritubular fluid, HCO_3^- is "bounced off" the epithelium (i.e., reflected) more readily than Cl^-. This fact would make it possible to have HCO_3^- and Cl^- in equal numbers (i.e., isosmolal) on the two sides of the epithelium, yet have HCO_3^- supply an effective osmotic force to cause net reabsorption of water. An analogous osmotic effect might be supplied by other substances, such as the organic solutes.

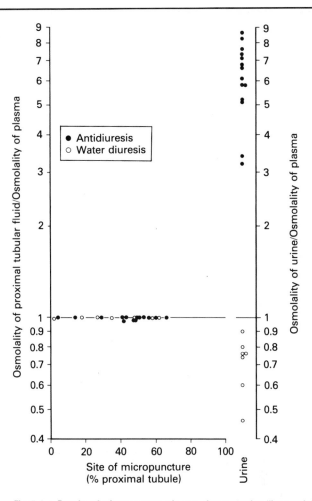

Fig. 7-4 : **Results of micropunctures in rats, demonstrating "isosmotic" fluid reabsorption from the proximal tubules. Within the sensitivity of methods currently used for measuring osmolality, proximal tubular fluid has the "same" osmolal concentration as plasma, whether the urine is more concentrated than plasma (antidiuresis) or less concentrated than plasma (water diuresis). The site of micropuncture was determined at the end of the experiment, through microdissection of the nephron. Only about the first 60% of the proximal tubule is accessible to micropuncture, since the last portion of the tubule dips beneath the surface of the kidney (see Fig. 1-2). Data from Gottschalk, C. W., and Mylle, M.** Am. J. Physiol. **196:927, 1959. The same type of results were obtained by A. M. Walker, P. A. Bott, J. Oliver, and M. C. MacDowell in some of the earliest renal micropuncture studies.** Am. J. Physiol. **134:580, 1941.**

A third possible mechanism for isosmotic reabsorption — no longer, however, championed by most workers — involves a postulated *standing osmotic gradient* within the lateral intercellular spaces. This theory proposes that the difference in osmolality exists not between tubular lumen and peritubular fluid but between these two solutions and fluid within the lateral intercellular space. The last, so the theory states, is rendered hyperosmotic by the active transport of Na^+, and water flows in response to this gradient via route A, B, E in Figure 7-3C, being driven into the peritubular area by bulk flow as hydraulic pressure builds up within the lateral intercellular space.

Na^+, Cl^-, and H_2O Reabsorption in Other Parts of Nephron

We mentioned above, under Heterogeneity, that structural and functional differences are being identified within parts of nephrons that we call by one name (as if they were single, homogeneous structures). As is the case with proximal tubules, so each of the subsequent parts of the nephron can be subdivided into two or more segments; to cite just one example, the thick ascending limb of Henle has a medullary and a cortical segment. The student should be aware of this fact, especially since heterogeneity is likely to play an increasing role in our understanding of renal function. For the sake of simplicity, however, such subdivisions will be largely ignored in the description that follows. Some reasonable average values for each part of the nephron are given in Table 7-1.

Table 7-1 : Some properties of various parts of the nephron.[a] In most instances, the electrical potential difference (P.D.) has a range of values along a given part; for the sake of clarity, only a single representative value is indicated.

Part of Nephron	Transepithelial P.D.[b] mV	Lumen	Ion That Is Actively Transported	Permeability to Water ADH[b] Present	ADH Absent
Proximal tubule					
Early	4	−	Na^+	+ + +	+ + +
Late	2	+	Na^+	+ + +	+ + +
Loop of Henle					
Thin descending	0 (?)		0	+ + + +	+ + + +
Thin ascending	0 (?)		0 (?); Na^+(?)	±	±
Thick ascending	10	+	Na^+	±	±
Distal tubule					
Early	10	−	Na^+; sometimes Cl^-	±	±
Late	40	−	Na^+; sometimes Cl^-	+ + +	±
Collecting duct					
Cortical	35	−	Na^+; sometimes Cl^-	+ + +	±
Medullary	7	−	Na^+; sometimes Cl^-	+ + +	±

[a]A more complete listing of the permeability characteristics of various parts of the nephron is given in tabular form in Jamison, R. L. Urine Concentration and Dilution. The Roles of Antidiuretic Hormone and Urea. In Brenner, B. M., and Rector, F. C., Jr. (Eds.), *The Kidney* (2nd ed.). Philadelphia: Saunders, 1981. Chap. 11.
[b]ADH = antidiuretic hormone (Chap. 8); P.D. = electrical potential difference.

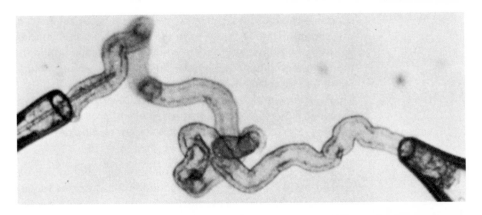

Fig. 7-5 : Preparation of the so-called *isolated, perfused renal tubule*. A segment of proximal convoluted tubule from a rabbit is held between two micropipets and suspended in a medium of varying composition. The segment is approximately 2 mm long. Fluid is perfused through the pipet on the left, and it is collected through the pipet on the right; electrical potential differences (P.D.'s) can also be measured. By this technique, valuable information has been gained on parts of the nephron that are not ordinarily accessible to micropuncture (e.g., pars recta, loop of Henle, medullary collecting duct, convolutions of juxtamedullary nephrons). From Burg, M. B., et al., *Am. J. Physiol.* 215:788, 1968, and reproduced from Valtin, H. *Renal Dysfunction: Mechanisms Involved in Fluid and Solute Imbalance.* Boston: Little, Brown, 1979.

Loops of Henle

THIN LOOPS. Partly because these structures are delicate, but more because they are not accessible to micropuncture except at the very tip of the papilla (see Fig. 1-2), it has been difficult to obtain conclusive information about them in situ. More recently, data have been obtained on isolated tubular segments that are perfused in vitro (Fig. 7-5); some of these data have disagreed with those obtained in vivo, in part for technical reasons and also, it appears, because of species variation. There seems to be no doubt, however, that the descending and ascending thin limbs have different transport properties, which are important for the mechanism by which urine is concentrated (discussed in Chap. 8).

Thin descending limbs. These may or may not have a slight transepithelial electrical P.D., of perhaps 3 mV; if there is a P.D., the lumen is negative with respect to peritubular fluid. The descending limbs are highly permeable to water and, depending on the species and the technique by which they are examined, either impermeable or moderately permeable to Na$^+$ and Cl$^-$ and to urea (discussed further in Chap. 8). Almost certainly, all solutes are transported passively in thin descending limbs.

Thin ascending limbs. These segments are impervious to water, highly permeable to Na$^+$ and Cl$^-$, and moderately permeable to urea. The transepithelial P.D. appears to be zero in some species although it has been reported to be approximately 10 mV, lumen negative, in other species. Again, in some species, the concentrations for both Na$^+$ and Cl$^-$ are greater within the tubular lumen than in peritubular fluid (by approximately 40 to 50 mEq/liter), which enables passive reabsorption of NaCl (see Chap. 8, Passive Model of Countercurrent Multiplication in Inner Medulla). If there is active reabsorption of Na$^+$ from thin ascending limbs, it is thought to constitute a minor portion of the total transport.

Thick ascending limbs. The situation here is similar to that described earlier for transport of chloride in the proximal tubule: Although analysis of the electrochemical gradient might suggest active Cl$^-$ transport, there is strong evidence that Na$^+$ transport is primary and active, and that Cl$^-$ is moved across the luminal membrane in cotransport with Na$^+$ as neutral NaCl. That is, it can be shown that movement of Na$^+$ and Cl$^-$ across the epithelium depends on Na-K-ATPase and on the presence of Na$^+$ within luminal fluid. In this part of the nephron, water does not follow solute except in negligible amounts because the thick limbs are virtually impervious to water (Table 7-1).

Distal Tubules

The distal tubule consists of at least four segments that are distinct morphologically and functionally; the following description and the values given in Table 7-1 and Figure 7-6 pertain to the two middle portions, namely, the distal convolutions and the part just beyond these convolutions.

The transepithelial P.D. increases along the length of the distal tubule, from approximately 10 mV to about 60 mV; the lumen is negative in respect to the peritubular fluid (Fig. 7-6 and Table 7-1). In analogy with the description for the proximal tubule (Fig. 7-2), Na$^+$ can diffuse passively down the electrochemical potential gradient from the lumen into the cell, but it must be transported actively against this gradient across the peritubular cell boundary, which probably includes the membrane lining the lateral intercellular spaces (Fig. 7-3C). That distal tubular cells can transport Na$^+$ against an electrochemical potential gradient has been shown by stop-flow microperfusion experiments (Fig. 7-1). The limiting steady-state Na$^+$ concentration (see p. 123) may be as low as 20 to 40 mEq/liter, indicating that distal tubular cells can transport Na$^+$ against a chemical concentration gradient of at least 100 mEq/liter (plasma Na$^+$ concentration in rats being about 140 mEq/liter).

The reabsorption of Cl$^-$ is usually passive across both the luminal and peritubular cell membranes. In severe Cl$^-$ deprivation, however, the concentration of Cl$^-$ in the distal tubular fluid may

Distal Tubule

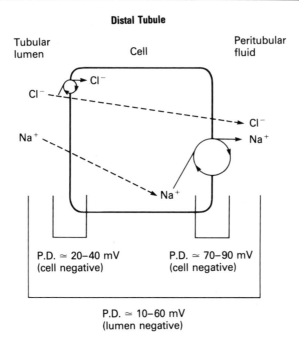

Fig. 7-6 : Electrical potential profile and transport of Na$^+$ and Cl$^-$ across a mammalian distal tubular cell. The electrical potential differences (P.D.'s) increase as the later portions of the distal tubule are approached.

be < 1.0 mEq/liter. The Nernst equation shows that under these circumstances a transepithelial P.D. of 186 mV would be required for Cl$^-$ reabsorption to be wholly passive; no P.D. of this magnitude has been recorded in any portion of the distal tubule. Thus, under certain circumstances, Cl$^-$ reabsorption in the distal tubule may be active, and this possibility has been indicated in Figure 7-6 by the Cl$^-$ "pump" at the luminal membrane.

Reabsorption of water from the early distal tubule is very low, whether or not antidiuretic hormone (ADH, or vasopressin; Chap. 8) is present. Toward the end of the distal tubule, however, the rate of water reabsorption varies with the concentration of ADH. In the presence of this hormone, water permeability and hence reabsorption are very high, whereas in the absence of ADH they are very low (Table 7-1).

Collecting Ducts

Qualitatively, the properties of the cortical and medullary collecting ducts are the same as those of the late distal tubule, and the analysis of NaCl transport is therefore analogous to that described in conjunction with Figure 7-6: The lumen is negative to peritubular fluid; reabsorption of Na$^+$ is active, with the pump being located in the basolateral membrane; and the reabsorption of Cl$^-$ is largely passive except under conditions of extreme

Cl$^-$ deprivation, when there may be active transport by a pump located in the luminal membrane.

There are, however, some quantitative differences. The transepithelial electrical P.D. declines along the length of the collecting duct, being highest in the cortical portion and lowest near the tip of the papilla. It is in this part of the nephron that final modulation of Na$^+$ and Cl$^-$ excretion takes place; whereas earlier parts of the nephron, especially the proximal tubules, reabsorb large amounts of these ions against a relatively small or no chemical concentration difference, the collecting ducts transport lesser amounts but can do so to a point where the concentrations of Na$^+$ and Cl$^-$ in the tubular fluid may become vanishingly small ($<$ 1.0 mEq/liter). As is the case in the late distal tubules, the rate of water reabsorption from collecting ducts varies with the concentration of ADH (Chap. 8; Table 7-1). When the concentration of ADH in blood is high, so is the rate of water reabsorption from collecting ducts, and vice versa.

Renal Regulation of Na$^+$ Balance

As pointed out at the beginning of this chapter (under Definitions, Na$^+$ balance), we often speak of "Na$^+$ balance" or "dietary intake of Na$^+$" when we really mean NaCl, or salt. It should be borne in mind that in all the body fluids, including blood and urine, as well as in food and drink, cationic Na$^+$ occurs in combination with anions so that electroneutrality exists. Although the predominant anion is usually Cl$^-$, that is not always the case; for example, patients being treated with NaHCO$_3$ may ingest a great deal of Na$^+$ that is not in the form of ordinary table salt, or NaCl. Because of these exceptions, because even normally intake of Na$^+$ is not exclusively in the form of the chloride salt, and because Na$^+$ and Cl$^-$ do not always move together in the nephron, we will continue to use the terms *Na$^+$ balance, Na$^+$ handling,* and *dietary Na$^+$* in the ensuing discussion.

The handling of Na$^+$ by the kidneys of a normal adult human is depicted in Figure 7-7, in which the single nephron represents the total function of both kidneys. With a glomerular filtration rate of 180 liters per day (see Table 1-1) and a plasma Na$^+$ concentration of 140 mEq/liter, the filtered load of Na$^+$ is 180 · 140, or 25,200 mEq per day. (Strictly speaking, this value should be lowered by the Donnan factor of about 0.95, but, as stated in Chapter 4, such corrections are customarily ignored; see p. 66.) Of the 25,200 mEq filtered, roughly 67%, or 16,800 mEq per day, is reabsorbed in the proximal tubules. Normal urine flow is about 1 ml per minute; since there are 1,440 minutes in 24 hours, normal urine flow is about 1,500 ml per day. At a normal urinary Na$^+$ concentration of about 100 mEq/liter (see Answer to Problem 11-1), the daily urinary excretion of Na$^+$ is about 150 mEq, or 0.6%

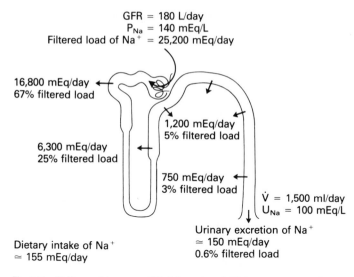

GFR = 180 L/day
P$_{Na}$ = 140 mEq/L
Filtered load of Na$^+$ = 25,200 mEq/day

16,800 mEq/day
67% filtered load

1,200 mEq/day
5% filtered load

6,300 mEq/day
25% filtered load

750 mEq/day
3% filtered load

$\dot{V}$ = 1,500 ml/day
U$_{Na}$ = 100 mEq/L

Urinary excretion of Na$^+$
$\simeq$ 150 mEq/day
0.6% filtered load

Dietary intake of Na$^+$
$\simeq$ 155 mEq/day

Fig. 7-7 : Daily renal turnover of Na$^+$ in a normal adult human. The diagram of the nephron represents the composite of the roughly two million nephrons of both kidneys. In the steady (equilibrium) state, the organism is by definition in "balance." For Na$^+$ this means that the daily output of Na$^+$ equals the daily intake. Obviously, Na$^+$ is excreted mainly by the kidneys; the difference between the rate of urinary excretion of Na$^+$ and the daily intake is made up by extrarenal routes, such as sweat, saliva, and other gastrointestinal secretions. Under normal circumstances, the extrarenal losses of Na$^+$ are negligible. GFR = glomerular filtration rate; P$_{Na}$ and U$_{Na}$ = plasma and urinary concentration of sodium, respectively.

of the filtered load. Hence, nearly 33% of the filtered load of Na$^+$ is reabsorbed beyond the proximal tubules. This is apportioned as follows: about 25% or 6,300 mEq per day in the loops of Henle; about 5% or 1,200 mEq per day in the distal tubules; and about 3% or 750 mEq per day in the collecting ducts.

Normally, then, about 99.4% of the filtered Na$^+$ is reabsorbed (see Table 1-1). It is obvious that, given a normal dietary intake of Na$^+$ of about 155 mEq per day, any change in the GFR or in the rate of tubular Na$^+$ reabsorption could seriously threaten Na$^+$ balance and hence the maintenance of the body fluid compartments (Chap. 2). Or, a change in the dietary intake of Na$^+$ would pose a similar threat unless the GFR or tubular reabsorptive rate were quickly adjusted. The fact that the plasma Na$^+$ concentration is normally carefully maintained in the narrow range of 136 to 146 mEq/liter shows that physiological adjustments must quickly come into play when Na$^+$ balance is challenged. These adjustments are discussed next.

Challenges to Na$^+$ Balance

SPONTANEOUS CHANGES IN GFR. Given a stable plasma concentration for Na$^+$, changes in GFR markedly alter the filtered load of Na$^+$. Hence, unless such changes were quickly accompanied by physiological adjustments, a decrease in GFR would lead to a surfeit of body Na^+, and an increase in GFR might lead to fatal Na^+ depletion. The following quantitative example will illustrate this point. Working with the values depicted in Figure 7-7: If GFR were to increase by just 2%, the filtered load of Na^+ would increase to $183.6 \cdot 140$, or 25,704 mEq per day. Note that the extra amount filtered because of this very small increase in GFR — 504 mEq per day — is three times greater than the daily intake of Na^+. Therefore, if the absolute amount of Na^+ reabsorbed *were* to remain at 25,050 mEq per day (Fig. 7-7), the daily excretion of Na^+ would rise to 654 mEq, an intolerably high value. In fact, this does not happen because two physiological compensations set in: glomerulotubular balance (G-T balance) and autoregulation of the GFR.

Glomerulotubular balance. It was pointed out in Chapter 4 that, when used in the context of Na^+ balance, G-T balance has a different connotation from the one that is derived from the glucose titration curve. In the present context, G-T balance refers to the fact that under steady-state conditions a constant fraction of the filtered Na^+ is reabsorbed in the proximal tubules despite variations in GFR. Normally, this fraction is about 0.67, or 67% (Fig. 7-7). In the hypothetical example described above, in which GFR had increased by 2%, G-T balance would have adjusted Na^+ reabsorption in the proximal tubules to $25,704 \cdot 0.67$, or approximately 17,222 mEq per day. This adjustment would therefore "recapture" all but 82 mEq of the extra amount of Na^+ filtered (504 mEq − 422 mEq), and this remainder is reabsorbed in the loops of Henle, distal tubules, and collecting ducts. As a general rule, the loops of Henle have a large capacity for reabsorbing extra Na^+ that is delivered to them from the proximal tubules. As pointed out above (under Collecting Ducts), final, fine adjustments of reabsorption to meet the requirements for Na^+ balance are effected beyond the loops of Henle. That is, the collecting ducts (and possibly the distal tubules) are the ultimate regulators of urinary Na^+ excretion, even though they process less than 10% of the glomerular filtrate (Fig. 7-7). The main mediator of the regulation is probably aldosterone, although other factors and other hormones may be involved as well (see also below, under Changes in Na^+ Intake. Decreased Aldosterone).

Despite a great deal of investigation, the mechanisms for proximal G-T balance have not been fully identified. There may be at least two processes: (1) One involves changes in the filtration fraction and hence in the oncotic pressure within peritubular capillaries. The dynamics of this effect are described in conjunction with Figure 7-9; the required resistances in the glomerular arterioles might be brought about by nervous or humoral influences (e.g., angiotensin, prostaglandins, kinins, and others). (2) Another possible mechanism may relate to the phenomenon of cotransport (described in Chap. 4), in which the reabsorption of Na$^+$ is linked to that of various organic solutes. The proposal is that, since these solutes are reabsorbed virtually completely in the early proximal tubule (Fig. 7-3C), an increased filtered load of organic solutes will be followed automatically by an equal increment in reabsorption, not only of the organic compounds but also, through cotransport, of Na$^+$.

Autoregulation of GFR. This phenomenon, which is illustrated in Figure 6-3, involves the relative constancy of the total filtration rate (GFR) and of the glomerular filtration rate of single nephrons (sGFR). Whenever there is a tendency for the GFR to increase, whether it be through increased renal arterial perfusion pressure (Fig. 6-3) or through some other means, a negative feedback mechanism is activated, which tends to return the GFR to the normal level. As discussed in Chapter 6 (under Autoregulation of RBF and GFR), at least part of this feedback appears to involve the juxtaglomerular apparatus (JGA). Whatever the mechanism, it seems likely that autoregulation, by tending to keep the filtered load of Na$^+$ constant, is a major means whereby serious Na$^+$ wastage is prevented.

Thus, the threat to Na$^+$ balance that would be occasioned by spontaneous changes in GFR is ordinarily combated by relative constancy of the so-called proximal fractional reabsorption (G-T balance), by adjustments of the reabsorptive rate in more distal parts, and by a feedback mechanism that tends quickly to return the GFR toward the normal level (autoregulation).

CHANGES IN Na$^+$ INTAKE. Changes in the acquisition of Na$^+$ pose a second major threat to Na$^+$ balance. For example, unless a decrease in Na$^+$ intake were accompanied by decreased excretion, depletion of Na$^+$ and hence of fluid volumes would quickly ensue. Conversely, a large increase in Na$^+$ intake might quickly lead to an augmentation of total body Na$^+$ followed by expansion of the fluid compartments and heart failure — unless there were a rapid increase in the urinary excretion of Na$^+$. Physiological adjustments (sometimes called *factors*) do in fact set in, and we shall now consider them from the point of view of compensating for increases in Na$^+$ intake.

Increase in GFR (first factor). An increase in Na$^+$ intake is often accompanied by an increase in GFR. This occurs partly because expansion of the extracellular fluid volume, which is brought about by increased Na$^+$ (see Fig. 2-4), is accompanied by decreased plasma oncotic pressure and often by increased arterial blood pressure, and partly for as yet unknown reasons. The increased GFR raises the filtered load of Na^+ and, other things being equal, the urinary excretion of Na^+. The argument may seem self-contradictory, since we have just reviewed physiological compensations that minimize Na^+ excretion when GFR is increased. The solution to this apparent paradox lies in the distinction between a spontaneous (primary) and a compensatory (secondary) increase in GFR. When the latter occurs, as in response to augmented Na^+ intake, it is usually not accompanied by G-T balance or by autoregulation. That is, whatever the mechanisms are that bring about G-T balance and autoregulation, these mechanisms appear to be attenuated or abolished by a high intake of Na^+.

Decreased aldosterone (second factor). The production of aldosterone is decreased as Na^+ intake is increased (see Appendix to this chapter). A low blood concentration of aldosterone leads to decreased tubular reabsorption of Na^+. This effect may involve mainly the cortical and medullary collecting ducts and ascending limbs of Henle, and even other parts of the nephron such as the proximal tubules. Aldosterone appears to exert its action by stimulating the formation of messenger ribonucleic acid (mRNA) and thereby the synthesis of specific proteins. These proteins may augment Na^+ transport by three means: (a) by increasing the permeability to Na^+ of the luminal membrane; (b) by increasing, within the peritubular membrane, the activity or amount of Na-K-ATPase, which may be the carrier for active Na^+ transport (Fig. 7-6); and (c) by increasing oxidative metabolism within mitochondria, thereby supplying more energy to the Na^+ pump.

Other factors. For many years it was thought that the first two factors cited above could wholly account for the increased urinary excretion of Na^+ that follows increased Na^+ intake. In 1961, however, H. E. de Wardener and his associates showed conclusively that under some experimental conditions these two factors did not suffice and that it was therefore necessary to invoke another factor or factors. An experiment of the type that led to this conclusion is shown in Figure 7-8. This experiment was carried out on a dog that was given high doses of aldosterone in order to rule out alterations in the blood concentration of this hormone as a cause of the observed changes. During the control periods, the dog filtered about 5 mEq of Na^+ per minute. He excreted about 0.04 mEq per minute; i.e., he reabsorbed about 99.2% of the filtered Na^+. He was then given an intravenous infusion of 0.9% NaCl, which has a Na^+ concentration of approximately 140 mEq/liter and therefore does not change the plasma concentration of Na^+. Ninety minutes later the urinary excretion of Na^+ had risen to 0.48 mEq per minute; however, at this point,

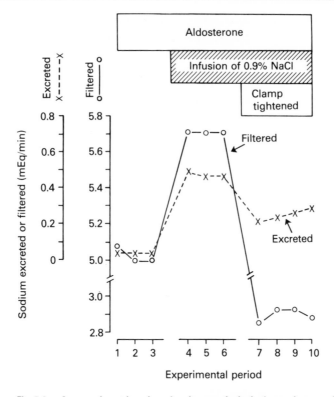

Fig. 7-8 : An experiment in a dog, showing conclusively that an increase in glomerular filtration rate (and hence in the filtered load of Na$^+$) and a decrease in aldosterone cannot fully account for the increased Na$^+$ excretion that follows an infusion of NaCl. This fact was first demonstrated conclusively by de Wardener and his associates in 1961; the experiment depicted here was taken from Levinsky, N. G. *Ann. N.Y. Acad. Sci.* 139:295, 1966. In addition to the aldosterone, the dog also received large amounts of antidiuretic hormone (ADH), thereby also ruling out alterations in the concentration of this hormone as a cause of the observed changes.

the increment in the filtered load of Na$^+$ (consequent to an increase in GFR) could more than account for the increment in Na$^+$ excretion. The GFR was then reduced by tightening a clamp around the aorta, just above the renal arteries. This maneuver greatly reduced the filtered load of Na$^+$ to about 2.9 mEq per minute. Nevertheless, with the continuance of the saline infusion, Na$^+$ excretion remained increased at about 0.25 mEq per minute.

The conclusion from this type of experiment is that the increased Na$^+$ excretion that follows saline loading cannot be fully accounted for by increased GFR (the first factor) and therefore must be due to decreased tubular reabsorption. Since high doses of aldosterone were given throughout this experiment, the decreased reabsorption could not be ascribed to a decreased blood concentration of aldosterone (the second factor) and was therefore ascribed to a third factor or factors. This conclusion has been confirmed by micropuncture techniques. It was found by analysis of tubular fluid to plasma (TF/P) ratios for Na$^+$ and inulin (see part 3 of Answer to Problem 6-1) that acute saline loading decreased the proportion of the filtered Na$^+$ (and often the absolute amount of Na$^+$) that is reabsorbed in proximal tubules, from the normal of about 67% to about 40%. The additional factor or factors also inhibit the reabsorption of Na$^+$ beyond the proximal tubules.

It is likely that there are several additional factors. (1) *Starling forces.* A possible scheme of how these so-called peritubular physical factors might change following increased Na$^+$ intake is diagrammed in Figure 7-9. It is proposed that an increased Na$^+$ intake raises the hydrostatic pressure within the peritubular capillaries. This change might come about directly as a result of expansion of the extracellular fluid volume and consequent increased systemic arterial pressure, as well as indirectly through decreases in resistances at the afferent and efferent arterioles,

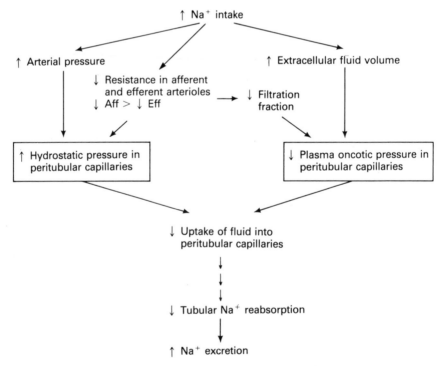

Fig. 7-9 : **Proposed scheme whereby increased Na$^+$ intake might lead to increased Na$^+$ excretion through changes in Starling forces across peritubular capillaries. Slightly modified from Earley, L. E., and Daugharty, T. M. *N. Engl. J. Med.* 281:72, 1969.**

with the decrease being greater in the former than in the latter. Such decreased resistances would permit greater transmission of the systemic arterial pressure into the peritubular capillaries. In addition, the RPF would increase and so would the GFR, since the change in resistance in the afferent arteriole is postulated to exceed that in the efferent. The simultaneous decrease in efferent resistance, however, would tend to decrease the GFR; thus, the net effect of the changes in arteriolar resistances would be that the GFR rises relatively less than the RPF. Consequently, the filtration fraction (Chap. 5) would decline and more plasma would be left in the postglomerular vessels, so that the concentration of protein in that plasma, and hence the oncotic pressure, would fall. As a result of the changes in the two major Starling forces, the uptake of fluid into peritubular capillaries will be decreased. It is uncertain just how this decreased uptake comes about or exactly how it is related to the simultaneous decrease in Na$^+$ reabsorption. Probably there are changes in the lateral intercellular spaces (Fig. 7-3C), such as their geometry, diffusion distances or permeabilities for Na$^+$, or Na$^+$ concentration gradients. But whatever the exact mechanisms may be, there is much experimental evidence that supports the general scheme shown in Figure 7-9. (2) *Natriuretic hormone(s).* Investigators have long searched for a humoral substance that increases Na$^+$ excretion, and some now have evidence for the existence of one or more such compounds, which are different from any known hormone. Neither the structure nor the site(s) of origin of these compounds is yet known. (3) *Changes in sGFR.* When animals are put on a high Na$^+$ intake, there may be a selective increase in the single nephron filtration rate (sGFR) of outer cortical nephrons (see Table 6-1). These nephrons have shorter proximal tubules than do juxtamedullary nephrons, and they may thus have a lesser capacity for reabsorbing Na$^+$ than do the deeper ones. It has been suggested that the selective increase in the filtered load to the outer nephrons may augment Na$^+$ excretion by placing the load principally into nephrons having a lesser capacity for reabsorbing Na$^+$. (4) *Sympathetic nervous activity.* This factor can influence the excretion of Na$^+$ indirectly, through various hemodynamic changes, as in GFR, sGFR, and hydrostatic pressure within peritubular capillaries. In addition, there appears to be a direct influence of sympathetic nerves on the rate of tubular Na$^+$ reabsorption, although investigators are not agreed on the contribution that this effect makes to the day-to-day balance for Na$^+$.

Tuners of Na$^+$ Balance

Various portions of the nephron appear to play different roles in the maintenance of Na$^+$ balance. It is useful to think of the proximal tubules as "coarse tuners," which recapture the bulk of filtered Na^+ and H_2O; of the loops of Henle as "medium tuners," which tend to compensate for failure of the proximal tubules to reabsorb the requisite amounts; and of the collecting ducts (and possibly the distal tubules) as "fine tuners," where precise adjustments of Na^+ and H_2O reabsorption, and hence of their excretion, are made.

Volume Contraction and Volume Expansion

In the foregoing descriptions, we have not considered how the body perceives that it contains too much or too little Na^+. Although there may be receptors that sense sodium as such, the main variable(s) that is monitored is some derivative of Na^+, such as the extracellular fluid volume. Not only is this fact inherent in Equation 2-1 (p. 25), which shows that the volume of a given compartment (say, extracellular fluid) depends on the amount of solute (mainly NaCl and $NaHCO_3$ — Fig. 2-2) within it, but the fact is also reasonable physiologically. When there is too little Na^+ aboard, the extracellular fluid volume will contract, sometimes to the point where decreases in blood volume, in cardiac output, and in blood pressure may threaten life. Conversely, too much NaCl will expand extracellular fluid and may lead to serious hypertension and heart failure. Thus, what the body appears to sense is one or more important physiological derivatives of sodium — plasma volume, the interstitial volume, venous pressure, atrial pressure, cardiac output, systemic arterial pressure, possibly blood flow through different organs, or others. Since all these derivatives are functions of volume, the structures that sense them are known as *volume receptors;* at least some of these receptors appear to be located in the thorax, as in the pulmonary veins and atria. It also follows that, if the perceived variable that regulates Na^+ excretion is the volume of extracellular fluid (or some function thereof), then contraction or expansion of this fluid by means other than changing the intake of Na^+ should lead to changes in Na^+ excretion. This is indeed the case; e.g., expansion with a solution of albumin that contains no salt will increase urinary Na^+ excretion. It is for this reason that many workers test the effects of "volume expansion" or "volume contraction" (brought about by maneuvers other than giving Na^+ or depriving the organism of it) in order to define the mechanisms that maintain Na^+ balance.

Summary

The amounts of H_2O, and of Na^+ with its attendant anions, that are filtered every day exceed their daily intakes by more than a hundredfold (see Table 1-1). For this reason, Na^+ and H_2O balance — i.e., the equality between intake and output — depends critically on the tubular reabsorption of these substances. In most parts of the nephron, Na^+ reabsorption is active, and it is the primary process that is followed by passive reabsorption of

H$_2$O. Exceptions include the thin descending limb of Henle, in which all solutes appear to be transported passively, and the thin ascending limb of Henle, in which Na$^+$ reabsorption may be partly or mostly passive.

In proximal tubules, Na$^+$ is reabsorbed mainly in three forms: as NaHCO$_3$, as NaCl, and in cotransport with organic solutes (Fig. 7-3C). Water is reabsorbed passively and "isosmotically" as a consequence of the reabsorption of the solutes. The driving force for isosmotic reabsorption — whether it depends on a small difference in osmolality between tubular and peritubular fluid, or on a difference in reflection coefficients, σ, or on a standing osmotic gradient within lateral intercellular spaces — has not been conclusively identified.

Net movement of Na$^+$ and H$_2$O in thin loops of Henle has not been fully defined. In thin descending limbs, the movement of both solute and water is passive (Table 7-1); Na$^+$ and Cl$^-$ (and urea) may be secreted into these limbs (at least in some species), and H$_2$O is reabsorbed from them. Reabsorption of Na$^+$ and Cl$^-$ from thin ascending limbs may be mainly passive, and in this part of the nephron H$_2$O does not follow the movement of solute.

In thick ascending limbs, Na$^+$ transport is primary and active, but, as in the thin ascending limbs, virtually no H$_2$O is reabsorbed because thick limbs of Henle are highly impermeable to H$_2$O.

Na$^+$ reabsorption from distal tubules and collecting ducts is active; Cl$^-$ reabsorption is largely passive, with a small active component when very low intratubular Cl$^-$ concentrations are attained. Virtually no H$_2$O is reabsorbed from the early parts of distal tubules, whether or not antidiuretic hormone (ADH) is present. In the late portions of the distal tubules, as well as in cortical and medullary collecting ducts, reabsorption of H$_2$O varies directly with the blood concentration of ADH, which can greatly increase the water permeability of these parts.

Normally, about 67% of the filtered Na$^+$ is reabsorbed in the proximal tubules, about 25% in the loops of Henle, about 5% in the distal tubules, and nearly 3% in the collecting ducts.

There are perhaps two major threats to Na$^+$ balance: (a) spontaneous (primary) changes in glomerular filtration rate (GFR) and hence in the filtered load of Na$^+$, and (b) changes in Na$^+$ intake. The first threat is countered by the physiological compensations of glomerulotubular (G-T) balance and autoregulation of the GFR. Balance for Na$^+$ is usually re-established in the presence of the second threat, namely, changes in Na$^+$ intake, by secondary alterations in GFR (first factor), changes in the blood concentration of aldosterone (second factor), and one or more additional factors. These factors may include, among others, changes in the Starling forces across the walls of peritubular capillaries, natriuretic hormone(s), changes in the filtration rate of single nephrons (sGFR), and possibly a direct effect of sympathetic nervous activity on the tubular reabsorption of Na^+.

Problem 7-1

What is a normal dietary intake of sodium for a normal adult human? How much sodium is contained in the salt-poor or low-salt diet that is prescribed for many patients? Express your answer as grams, millimoles, and milliequivalents per day.

Problem 7-2

A hospitalized patient has a plasma Na^+ concentration of 112 mEq/liter (normal, 136 to 146 mEq/liter; Table 1-2). It is decided that this abnormality should be quickly corrected, at least partially. If it is desired to raise the plasma Na^+ concentration to 132 mEq/liter, how much 5% NaCl solution should be infused intravenously? The patient weighs 53 kg; atomic weights are given in Table 1-5.

[*Note:* Since a low plasma Na^+ concentration (called *hyponatremia*) represents a relative abundance of H_2O over Na^+, most patients with hyponatremia are treated through restriction of fluid intake. Occasionally, however, a very low plasma Na^+ concentration (as in this instance) is treated by giving NaCl.]

Appendix

The Renin-Angiotensin-Aldosterone System

The fine adjustments of Na^+ reabsorption in the distal tubules and collecting ducts are probably mediated mainly by aldosterone. In turn, the secretion of aldosterone in response to a change in Na^+ intake is regulated primarily by the plasma level of angiotensin II, which itself depends on the production of renin by the kidneys. Thus, not only is urinary excretion the principal route by which balance for Na^+ is adjusted, but the main regulating mechanism appears also to lie within the kidneys. This appendix describes the so-called renin-angiotensin-aldosterone system, which, in a multifaceted and interrelated manner, regulates some of the most vital physiological variables, such as the volume of extracellular fluid and the systemic arterial pressure.

The renin-angiotensin-aldosterone system is shown in Figure 7-10. *Renin* is secreted by the juxtaglomerular apparatus (JGA) in the kidney, probably from granular cells that are located mainly or exclusively in the afferent arterioles. Renin is a proteolytic enzyme that splits a decapeptide from *angiotensinogen,* an α_2-globulin substrate that is produced by the liver. The decapeptide, *angiotensin I,* may have little physiological action of its own; it is

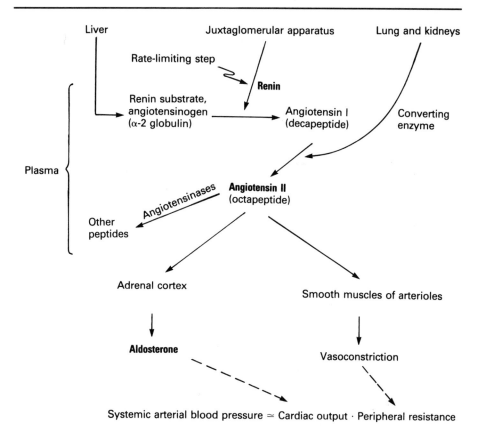

Fig. 7-10 : Dynamics of the renin-angiotensin-aldosterone system and its possible relation to the systemic arterial blood pressure. Slightly modified from Valtin, H. *Renal Dysfunction: Mechanisms Involved in Fluid and Solute Imbalance.* Boston: Little, Brown, 1979.

converted to an active principle, *angiotensin II,* through the loss of two terminal amino acids under the influence of *converting enzyme.* The conversion occurs mainly in the lungs, but also in the kidneys and perhaps in other organs.

Angiotensin II has two principal actions: (1) It is an extremely potent vasoconstrictor, and this action when exerted on the smooth muscles of the peripheral arterioles increases the total peripheral resistance. (2) It stimulates the zona glomerulosa of the adrenal cortex to secrete aldosterone, which tends to increase the extracellular fluid volume and hence cardiac output. Through both actions, angiotensin II influences the systemic arterial pressure.

CONTROL OF RENIN RELEASE. The plasma concentration of angiotensin II is controlled primarily by the rate at which renin is released from the JGA; and the level of renin is itself regulated by a feedback system that involves the various components

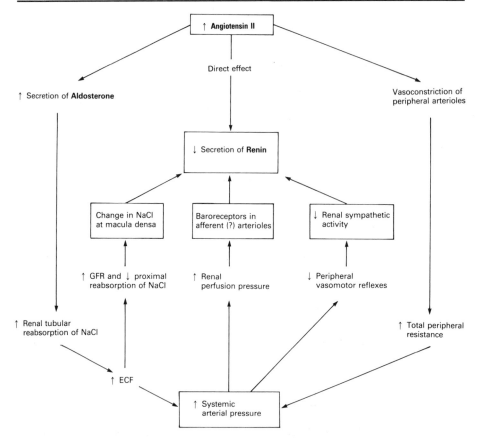

**Fig. 7-11 : Direct and indirect means by which the plasma concentration of an-
giotensin II exerts negative feedback control on the renal secretion of renin.
Modified from Schrier, R. W. (Ed.),** *Renal and Electrolyte Disorders* **(2nd ed.). Boston:
Little, Brown, 1980, and reproduced from Valtin, H.** *Renal Dysfunction: Mechanisms
Involved in Fluid and Solute Imbalance.* **Boston: Little, Brown, 1979.**

shown in Figure 7-10. In addition to a direct effect, angiotensin II
indirectly regulates the release of renin by three major mechanisms (Fig. 7-11): (a) baroreception in the afferent arterioles, (b)
alteration of the amount of NaCl flowing at the macula densa,
and (c) the influence of sympathetic nerves on the arterioles of
the JGA. Depending on the circumstances, these three may act
together in a coordinated manner, or one or more may predominate over the others.

Baroreceptor mechanism. Figure 7-11 shows a negative feedback system whereby an increase in renal perfusion pressure
decreases the release of renin. The opposite is also true: A moderate to marked decrease in renal perfusion pressure, whether
induced by hemorrhage or by constriction of the aorta above the
renal arteries, stimulates the release of renin.

Macula densa mechanism. Experiments in which the intratubular load of NaCl to the area of the macula densa is varied independently of changes in renal perfusion pressure leave little doubt that NaCl in the region of the JGA can influence the release of renin. Major controversy remains, however, about the details of this mechanism. It is not known whether Na$^+$, Cl$^-$, or both are sensed; whether it is their concentration or amount that is sensed; whether their presence within the tubular fluid or in the reabsorbate is the perceived variable; whether the macula densa cells, the lacis cells, or the granular cells are the sensors; and most important, whether an increase in NaCl at the macula densa leads to a decrease or an increase in the release of renin. It is because of these unresolved issues that Figure 7-11 speaks only of a "change in NaCl at the macula densa" and does not specify the direction or the nature of the change.

Sympathetic nervous system and catecholamines. The arterioles of the JGA are innervated by sympathetic nerve fibers. Electrical stimulation of the renal nerves, as well as stimulation of β-adrenergic receptors by isoproterenol, increases the release of renin, whereas renal denervation and β-adrenergic blockade by propranolol have the opposite effect. It can be shown experimentally that these effects are distinct from those that act via baroreceptors or the macula densa.

Other influences. At least three other factors, in addition to those shown in Figure 7-11, may play a physiological role in the control of renin release. (1) There is an inverse correlation between the plasma concentration of K$^+$ and the release of renin. It is possible that this effect is exerted through changes in the delivery of NaCl to the macula densa. (2) Vasopressin, even at physiological doses, inhibits the release of renin. This effect is apparently independent of changes in the three major mechanisms listed above. (3) Prostaglandin E$_2$ stimulates the production or release of renin.

Selected References

General

Andreoli, T. E., Hoffman, J. F., and Fanestil, D. D. (Eds.). *Physiology of Membrane Disorders.* New York: Plenum, 1978.
A very useful, thorough, and authoritative treatise on both the physiology and pathophysiology of transport mechanisms. The first section of this book has been published separately, in paperback form, under the title Membrane Physiology *(Plenum, 1980).*

Berry, C. A. Heterogeneity of tubular transport processes in the nephron. *Annu. Rev. Physiol.* 44:181, 1982.

Boulpaep, E. L. (Ed.). Cellular mechanisms of renal tubular ion transport. *Curr. Top. Membr. Transp.* 13:3, 1980.
An authoritative and useful collection of papers presented at a symposium held at Yale University School of Medicine in 1978.

Brodsky, W. A., Rehm, W. S., Dennis, W. H., and Miller, D. G. Thermodynamic analysis of the intracellular osmotic gradient hypothesis of active water transport. *Science* 121:302, 1955.

Burg, M. B. Renal Handling of Sodium, Chloride, Water, Amino Acids, and Glucose. In B. M. Brenner and F. C. Rector, Jr. (Eds.), *The Kidney* (2nd ed.). Philadelphia: Saunders, 1981.

Civan, M. M. Intracellular activities of sodium and potassium. *Am. J. Physiol.* 234 (Renal Fluid Electrolyte Physiol. 3):F261, 1978.

Curran, P. F., and Schultz, S. G. Some Thermodynamic and Kinetic Principles Governing Solvent and Solute Transport Across Membranes. In B. M. Brenner and F. C. Rector, Jr. (Eds.), *The Kidney.* Philadelphia: Saunders, 1976.

Fishman, A. P. (Ed.). Symposium on salt and water metabolism. *Circulation* 21:803, 1960.
Although in some respects outdated, this excellent symposium contains valuable material. It is, in many places, enlivened by discussion that is still remembered by those who attended the meeting.

Giebisch, G. (Ed.). *Transport Organs,* vols. IVA and IVB. New York: Springer-Verlag, 1979.
This superb reference work includes authoritative, up-to-date reviews. Volumes IVA and B are part of a four-volume series, entitled Membrane Transport in Biology *and edited by G. Giebisch, D. C. Tosteson, and H. H. Ussing.*

Gottschalk, C. W. Renal tubular function: Lessons from micropuncture. *Harvey Lect.* 58:99, 1963.

Graf, J., and Giebisch, G. Intracellular sodium activity and sodium transport in *Necturus* gallbladder epithelium. *J. Membr. Biol.* 47:327, 1979.

Heinz, E. *Mechanics and Energetics of Biological Transport.* Berlin: Springer-Verlag, 1978.

Kinne, R. A membrane-molecular approach to renal physiology. In L. Takács, (Ed.), *Advances in Physiological Sciences,* vol. 11, *Kidney and Body Fluids.* Budapest: Akadémiai Kiadó, 1981.

Koefoed-Johnsen, V., and Ussing, H. H. Ion Transport. In C. L. Comar and F. Bronner (Eds.), *Mineral Metabolism. An Advanced Treatise,* vol. I, part A. New York: Academic, 1960.

Lichardus, B., Schrier, R. W., and Ponec, J. (Eds.). *Hormonal Regulation of Sodium Excretion.* Amsterdam: Elsevier/North Holland, 1980.
A very useful summary on the status of the natriuretic hormone(s) and other humoral substances or factors that influence the urinary excretion of sodium.

Schmidt, U., Horster, M., Schmid, H., and Dubach, U. C. Enzymes of Cation Pumps Along the Nephron. In M. Bergeron et al. (Eds.), *Proceedings VII International Congress of Nephrology.* Basel: Karger, 1978.

Schultz, S. G. Transport across epithelia: Some basic principles. *Kidney Int.* 9:65, 1976.

Sullivan, L. P. *Physiology of the Kidney.* Philadelphia: Lea & Febiger, 1975, Chap. 1.

Sweadner, K. J., and Goldin, S. M. Active transport of sodium and potassium ions. Mechanism, function, and regulation. *N. Engl. J. Med.* 302:777, 1980.

Taylor, A., and Windhager, E. E. Possible role of cytosolic calcium and Na-Ca exchange in regulation of transepithelial sodium transport. *Am. J. Physiol.* 236 (Renal Fluid Electrolyte Physiol. 5):F505, 1979.

Walser, M. Sodium Excretion. In C. Rouiller and A. F. Muller (Eds.), *The Kidney,* vol. III. New York: Academic, 1971.

Wright, E. M. General Physiology. In G. Ross (Ed.), *Essentials of Human Physiology.* Chicago: Year Book, 1978.

Na$^+$ and H$_2$O Transport in Various Tubular Segments

Note: Also see references under Cotransport (Chap. 4, p. 81).

Andreoli, T. E., and Schafer, J. A. Volume absorption in the pars recta: III. Luminal hypotonicity as a driving force for isotonic volume absorption. *Am. J. Physiol.* 234 (Renal Fluid Electrolyte Physiol. 3):F349, 1978.

Burg, M. B., and Green, N. Function of the thick ascending limb of Henle's loop. *Am. J. Physiol.* 224:659, 1973.

Burg, M. B., and Stoner, L. Renal tubular chloride transport and the mode of action of some diuretics. *Annu. Rev. Physiol.* 38:37, 1976.

Costanzo, L. S., and Windhager, E. E. Calcium and sodium transport by the distal convoluted tubule of the rat. *Am. J. Physiol.* 235 (Renal Fluid Electrolyte Physiol. 4):F492, 1978.

Dennis, V. W., and Brazy, P. C. Sodium, phosphate, glucose, bicarbonate, and alanine interactions in the isolated proximal convoluted tubule of the rabbit kidney. *J. Clin. Invest.* 62:387, 1978.

Epstein, F. H. The Role of Sodium and Potassium ATPase in Renal Sodium Reabsorption. In K. Thurau and H. Jahrmärker (Eds.), *Renal Transport and Diuretics.* Berlin: Springer-Verlag, 1969.

Frömter, E. Magnitude and Significance of the Paracellular Shunt Path in Rat Kidney Proximal Tubule. In M. Kramer and F. Lauterbach (Eds.), *Intestinal Permeation.* Amsterdam: Excerpta Medica, 1977.

Giebisch, G., Boulpaep, E. L., and Whittembury, G. Electrolyte transport in kidney tubule cells. *Philos. Trans. R. Soc. Lond.* Series B. [Biol.] 262:175, 1971.

Giebisch, G., and Windhager, E. E. Electrolyte Transport Across Renal Tubular Membranes. In J. Orloff and R. W. Berliner (Eds.), *Handbook of Physiology,* section 8, Renal Physiology. Washington, D.C.: American Physiological Society, 1973.

Grantham, J. J., and Irish, J. M., III. Variations in Permeability and Transport Along the Proximal Convoluted Tubule and Pars Recta. In M. Bergeron et al. (Eds.), *Proceedings VII International Congress of Nephrology.* Basel: Karger, 1978.

Grantham, J. J., Irish, J. M., III, and Hall, D. A. Studies of isolated renal tubules in vitro. *Annu. Rev. Physiol.* 40:249, 1978.

Greger, R. Chloride reabsorption in the rabbit cortical thick ascending limb of the loop of Henle. A sodium dependent process. *Pflügers Arch. Eur. J. Physiol.* 390:38, 1981.

152

Greger, R. Presence of luminal K$^+$, a prerequisite for active NaCl transport in the cortical thick ascending limb of Henle's loop of rabbit kidney. *Pflügers Arch. Eur. J. Physiol.* 392:92, 1981.

Gross, J. B., Imai, M., and Kokko, J. P. A functional comparison of the cortical collecting tubule and the distal convoluted tubule. *J. Clin. Invest.* 55:1284, 1975.

Hilger, H. H., Klümper, J. D., and Ullrich, K. J. Wasserrückresorption und Ionentransport durch die Sammelrohrzellen der Säugetierniere. *Pflügers Arch. Ges. Physiol.* 267:218, 1958.

Jacobson, H. R. Characteristics of volume reabsorption in rabbit superficial and juxtamedullary proximal convoluted tubules. *J. Clin. Invest.* 63:410, 1979.

Katz, A. I., Doucet, A., and Morel, F. Na-K-ATPase activity along the rabbit, rat, and mouse nephron. *Am. J. Physiol.* 239 (Renal Fluid Electrolyte Physiol. 8):F114, 1979.

Kokko, J. P. Sodium chloride and water transport in the descending limb of Henle. *J. Clin. Invest.* 49:1838, 1970.

Kokko, J. P. Membrane characteristics governing salt and water transport in the loop of Henle. *Fed. Proc.* 33:25, 1974.

Marsh, D. J., and Solomon, S. Analysis of electrolyte movement in thin Henle's loops of hamster papilla. *Am. J. Physiol.* 208:1119, 1965.

Sasaki, S., and Imai, M. Effects of vasopressin on water and NaCl transport across the in vitro perfused medullary thick ascending limb of Henle's loop of mouse, rat, and rabbit kidneys. *Pflügers Arch. Eur. J. Physiol.* 383:215, 1980.

Schafer, J. A. Salt and water absorption in the proximal tubule. *Physiologist* 25(2):95, 1982.

Schafer, J. A., and Andreoli, T. E. Rheogenic and passive Na$^+$ absorption by the proximal nephron. *Annu. Rev. Physiol.* 41:211, 1979.

Ullrich, K. J., and Frömter, E. Active and Passive Transtubular Transport in the Proximal Convolution. In M. Bergeron et al. (Eds.), *Proceedings VII International Congress of Nephrology.* Basel: Karger, 1978.

Vogel, H. G., and Ullrich, K. J. (Eds.). *New Aspects of Renal Function.* Amsterdam: Excerpta Medica, 1978.
This international symposium was organized to summarize recent findings in all parts of the nephron, going from the glomerulus to the collecting duct.

Walker, A. M., Bott, P. A., Oliver, J., and MacDowell, M. C. The collection and analysis of fluid from single nephrons of the mammalian kidney. *Am. J. Physiol.* 134:580, 1941.

Warnock, D. G., and Eveloff, J. NaCl entry mechanisms in the luminal membrane of the renal tubule. *Am. J. Physiol.* 242 (Renal Fluid Electrolyte Physiol. 11):F561, 1982.

Welling, D. J., Welling, L. W., and Hill, J. J. Phenomenological model relating cell shape to water reabsorption in proximal nephron. *Am. J. Physiol.* 234 (Renal Fluid Electrolyte Physiol. 3):F308, 1978.

Windhager, E. E. Electrophysiological study of renal papilla of golden hamsters. *Am. J. Physiol.* 206:694, 1964.

Windhager, E. E., and Giebisch, G. Proximal sodium and fluid transport. *Kidney Int.* 9:121, 1976.

Windhager, E. E., Whittembury, G., Oken, D. E., Schatzmann, H. J., and Solomon, A. K. Single proximal tubules of the *Necturus* kidney: III. Dependence of H$_2$O movement on NaCl concentration. *Am. J. Physiol.* 197:313, 1959.

Fluid and Solute Transport in Epithelia. Isosmotic Reabsorption

Andreoli, T. E., Schafer, J. A., and Troutman, S. L. Perfusion rate-dependence of transepithelial osmosis in isolated proximal convoluted tubules: Estimation of the hydraulic conductance. *Kidney Int.* 14:263, 1978.

Bishop, J. H. V., Green, R., and Thomas, S. Free-flow reabsorption of glucose, sodium, osmoles and water in rat proximal convoluted tubule. *J. Physiol.* (Lond.) 288:331, 1979.

Boulpaep, E. L. (Chairman). Symposium on isotonic water movement. *Yale J. Biol. Med.* 50:97, 1977.

Carvounis, C. P., Franki, N., Levine, S. D., and Hays, R. M. Membrane pathways for water and solute in the toad bladder: I. Independent activation of water and urea transport. *J. Membr. Biol.* 49:253, 1979.

Civan, M. M., and DiBona, D. R. Pathways for movement of ions and water across toad urinary bladder: III. Physiologic significance of the paracellular pathway. *J. Membr. Biol.* 38:359, 1978.

Curran, P. F. Ion transport in intestine and its coupling to other transport processes. *Fed. Proc.* 24:993, 1965.

Curran, P. F., and MacIntosh, J. R. A model system for biological water transport. *Nature* 193:347, 1962.

Diamond, J. M., and Bossert, W. H. Standing-gradient osmotic flow. A mechanism for coupling of water and solute transport in epithelia. *J. Gen. Physiol.* 50:2061, 1967.

Evan, A. P., Hay, D. A., and Dail, W. G. SEM of the proximal tubule of the adult rabbit kidney. *Anat. Rec.* 191:397, 1978.

Ganote, C. E., Grantham, J. J., Moses, H. L., Burg, M. B., and Orloff, J. Ultrastructural studies of vasopressin effect on isolated perfused renal collecting tubules of the rabbit. *J. Cell Biol.* 36:355, 1968.

Giebisch, G. H., and Purcell, E. F. (Eds.). *Renal Function.* New York: Josiah Macy, Jr. Foundation, 1978.
Sections II and III of this book, entitled "Basic Mechanisms of Epithelial Transport" and "Mechanisms of Proximal Tubular Ion Transport," respectively, offer authoritative reviews.

Kinne, R., Murer, H., Kinne-Saffran, E., Thees, M., and Sachs, G. Sugar transport by renal plasma membrane vesicles. Characterization of the systems in the brush-border microvilli and basal-lateral plasma membranes. *J. Membr. Biol.* 21:375, 1975.

Kyte, J. Immunoferritin determination of the distribution of (Na$^+$ + K$^+$)ATPase over the plasma membranes of renal convoluted tubules: II. Proximal segment. *J. Cell Biol.* 68:304, 1976.

154

Loewenstein, W. R. (Chairman). Symposium on membrane channels. *Fed. Proc.* 37:2626, 1978.

Marsh, D. J. (Chairman). Symposium on theoretical aspects of epithelial transport. *Fed. Proc.* 38:2023, 1979.

Morel, F. La réabsorption isoosmotique proximale du rein. Mécanisme et régulation. *J. Physiol.* (Paris) 72:515, 1976.

Sachs, G., and Kinne, R. Isolation and Characterization of Biological Membranes. In T. E. Andreoli, J. F. Hoffman, and D. D. Fanestil (Eds.), *Physiology of Membrane Disorders.* New York: Plenum, 1978.

Sackin, H., and Boulpaep, E. L. Models for coupling of salt and water transport. Proximal tubular reabsorption in *Necturus* kidney. *J. Gen. Physiol.* 66:671, 1975.

Schafer, J. A. (Chairman). Symposium on water transport in epithelia. *Fed. Proc.* 38:119, 1979.
A very useful summary.

Schafer, J. A., Patlak, C. S., and Andreoli, T. E. Fluid absorption and active and passive ion flows in the rabbit superficial pars recta. *Am. J. Physiol.* 233 (Renal Fluid Electrolyte Physiol. 2):F154, 1977.

Tisher, C. C., Bulger, R. E., and Valtin, H. Morphology of renal medulla in water diuresis and vasopressin-induced antidiuresis. *Am. J. Physiol.* 220:87, 1971.

Tisher, C. C., and Yarger, W. E. Lanthanum permeability of the tight junction (zonula occludens) in the renal tubule of the rat. *Kidney Int.* 3:238, 1973.

Ullrich, K. J., Rumrich, G., and Fuchs, G. Wasserpermeabilität und transtubulärer Wasserfluss corticaler Nephronabschnitte bei verschiedenen Diuresezuständen. *Pflügers Arch. Ges. Physiol.* 280:99, 1964.

Welling, L. W., and Welling, D. J. Shape of epithelial cells and intercellular channels in the rabbit proximal nephron. *Kidney Int.* 9:385, 1976.

Electrophysiology

Boulpaep, E. L. Mechanisms of Proximal Tubular Ion Transport. In G. H. Giebisch and E. F. Purcell (Eds.), *Renal Function.* New York: Josiah Macy, Jr. Foundation, 1978.

Boulpaep, E. L. Electrophysiology of the Kidney. In G. Giebisch, D. C. Tosteson, and H. H. Ussing (Eds.), *Membrane Transport in Biology,* vol. IVA. New York: Springer-Verlag, 1979.

Frömter, E. Electrophysiology and isotonic fluid absorption of proximal tubules of mammalian kidney. *Int. Rev. Physiol.* 6:1, 1974.

Frömter, E., and Gessner, K. Free-flow potential profile along rat kidney proximal tubule. *Pflügers Arch. Eur. J. Physiol.* 351:69, 1974.

Hanley, M. J., Kokko, J. P., Gross, J. B., and Jacobson, H. R. Electrophysiologic study of the cortical collecting tubule of the rabbit. *Kidney Int.* 17:74, 1980.

Hayslett, J. P., Boulpaep, E. L., Kashgarian, M., and Giebisch, G. H. Electrical characteristics of the mammalian distal tubule: Comparison of Ling-Gerard and macroelectrodes. *Kidney Int.* 12:324, 1977.

Kokko, J. P. Proximal tubule potential difference. Dependence on glucose, HCO$_3$, and amino acids. *J. Clin. Invest.* 52:1362, 1973.

Maffly, R. H. The Body Fluids: Volume, Composition, and Physical Chemistry. In B. M. Brenner and F. C. Rector, Jr. (Eds.), *The Kidney* (2nd ed.). Philadelphia: Saunders, 1981.

Reuss, L. (Chairman). Symposium on electrophysiology of epithelial transport. *Fed. Proc.* 38:2720, 1979.

Spring, K. R., and Giebisch, G. Kinetics of Na$^+$ transport in *Necturus* proximal tubule. *J. Gen. Physiol.* 70:307, 1977.

Ussing, H. H., and Windhager, E. E. Nature of shunt path and active sodium transport path through frog skin epithelium. *Acta Physiol. Scand.* 61:484, 1964.

Ussing, H., and Zerahn, K. Active transport of sodium as the source of electric current in the short-circuited frog skin. *Acta Physiol. Scand.* 23:110, 1951.

Windhager, E. E. Electrophysiological study of renal papilla of golden hamsters. *Am. J. Physiol.* 206:694, 1964.

Windhager, E. E., and Giebisch, G. Electrophysiology of the nephron. *Physiol. Rev.* 45:214, 1965.

Wright, F. S. Increasing magnitude of electrical potential along the renal distal tubule. *Am. J. Physiol.* 220:624, 1971.

Na$^+$ Balance

Note: Also see references under Autoregulation and Tubuloglomerular Feedback (Chap. 6, p. 115).

Arrizurieta-Muchnik, E. E., Lassiter, W. E., Lipham, E. M., and Gottschalk, C. W. Micropuncture study of glomerulotubular balance in the rat kidney. *Nephron* 6:418, 1969.

Blair-West, J. R. Renin-angiotensin system and sodium metabolism. *Int. Rev. Physiol.* 11:95, 1976.

Blythe, W. B., D'Avila, D., Gitelman, H. J., and Welt, L. G. Further evidence for a humoral natriuretic factor. *Circ. Res.* 28 (Suppl. 2):II-21, 1971.

Brenner, B. M., Bennett, C. M., and Berliner, R. W. The relationship between glomerular filtration rate and sodium reabsorption by the proximal tubule of the rat nephron. *J. Clin. Invest.* 47:1358, 1968.

Brenner, B. M., and Stein, J. H. (Eds.). Sodium and Water Homeostasis. *Contemporary Issues in Nephrology,* vol. 1. New York: Churchill Livingstone, 1978.
In this symposium, the various contributors apply basic scientific principles to the explanation of imbalances of water and sodium in various pathological states.

Cort, J. H., Dousa, T., Pliska, V., Lichardus, B., Safarova, J., Vranesic, M., and Rudinger, J. Saluretic activity of blood during carotid occlusion in the cat. *Am. J. Physiol.* 215:921, 1968.

Davis, J. M., Brechtelsbauer, H., Prucksunand, P., Weigl, J., Schnermann, J., and Kramer, K. Relationship between salt loading and distribution of nephron filtration rates in the dog. *Pflügers Arch. Eur. J. Physiol.* 350:259, 1974.

de Wardener, H. E. The control of sodium excretion. *Am. J. Physiol.* 235 (Renal Fluid Electrolyte Physiol. 4):F163, 1978.

Edelman, I. S., and Marver, D. Mediating events in the action of aldosterone. *J. Steroid Biochem.* 12:219, 1980.

Gertz, K. H. Glomerular Tubular Balance. In J. Orloff and R. W. Berliner (Eds.), *Handbook of Physiology,* section 8, Renal Physiology. Washington, D.C.: American Physiological Society, 1973.

Gottschalk, C. W. Renal nerves and sodium excretion. *Annu. Rev. Physiol.* 41:229, 1979.

Guyton, A. C., Coleman, T. G., Young, D. B., Lohmeier, T. E., and DeClue, J. W. Salt balance and long-term blood pressure control. *Annu. Rev. Med.* 31:15, 1980.

Häberle, D. A., Shiigai, T. T., Maier, G., Schiffl, H., and Davis, J. M. Dependency of proximal tubular fluid transport on the load of glomerular filtrate. *Kidney Int.* 20:18, 1981.

Hollenberg, N. K. Set point for sodium homeostasis: Surfeit, deficit, and their implications. *Kidney Int.* 17:423, 1980.
This editorial review was followed by the presentation of a contrary point of view, set forth by Drs. J. V. Bonventre and A. Leaf: Kidney Int. *21:880–885, 1982.*

Kramer, K., Boylan, J. W., and Keck, W. Regulation of total body sodium in the mammalian organism. *Nephron* 6:379, 1969.

Lancet Editorial. Natriuretic hormone. *Lancet* 2:537, 1977.

Michell, A. R. Salt appetite, salt intake, and hypertension: A deviation of perspective. *Perspect. Biol. Med.* 21:335, 1978.

Navar, L. G., Bell, P. D., and Burke, T. J. Autoregulatory responses of superficial nephrons and their association with sodium excretion during arterial pressure alterations in the dog. *Circ. Res.* 41:487, 1977.

Oomen, H. A. P. Salt and hypertension (Letter to the Editor). *Lancet* 2:260, 1980.

Osgood, R. W., Reineck, H. J., and Stein, J. H. Effect of Hyperoncotic albumin on superficial and juxtamedullary nephron sodium transport. *Am. J. Physiol.* 237 (Renal Fluid Electrolyte Physiol. 6):F34, 1979.

Schafer, J. A. Response of the collecting duct to the demands of homeostasis. *Physiologist* 22 (No. 5):44, 1979.

Seely, J. F., and Levy, M. Control of Extracellular Fluid Volume. In B. M. Brenner and F. C. Rector, Jr. (Eds.), *The Kidney* (2nd ed.). Philadelphia: Saunders, 1981.

Stein, J. H., Osgood, R. W., and Kunau, R. T., Jr. Direct measurement of papillary collecting duct sodium transport in the rat. Evidence for heterogeneity of nephron function during Ringer loading. *J. Clin. Invest.* 58:767, 1976.

Tucker, B. J., Steiner, R. W., Gushwa, L. C., and Blantz, R. C. Studies on the tubulo-glomerular feedback system in the rat. The mechanism of reduction in filtration rate with benzolamide. *J. Clin. Invest.* 62:993, 1978.

Wright, F. S., Brenner, B. M., Bennett, C. M., Keimowitz, R. I., Berliner, R. W., Schrier, R. W., Verroust, P. J., de Wardener, H. E., and Holzgreve, H. Failure to demonstrate a hormonal inhibitor of proximal sodium reabsorption. *J. Clin. Invest.* 48:1107, 1969.

Renin-Angiotensin-
Aldosterone

Crabbé, J. The Mechanism of Action of Aldosterone. In J. R. Pasqualini (Ed.), *Receptors and Mechanism of Action of Steroid Hormones,* part II. New York: Dekker, 1977.

Davis, J. O., and Freeman, R. H. Mechanisms regulating renin release. *Physiol. Rev.* 56:1, 1976.

Edelman, I. S., and Marver, D. Mediating events in the action of aldosterone. *J. Steroid Biochem.* 12:219, 1980.

Fanestil, D. D., and Park, C. S. Steroid hormones and the kidney. *Annu. Rev. Physiol.* 43:637, 1981.

Hierholzer, K., and Lange, S. The effects of adrenal steroids on renal function. *Int. Rev. Physiol.* 6:273, 1974.

Horster, M., Schmid, H., and Schmidt, U. Aldosterone in vitro restores nephron Na-K-ATPase of distal segments from adrenalectomized rabbits. *Pflügers Arch. Eur. J. Physiol.* 384:203, 1980.

Keeton, T. K., and Campbell, W. B. The pharmacologic alteration of renin release. *Pharmacol. Rev.* 32:81, 1980.

Laragh, J. H., and Sealey, J. E. The Renin-Angiotensin-Aldosterone Hormonal System and Regulation of Sodium, Potassium, and Blood Pressure Homeostasis. In J. Orloff and R. W. Berliner (Eds.), *Handbook of Physiology,* section 8, Renal Physiology. Washington, D.C.: American Physiological Society, 1973.

Rabinowitz, L. Aldosterone and renal potassium excretion. *Renal Physiol.* 2:229, 1980.

Schwartz, G. J., and Burg, M. B. Mineralocorticoid effects on cation transport by cortical collecting tubules in vitro. *Am. J. Physiol.* 235 (Renal Fluid Electrolyte Physiol. 4):F576, 1978.

Sharp, G. W. G., and Leaf, A. Aldosterone. In J. Orloff and R. W. Berliner (Eds.), *Handbook of Physiology,* section 8, Renal Physiology. Washington, D.C.: American Physiological Society, 1973.

Stokes, J. B., Ingram, M. J., Williams, A. D., and Ingram, D. Heterogeneity of the rabbit collecting tubule: Localization of mineralocorticoid hormone action to the cortical portion. *Kidney Int.* 20:340, 1981.

Tait, S. A. S., and Tait, J. F. (Eds.). Symposium on aldosterone. *J. Endocrinol.* 81:1P, 1979.

Thölen, H. (Chairman). Symposium on aldosterone and active sodium transport across epithelia. *J. Steroid Biochem.* 3:105, 1972.

Thurau, K., and Mason, J. The intrarenal function of the juxtaglomerular apparatus. *Int. Rev. Physiol.* 6:357, 1974.

Vander, A. J. *Renal Physiology* (2nd ed.). New York: McGraw-Hill, 1980. Chap. 7.

Peritubular Control
of Fluid
Reabsorption.
Starling Forces.
Natriuretic
Hormone(s)

Berry, C. A., and Cogan, M. G. Influence of peritubular protein on solute absorption in the rabbit proximal tubule. *J. Clin. Invest.* 68:506, 1981.

Brenner, B. M., and Troy, J. L. Postglomerular vascular protein concentration: Evidence for a causal role in governing fluid reabsorption and glomerulotubular balance by the renal proximal tubule. *J. Clin. Invest.* 50:336, 1971.

Bricker, N. S., Schmidt, R. W., Favre, H., Fine, L., and Bourgoignie, J. J. On the biology of sodium excretion: The search for a natriuretic hormone. *Yale J. Biol. Med.* 48:293, 1975.

Burg, M. B. The Renal Handling of Sodium Chloride, Water, Amino Acids, and Glucose. In B. M. Brenner and F. C. Rector, J. (Eds.), *The Kidney* (2nd ed.). Philadelphia: Saunders, 1981.

de Wardener, H. E., Mills, I. H., Clapham, W. F., and Hayter, C. J. Studies on the efferent mechanism of the sodium diuresis which follows the administration of intravenous saline in the dog. *Clin. Sci. Mol. Med.* 21:249, 1961.

DiBona, G. F. Neural control of renal tubular sodium reabsorption in the dog. *Fed. Proc.* 37:1214, 1978.

Earley, L. E. Influence of hemodynamic factors on sodium reabsorption. *Ann. N.Y. Acad. Sci.* 139:312, 1966.

Earley, L. E., and Schrier, R. W. Intrarenal Control of Sodium Excretion by Hemodynamic and Physical Factors. In J. Orloff and R. W. Berliner (Eds.), *Handbook of Physiology,* section 8, Renal Physiology. Washington, D.C.: American Physiological Society, 1973.

Falchuk, K. H., Brenner, B. M., Tadokoro, M., and Berliner, R. W. Oncotic and hydrostatic pressures in peritubular capillaries and fluid reabsorption by proximal tubule. *Am. J. Physiol.* 220:1427, 1971.

Grantham, J. J., Qualizza, P. B., and Welling, L. W. Influence of serum proteins on net fluid reabsorption of isolated proximal tubules. *Kidney Int.* 2:66, 1972.

Green, R., Windhager, E. E., and Giebisch, G. Protein oncotic pressure effects on proximal tubular fluid movement in the rat. *Am. J. Physiol.* 226:265, 1974.

Howards, S. S., Davis, B. B., Knox, F. G., Wright, F. S., and Berliner, R. W. Depression of fractional sodium reabsorption by the proximal tubule of the dog without sodium diuresis. *J. Clin. Invest.* 47:1561, 1968.

Imai, M., and Kokko, J. P. Transtubular oncotic pressure gradients and net fluid transport in isolated proximal tubules. *Kidney Int.* 6:138, 1974.

Jacobson, H. R., and Seldin, D. W. Proximal tubular reabsorption and its regulation. *Annu. Rev. Pharmacol. Toxicol.* 17:623, 1977.

Levy, M., and Levinsky, N. G. Proximal reabsorption and intrarenal pressure during colloid infusions in the dog. *Am. J. Physiol.* 220:415, 1971.

Lichardus, B., Schrier, R. W., and Ponec, J. *Hormonal Regulation of Sodium Excretion.* Amsterdam: Elsevier/North Holland, 1980.
A very useful summary on the status of the natriuretic hormone(s) and other humoral substances or factors that influence the urinary excretion of sodium.

Nizet, A. Quantitative influence of non-hormonal blood factors on the control of sodium excretion by the isolated dog kidney. *Kidney Int.* 1:27, 1972.

Windhager, E. E., Lewy, J. E., and Spitzer, A. Intrarenal control of proximal tubular reabsorption of sodium and water. *Nephron* 6:247, 1969.

Ziegler, T. W. A new model for regulation of sodium transport in high resistance epithelia. *Med. Hypotheses* 2:85, 1976.

Divalent Cations

Note: Also see references under Phosphate and Calcium (Chap. 4, p. 83).

Costanzo, L. S., and Windhager, E. E. Calcium and sodium transport by the distal convoluted tubule of the rat. *Am. J. Physiol.* 235 (Renal Fluid Electrolyte Physiol 4):F492, 1978.

Edwards, B. R., Baer, P. G., Sutton, R. A. L., and Dirks, J. H. Micropuncture study of diuretic effects on sodium and calcium reabsorption in the dog nephron. *J. Clin. Invest.* 52:2418, 1973.

Kinne, R., Keljo, D., Gmaj, P., and Murer, H. The Energy Source of Glucose and Calcium Transport in the Renal Proximal Tubule. In H. G. Vogel and K. J. Ullrich (Eds.), *New Aspects of Renal Function.* Amsterdam: Excerpta Medica, 1978.

Lemann, J., Jr., Adams, N. D., and Gray, R. W. Urinary calcium excretion in human beings. *N. Engl. J. Med.* 301:535, 1979.

Parfitt, A. M., and Kleerekoper, M. The Divalent Ion Homeostatic System — Physiology and Metabolism of Calcium, Phosphorus, and Bone. In M. H. Maxwell and C. R. Kleeman (Eds.), *Clinical Disorders of Fluid and Electrolyte Metabolism* (3rd ed.). New York: McGraw-Hill, 1980. Chap. 8. *Clinical disorders involving divalent ions are discussed in Chapters 19 and 20 of this volume.*

Sutton, R. A. L., Quamme, G. A., and Dirks, J. H. Transport of Calcium, Magnesium and Inorganic Phosphate in the Kidney. In G. Giebisch, D. C. Tosteson, and H. H. Ussing (Eds.), *Membrane Transport in Biology,* vol. IVA. New York: Springer-Verlag, 1979.

Walser, M. Divalent Cations: Physicochemical State in Glomerular Filtrate and Urine, and Renal Excretion. In J. Orloff and R. W. Berliner (Eds.), *Handbook of Physiology,* section 8, Renal Physiology. Washington, D.C.: American Physiological Society, 1973.

Heterogeneity of Nephrons

Berry, C. A. Heterogeneity of tubular transport processes in the nephron. *Annu. Rev. Physiol.* 44:181, 1982.

Bonvalet, J. P., and de Rouffignac, C. Hétérogénéité fonctionnelle des nephrons. *J. Physiol.* (Paris) 71:73A, 1975.

Bowman, W. On the structure and use of the Malpighian bodies of the kidney, with observations on the circulation through that gland. *Philos. Trans. R. Soc. Lond.* Series B. [Biol.] 132:57, 1842.

Bulger, R. E., and Dobyan, D. C. Recent advances in renal morphology. *Annu. Rev. Physiol.* 44:147, 1982.

Jacobson, H. R. Functional segmentation of the mammalian nephron. *Am. J. Physiol.* 241 (Renal Fluid Electrolyte Physiol. 10):F203, 1981.

Morel, F. Sites of hormone action in the mammalian nephron. *Am. J. Physiol.* 240 (Renal Fluid Electrolyte Physiol. 9):F159, 1981.

Peter, K. *Untersuchungen über Bau und Entwickelung der Niere.* Jena: Fischer, 1909.

Stokes, J. B., Tisher, C. C., and Kokko, J. P. Structural-functional heterogeneity along the rabbit collecting tubule. *Kidney Int.* 14:585, 1978.

Valtin, H. Structural and functional heterogeneity of mammalian nephrons. *Am. J. Physiol.* 233 (Renal Fluid Electrolyte Physiol. 2):F491, 1977.

Walker, L. A., and Valtin, H. Biological importance of nephron heterogeneity. *Annu. Rev. Physiol.* 44:203, 1982.

8 : Concentration and Dilution of Urine: H₂O Balance

Even though water reabsorption is a passive event that follows the reabsorption of Na^+, water balance can be regulated independently of Na^+ balance. This is accomplished through changes in the blood concentration of the antidiuretic hormone (ADH or vasopressin), which adjusts the amount of water that is reabsorbed from the late distal tubules and collecting ducts. When the concentration of ADH is high, so is the water permeability of these parts of the nephron (Table 7-1). Consequently, much water is reabsorbed and hyperosmotic urine is formed — up to about 1,200 mOsm/kg H_2O in humans (the state of antidiuresis, defined on p. 119). Conversely, a low concentration of ADH reduces the water permeability of late distal tubules and collecting ducts. This results in little water reabsorption from these parts and the formation of hyposmotic urine — down to about 50 mOsm/kg H_2O in man (water diuresis). (The terms *isosmotic, hyperosmotic,* and *hyposmotic* are defined at the beginning of Chapter 7. Except when specified, the comparison in the present chapter is with the osmolality of plasma.)

The Countercurrent Mechanism

As we have seen (Table 7-1), in all components of the nephron except the thin limbs of the loops of Henle, the transport of Na^+ is active, while water reabsorption is passive. Given these prerequisites, it is conceptually easy to form hyposmotic urine: The kidneys actively reabsorb Na^+ (and its anions) from an isosmotic glomerular filtrate while much of the water is retained within the tubules. It proved more difficult, however, to conceive a system that will produce hyperosmotic urine through the passive reabsorption of water, as this requires the buildup of hyperosmotic fluid in the tissues that surround the tubules. The problem of hyperosmotic urine formation through passive water reabsorption puzzled renal physiologists for many years until W. Kuhn and K. Ryffel proposed the countercurrent mechanism. The principle of this mechanism in a normal human being concentrating urine to 1,200 mOsm/kg H_2O is illustrated in Figure 8-1A.

Antidiuresis

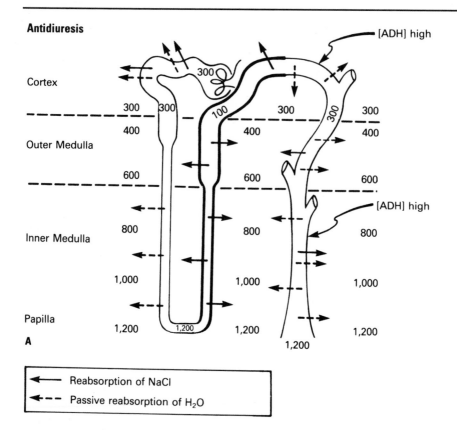

Water Diuresis

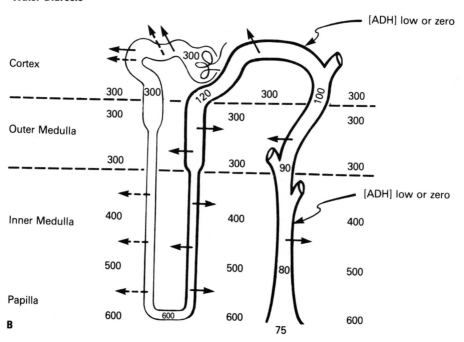

Formation of Hyperosmotic (Concentrated) Urine

This is thought to occur through the following sequence of events:

1. The fluid in Bowman's capsule, being an ultrafiltrate of plasma, has an osmolality of about 300 mOsm/kg H_2O.

2. About two-thirds of the glomerular filtrate is reabsorbed isosmotically in the proximal tubule (Figs. 7-4 and 7-7). Hence, intratubular fluid at the end of the proximal tubule still has an osmolality of 300 mOsm/kg H_2O.

3. The wall of the ascending limb of Henle is thought to be relatively impermeable to water. Therefore, in this segment NaCl is reabsorbed to the virtual exclusion of water, a process that renders the medullary and papillary interstitium hyperosmotic to plasma. This process is abetted by the loops of Henle acting as countercurrent multipliers (see below). Since isosmotic fluid entered the loops of Henle and NaCl was withdrawn, intratubular fluid at the beginning of the distal tubule is hyposmotic.

4. With a high concentration of ADH in the blood, the membranes lining the late distal tubules and collecting ducts are highly permeable to water. Hence, all along these tubular segments, water diffuses passively down the osmotic gradient between intratubular fluid and cortical, medullary, and papillary interstitium. The tubular fluid is thereby concentrated until osmotic equilibrium with the interstitium is reached, and this progressive concentration of intratubular fluid takes place even though some NaCl continues to be reabsorbed from the distal tubules and collecting ducts.

This is called the countercurrent system, for at least three reasons: (a) the loops of Henle act as countercurrent multipliers; (b) the vasa recta act as countercurrent exchangers (see below); and

Fig. 8-1 : Operation of the renal countercurrent system in a normal human being. Heavy boundaries indicate very low permeability to water. The numbers refer to the osmolality (mOsm/kg H_2O) of either intratubular or interstitial fluid. Solid arrows denote reabsorption of NaCl, which is active except in the thin ascending limbs of Henle, where it may be largely passive (see Passive Model of Countercurrent Multiplication in Inner Medulla, below); arrows with dashed line denote passive reabsorption of water. The number of arrows in each part of the nephron signifies semiquantitatively the amounts of solute transported relative to water. For example, in ascending limbs of Henle, solute is reabsorbed to the virtual exclusion of water (but not complete exclusion, since renal membranes are not wholly impervious to water).

A. During antidiuresis.

B. During water diuresis. It is possible (but not known for certain) that the osmolality of tubular fluid at the early distal tubule is slightly higher in water diuresis than in antidiuresis. The important changes from antidiuresis are: (1) the lower interstitial osmolality in the medulla and papilla; (2) the virtual absence of ADH; and hence (3) the lack of osmotic equilibration between fluid in the collecting duct and the surrounding interstitium.

(c) it is the countercurrent arrangement of the entire nephron that gives the tubular fluid in collecting ducts a chance to flow through an area of hyperosmolality, thereby permitting concentration of urine through the passive reabsorption of water.

Formation of Hyposmotic (Dilute) Urine

During the formation of dilute urine (Fig. 8-1B), the sequence is qualitatively identical up to the beginning of the distal tubule. (For reasons cited in part 4 of Table 8-1, there is a quantitative difference in that the osmolality of the papillary interstitium is only about one-half the value that it is during antidiuresis.) Now, in water diuresis, the blood concentration of ADH is low or zero, so that the membranes lining the late distal tubules and collecting ducts are relatively impermeable to water (see Table 7-1). Hence, very little water is reabsorbed even though an osmotic gradient between tubular lumen and interstitium persists. Some NaCl continues to be reabsorbed, which accounts for the further dilution of tubular fluid from approximately 120 mOsm/kg H_2O at the beginning of the distal tubule to perhaps 75 mOsm/kg H_2O in the urine.

Historical Hints

It is of interest that although the countercurrent hypothesis became accepted as the mechanism only around 1960, strong hints on where to search for the mechanism were extant in the literature for at least 50 years. In 1909, K. Peter pointed to the correlation between the length of thin loops of Henle in different species of mammals and the degree to which they could concentrate the urine. For example, in the Australian hopping mouse, which lives in the desert near Alice Springs and can concentrate its urine to at least 9,000 mOsm/kg H_2O, some long loops of Henle reach all the way into the ureter, whereas in rodents that do not live in an arid habitat and concentrate their urine to about 2,500 mOsm/kg H_2O the long loops are not nearly so extended, reaching only to the tip of the papilla. In 1925, E. H. Starling and E. B. Verney pointed out (albeit in a footnote) that there is a correspondence between the ability to make urine hyperosmotic to plasma, and the presence of medullary loops of Henle. This point was again made by E. K. Marshall, Jr., in 1934, when he emphasized in a review that only birds and mammals could render urine hyperosmotic to plasma, and only in these animals did one find medullary thin loops of Henle (see Fig. 1-4).

All this evidence suggested to investigators that urine must be concentrated within the loops of Henle. Then micropuncture studies showed that tubular fluid even in late portions of the distal tubules is either hyposmotic or isosmotic, but not hyperosmotic. It therefore was clear that the fluid must become hyperosmotic in the collecting ducts.

The correct role of the loops of Henle was first suggested in 1942 by two Swiss workers, W. Kuhn and K. Ryffel, who published a paper entitled "Production of concentrated solutions from diluted ones solely by membrane effects: A model for renal function." However, their countercurrent theory was largely ignored because it seemed unnecessarily complicated compared to active reabsorption of water. Nevertheless, the Swiss group persisted, and in 1951 H. Wirz, B. Hargitay, and W. Kuhn reproposed the countercurrent theory and presented preliminary experimental evidence (discussed below) supporting their hypothesis. By 1960 the experimental evidence in its favor became so overwhelming that the hypothesis was accepted.

Countercurrent Multiplication in Loops of Henle

One form of countercurrent multiplication is depicted in Figure 8-2. (It is to be stressed that the process of multiplication takes place in the loops of Henle, whereas that of countercurrent exchange, discussed later, occurs in the vasa recta.) We will illustrate the buildup of the so-called *corticomedullary interstitial osmotic gradient* by showing schematic, stepwise events as they are thought to occur in the thick ascending limb of Henle.

1. The loop is filled with isosmotic fluid coming out of the proximal tubule.
2. NaCl is reabsorbed actively from the thick ascending limb of Henle (Table 7-1). Since this part of the nephron has a very low permeability for water (Table 7-1), NaCl is reabsorbed virtually without water; this separation of solute transport from water transport — known as the *single effect* of the countercurrent multiplier — renders the osmolality of the interstitium hypertonic to the fluid within the ascending limb and to plasma. In the present example, the ascending limb can pump NaCl actively until a difference of 200 mOsm/kg H₂O has been established at each horizontal level. Since the thin descending limb is highly permeable to water (Table 7-1), fluid in that limb comes into osmotic equilibrium with the interstitium. This last process does not dissipate the high osmolality of the interstitium because the ascending limb continues to pump NaCl until the steady-state differences shown in step 2 have been established.
3. More isosmotic fluid comes out of the proximal tubule into the descending limb, pushing hyposmotic fluid out of the ascending limb and into the early distal tubule. (In the stepwise schema shown in Figure 8-2, step 3 dilutes part of the interstitium; in reality, this much dilution probably does not occur because reabsorption of more solute from the ascending limb, shown in step 4, takes place simultaneously.)

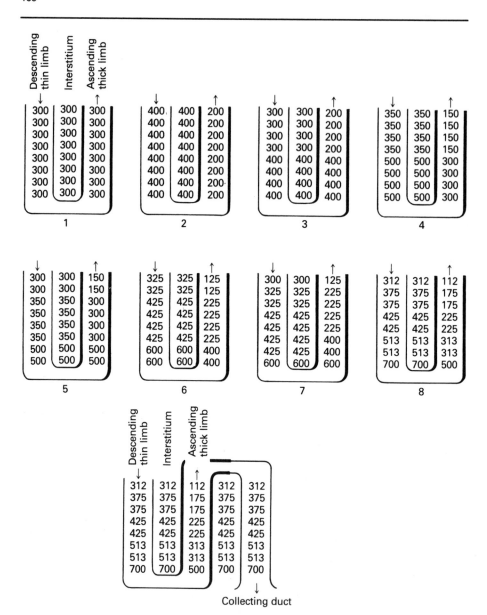

Fig. 8-2 : Schematic, stepwise operation by which a countercurrent multiplier system in the loops of Henle increases the osmolality of the medullary interstitium. The heavy boundaries of the ascending limb and early distal tubule indicate that these parts of the nephron are impermeable to water, even in the presence of ADH (see Table 7-1). Numbers refer to osmolalities (mOsm/kg H_2O) of tubular fluid and interstitium. Detailed description in text. Adapted from Pitts, R. F. *Physiology of the Kidney and Body Fluids* (3rd ed.). Chicago: Year Book, 1974.

4. The process described in step 2 is repeated, again building up a difference of 200 mOsm/kg H_2O between the descending limb and interstitium, on the one hand, and fluid in the ascending limb, on the other.
5. More isosmotic fluid enters the descending limb, pushing hyposmotic fluid into the distal tubule (and so on through steps 6, 7, and 8).

Note the following points. (1) By step 8, the interstitial concentration near the bend of the loop is nearly 400 mOsm/kg H_2O higher than that near the beginning of the descending limb, and this increase is much greater than that of 200 mOsm/kg H_2O which can be generated at any horizontal level through the active reabsorption of NaCl. That is, the "single effect" gets multiplied in this kind of system — by a factor of 2 in the present example. (2) The longer the loops of Henle, the greater will be the concentration of the interstitium — and hence of the tubular fluid — at the bend of the loop. (3) By themselves, the two limbs of Henle actually dilute the tubular fluid. It is only when a collecting duct is added to the system (lowest panel of Fig. 8-2), thereby giving the tubular fluid a second chance, so to speak, to flow past the hyperosmotic interstitium, that the urine can be rendered hyperosmotic. (4) The events described above and shown in Figure 8-2 occur in the thick ascending limb. Analogous countercurrent multiplication occurs as well in the thin ascending limbs of Henle, although the single effect may involve mainly passive, rather than active, reabsorption of NaCl (see Passive Model of Countercurrent Multiplication in Inner Medulla, below).

Countercurrent Exchange in Vasa Recta

Only about 5% of the total renal blood flow (RBF) (see Table 6-2), and hence of the total renal plasma flow (RPF), courses through the outer and inner medulla. Nevertheless, the amount of plasma that flows at the beginning of the outer medulla exceeds the flow of tubular fluid at the same point by a factor of about 10; i.e., approximately 10 times more plasma than tubular fluid enters the area of interstitial hyperosmolality (Fig. 8-1A), as the following numerical example makes clear. A normal RPF in man is about 660 ml per minute (p. 92), and 5% of this value, or 33 ml per minute, is the amount of plasma that flows in the descending vasa recta at the beginning of the outer medulla (Fig. 1-2B). A normal GFR in the same person might be approximately 125 ml per minute, and roughly 3% of this amount (see Answer to Problem 8-2a), or 3.8 ml per minute, enters the outer medullary collecting ducts (Fig. 1-2A). Since the vasa recta are highly permeable to water and, like the collecting ducts, are also surrounded by hyperosmotic interstitium, it would seem at first glance that the countercurrent mechanism might concentrate about 10 ml of

Countercurrent Exchange in Vasa Recta

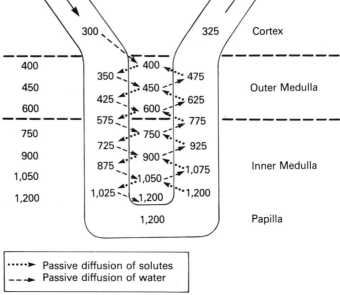

Fig. 8-3 : The countercurrent exchange system in the vasa recta. Arrows with dotted lines denote passive transport of solutes; arrows with dashed lines denote passive movement of water. The numbers refer to osmolalities (mOsm/kg H_2O) in the blood or interstitial fluid. Adapted from Berliner, R. W., Levinsky, N. G., Davidson, D. G., and Eden, M. *Am. J. Med.* 24:730, 1958.

plasma for every 1 ml of urine. In fact, this seemingly inefficient system for concentrating urine is prevented by the countercurrent flow of blood in the vasa recta.

The countercurrent exchange system in the vasa recta is illustrated in Figure 8-3. This system prevents undue concentration of plasma as it leaves the kidney, in the following manner:

1. Blood enters the vasa recta at a concentration of about 300 mOsm/kg H_2O.
2. As this blood flows through medullary interstitium of increasing osmolality, solute diffuses passively down its concentration gradient into the descending limb of the vasa recta, and water passively diffuses out of this limb in response to the osmotic gradient. This process results in increasing osmolality of plasma within the vasa recta as the bend is approached.
3. As the blood rises in the ascending limb of the vasa recta, it encounters less and less concentrated medullary interstitium.

Hence solutes passively diffuse into the interstitium and water diffuses back into the vasa recta.

As a result of this passive countercurrent exchange, blood leaves the kidneys not at 1,200 mOsm/kg H$_2$O (as it would if blood exited at the papilla) but at about 325 mOsm/kg H$_2$O. Thus, concentration of blood, and hence depletion of medullary solutes by the blood flow, is greatly minimized although not wholly prevented. Note that any blood flow would tend to deplete the medullary interstitium of solute unless countercurrent exchange were 100% efficient; but the lower the blood flow through this area, the less the depletion, and vice versa.

It might be asked why, if blood flow is such a threat to the renal concentrating mechanism, blood must course through the medulla and papilla at all. There are at least two reasons: (1) There must be nutrient blood flow to the medullary and papillary tissues. (2) The water that is reabsorbed from the descending limbs of Henle and the collecting ducts must be removed from the inner regions of the kidney by the vasa recta, lest these regions swell uncontrollably. This necessity is reflected in the finding that blood flow is approximately twice as great in the ascending vasa recta as in the descending vasa recta.

Experimental Evidence for the Countercurrent System

Table 8-1 lists some conditions that must be met if the countercurrent hypothesis is correct, and the experimental proof that the conditions are met.

Role of Urea in the Countercurrent System

The principles of the countercurrent mechanism can be understood by considering the transport merely of Na$^+$, Cl$^-$, and water, as we have done. Urea, however, plays an additional and important role.

Deposition of Urea in the Medullary Interstitium

The medullary interstitial osmolality is higher in antidiuresis than in water diuresis (Fig. 8-1). The difference is due largely to urea (see proof for item 4 in Table 8-1), which is deposited in the medullary interstitium by the following mechanisms. In conjunction with Figure 4-4, we presented the fact that more urea is reabsorbed from the collecting ducts at low urine flows, when hyperosmotic urine is formed, than at high flows. Urea deposition into the medullary interstitium is also aided by the process of medullary recycling of urea (Fig. 4-5), which delivers more urea to the collecting ducts than would be the case if recycling did not occur. Finally, urea reabsorption from collecting ducts is abetted at low urine flows (antidiuresis) by a differential effect of ADH on the urea and water permeabilities of the distal tubules

Table 8-1 : Experimental proof for the countercurrent mechanism.

Condition	Proof
1. The osmolality of the interstitium must increase as the renal papilla is approached; i.e., there must be a so-called corticopapillary osmotic gradient	Cryoscopy of renal tissue slices, and chemical analysis of tissue homogenates. The cryoscopic data constituted the first experimental support for the hypothesis; they were published by Wirz, Hargitay, and Kuhn in 1951
2. Osmolalities of the tubular fluid along the nephron are as follows:	
During formation of hyperosmotic urine:	
Isosmotic in Bowman's space	Micropuncture (Fig. 8-1A)
Isosmotic at end of proximal tubule	Micropuncture (Fig. 8-1A)
Hyperosmotic at bend of loop of Henle	Micropuncture (Fig. 8-1A)
Hyposmotic at beginning of distal tubule	Micropuncture (Fig. 8-1A)
Isosmotic at end of distal tubule	Micropuncture (Fig. 8-1A)
Hyperosmotic at end of collecting duct	Micropuncture (Fig. 8-1A)
During formation of hyposmotic urine:	
Same as above through beginning of distal tubule; however, note quantitative differences (point 4 in this table)	Micropuncture (Fig. 8-1B)
Hyposmotic at end of distal tubule	Micropuncture (Fig. 8-1B)
Hyposmotic at end of collecting duct	Micropuncture (Fig. 8-1B)
3. During antidiuresis, osmolalities at any given level perpendicular to the corticopapillary axis should be about equal	Micropuncture, and cryoscopy of renal tissue slices. At any given horizontal level, the osmolality is about the same in the loops of Henle, collecting ducts, interstitium, and vasa recta; the only exceptions are the ascending limbs of Henle and early distal tubules, where osmolalities are lower than in the interstitium. During water diuresis (formation of hyposmotic urine), fluid in distal tubules and collecting ducts is hyposmotic to plasma and to fluid in the other structures
4. If the major change in the system between forming hyperosmotic rather than hyposmotic urine is the water permeability of the late distal tubules and collecting ducts, the medullary and papillary interstitium should be hyperosmotic even during water diuresis	Micropuncture, cryoscopy of renal tissue slices, and chemical analysis of tissue homogenates. The condition is met, but the degree of interstitial hyperosmolality is much less in water diuresis than in antidiuresis. For example, in water diuresis the papillary interstitium has an osmolality of 500 to 600 mOsm/kg H_2O (Fig. 8-1B). Not all the reasons for the difference have been identified; they include decreased reabsorption of urea into the medullary and papillary interstitium (see below), and probably depletion of interstitial solutes (so-called washout) by increased blood flow through the medulla and papilla

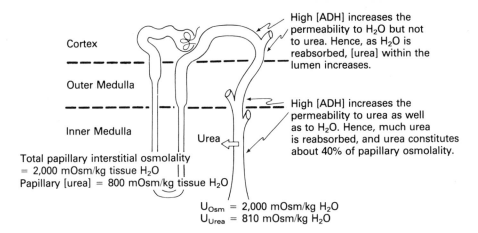

Cortex

Outer Medulla

Inner Medulla

Urea

High [ADH] increases the permeability to H$_2$O but not to urea. Hence, as H$_2$O is reabsorbed, [urea] within the lumen increases.

High [ADH] increases the permeability to urea as well as to H$_2$O. Hence, much urea is reabsorbed, and urea constitutes about 40% of papillary osmolality.

Total papillary interstitial osmolality = 2,000 mOsm/kg tissue H$_2$O

Papillary [urea] = 800 mOsm/kg tissue H$_2$O

U_{Osm} = 2,000 mOsm/kg H$_2$O
U_{Urea} = 810 mOsm/kg H$_2$O

Fig. 8-4 : Some of the major mechanisms whereby urea is deposited in the medullary interstitium, and hence aids the conservation of water. Brackets denote concentrations. The data were obtained in rats, and have been adapted from Valtin, H. *J. Clin. Invest.* 45:337, 1966.

and collecting ducts (Fig. 8-4). ADH increases the *water* permeability of the late distal tubule and the *entire* collecting duct (Table 7-1); however, it increases the *urea* permeability only of those portions of the collecting duct that pass through the inner medulla, the so-called inner medullary collecting ducts. Even in the presence of ADH, the distal tubule and cortical collecting duct have a very low permeability for urea. Consequently, as water is withdrawn from these structures during the formation of hyperosmotic urine, the urea, unable to diffuse out of the lumen as readily as water, is progressively concentrated. When the fluid reaches the medullary collecting ducts, the concentrated urea diffuses into the medullary and papillary interstitium until its concentration at any given level in the interstitium is equal to its concentration at the same level in the collecting ducts. As a result of these processes that promote its reabsorption, urea constitutes about 40% of the total medullary and papillary solute concentration during antidiuresis, whereas it contributes less than 10% to the interstitial osmolality during water diuresis.

Excretion of Urea with Minimal Water

It is of considerable interest, from an evolutionary point of view, that urea is the only endogenous solute that is handled by the kidneys in the above-described manner. As the major end product of protein catabolism in mammals, urea must be excreted by the kidneys largely unmetabolized, in order to preserve urea balance. Usually when a solute is excreted in the urine, it obligates the simultaneous excretion of water. This is so because the solute contributes to the osmolality of the tubular fluid and thereby decreases the osmotic gradient (which governs the passive reabsorption of water) between tubular lumen and interstitium. The classic example is osmotic diuresis, as induced by mannitol. Mannitol is a six-carbon sugar (i.e., a small, freely filterable solute) that, for practical purposes, is not reabsorbed by the tubules. When mannitol is given intravenously, and thence filtered, it raises the osmolality of tubular fluid and decreases the reabsorption of water, so that a diuresis ensues. In the case of urea, however, that portion of the osmolality within late collecting ducts that is due to urea is balanced by an equal concentration of urea in the interstitium surrounding the collecting ducts (Fig. 8-4). Hence, urea can be excreted in the urine without obligating the simultaneous excretion of large amounts of water. This fact was described in 1934 by J. L. Gamble and his associates as a feature that is unique to urea. They noticed that rats had a much lower rate of urinary flow if they excreted urea than if they had to excrete any other solute in equimolar amounts. Such "economy of water," as they called it, is of obvious advantage for organisms that must avidly conserve water in order to survive.

Note that the process that we have described is not one primarily suited to raising the osmolality of urine. Urine with a high content of urea does indeed have a higher osmolality than urine without urea (Fig. 8-4). But that higher osmolality is achieved not by greater abstraction of water from collecting ducts but by the fact that urea balances itself, so to speak, through equal concentration in the interstitium. As a matter of fact, greater abstraction of water also occurs when urea is the main solute in urine, but this effect contributes less to the higher osmolality than does the urea per se. The mechanisms by which more urea presented to the kidneys results in greater reabsorption of water from collecting ducts — noted by Gamble and his co-workers as an increase in the concentration of "non-urea solutes" in the urine — are not yet fully understood. It is possible that they involve the so-called *passive model* of countercurrent multiplication, which is described next.

Passive Model of Countercurrent Multiplication in Inner Medulla

Very similar theories to explain countercurrent multiplication through passive transport of solute were proposed independently and simultaneously in 1972 by J. L. Stephenson and by J. P. Kokko and F. C. Rector, Jr. Analogous suggestions had also been published some years earlier by others. The theories addressed an old problem, namely, how an interstitial osmotic gradient could be built up within the *inner medulla* — i.e., from the junction of outer and inner medulla to papilla (Fig. 8-1) — when there might be no active transport of solute in the thin limbs of Henle's loops (see Table 7-1). Phrased differently: As depicted in Figure 8-2, the "single effect" that is prerequisite to countercurrent multiplication begins with active reabsorption of NaCl from thick ascending limbs of Henle; but can there be a single effect when neither solute nor water is transported actively? The theories say "yes," through the intermediation of urea, as outlined in the next paragraph.

The essential features of the passive model are shown in Figure 8-5. The fact that only events in the inner medulla are depicted emphasizes that the passive model pertains only to that area of the kidney. (1) By the mechanisms discussed in connection with Figure 8-4, urea is deposited selectively in the inner medulla, thereby raising the interstitial concentration of urea (I_{Urea}). (2) The thin descending limb of Henle is relatively impermeable to urea, it has a high reflection coefficient (defined on p. 130) for urea, and it is highly permeable to water (Table 7-1). Hence, water is reabsorbed from the descending limb in response to an osmotic gradient set up by urea. (3) The thin descending limb also has a low permeability for NaCl. Therefore, as water, but not NaCl, is withdrawn from this limb, the concentration of NaCl

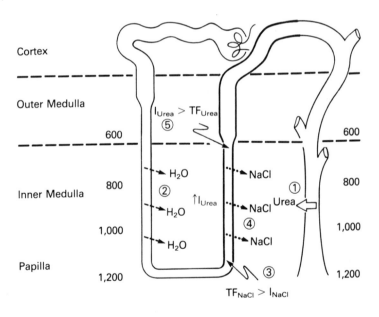

Fig. 8-5 : Schema for the passive model of countercurrent multiplication in the inner medulla, which assigns a critical role to urea. The encircled numbers refer to steps that are described in the text. The other numbers denote osmolalities within the interstitium. I_{Urea}, I_{NaCl} and TF_{Urea}, TF_{NaCl} = concentrations of these solutes in the interstitium and tubular fluid, respectively.

within the tubular fluid (TF_{NaCl}) increases to the point where it exceeds the concentration of NaCl in the interstitium (I_{NaCl}). (4) The last step supplies the potential energy that enables passive reabsorption of NaCl from the thin ascending limb of Henle. Since this limb is virtually impermeable to water (Table 7-1), the single effect of separating solute from water is now brought about through passive transport of solute. (5) Since tubular fluid leaving the inner medulla at the end of collecting ducts has a higher osmolality than that entering this area, osmotic work has been accomplished. This fact, coupled with the requirement for mass balance in the inner medulla, means that tubular fluid leaving this region at the end of the thin ascending limb must be hyposmotic to the interstitium. This requirement, which cannot be satisfied by passive reabsorption of NaCl alone (since it can diffuse only to equilibrium), is met by the concentration for urea in the interstitium (I_{Urea}) exceeding that in tubular fluid (TF_{Urea}). Point 5 thus emphasizes the fact that the passive model will work only if two solutes, NaCl and urea, are involved.

SOURCE OF ENERGY. Ultimately, all work requires energy. One must ask, therefore, where the energy comes from that makes it possible to accomplish osmotic work by the passive model. We can find the answer by retracing our steps: Creation of the single effect by passive reabsorption of NaCl is possible because the intratubular concentration of NaCl was raised through abstraction of water from the descending limb; this abstraction occurred because urea was selectively deposited in the inner medulla; and that deposition arose because water — but not urea — was reabsorbed from the late distal tubule and the cortical collecting duct; finally, that reabsorption of water took place because active transport of NaCl from the thick limb, distal tubule, and cortical collecting duct generated an osmotic gradient between these parts of the nephron and the surrounding interstitium. Thus, the source of energy is active transport of NaCl in the cortex and outer medulla, which is transferred by urea to the inner medulla, where it is "translated" into potential energy by generating a concentration difference for NaCl.

One criterion for the passive model that has been met is the requisite concentration difference for Na^+ and for Cl^- between tubular fluid at the beginning of the thin ascending limb and the interstitium (step 3 in Fig. 8-5). Another requirement — of strikingly different permeabilities for water, urea, Na^+, and Cl^- in the thin descending as opposed to the thin ascending limb — has been found by some investigators in some species but not by other investigators in other species (see Chap. 7, under Loops of Henle). Finally, it should be emphasized that countercurrent multiplication in the inner medulla need not be exclusively by the passive mode; it might well arise through some combination of both active and passive transport of NaCl.

Water Balance

There are two major mechanisms by which total body water is maintained at a normal level: (a) alteration in the rate of secretion of ADH and (b) regulation of thirst.

Secretion of ADH

OSMORECEPTORS. The classic experiments of E. B. Verney in the early 1940s elucidated the principal means by which the secretion of ADH from the posterior pituitary gland is regulated. These experiments are diagrammed in Figure 8-6A. Verney worked with trained, unanesthetized dogs in which he had exteriorized loops of both common carotid arteries, prior to carrying out the experiments. He observed that within 60 to 90 minutes after receiving a large oral load of tap water, these dogs excreted large amounts of hyposmotic urine. This water diuresis could be abruptly interrupted by infusing a bolus of hyperosmotic solution into the exteriorized carotid loop, but not if the posterior pituitary gland had been removed. If posterior pituitary extract was given to an hypophysectomized animal, the water diuresis was also interrupted.

On the basis of these results, Verney proposed the scheme outlined in Figure 8-6B. When an individual is deprived of water, continued obligatory excretion of water renders his plasma hyperosmotic. This change stimulates osmoreceptors that generate afferent signals calling for the secretion of ADH. The resulting high concentration of ADH in the blood then leads to antidiuresis, which is mediated mainly through increased water permeability of the late distal tubules and collecting ducts.

Conversely, when an individual drinks a large amount of dilute fluid, the plasma becomes hyposmotic. This, Verney proposed, sets off the opposite chain of events, leading to a decreased concentration of ADH in the blood, decreased water permeability of the late distal tubules and collecting ducts, and water diuresis.

Since prior removal of the pars nervosa abolished the response to hyperosmotic solutions, Verney surmised that ADH came from the posterior pituitary gland. This suspicion was supported by the antidiuretic response to posterior pituitary extract. The osmoreceptors have never been identified anatomically; they presumably lie within the distribution of the internal carotid artery.

As is shown in Figure 8-6A, modulations in ADH secretion, and hence in urine flow, occur very rapidly, within a few minutes. Thus, both the pituitary and the renal components of this system

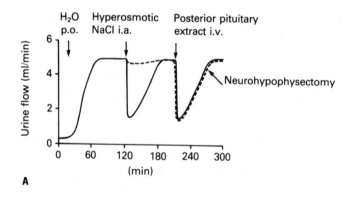

A

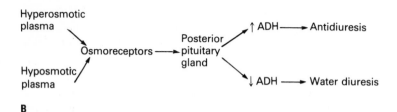

B

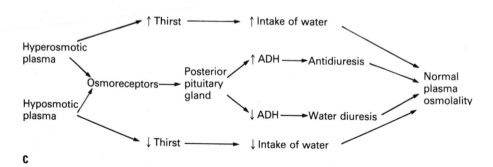

C

Fig. 8-6

A. Summary of some of the important results obtained on unanesthetized dogs by E. B. Verney. *Proc. Roy. Soc. London,* Series B. 135:25, 1947. Solid line graph represents results on a dog prior to removal of the neurohypophysis; the dashed line represents results on the same dog after neurohypophysectomy. p.o. = per os (by mouth); i.a. = intra-arterially (into the exteriorized loop of the common carotid artery); i.v. = intravenously.

B. Chain of events whereby changes in plasma osmolality regulate the secretion of antidiuretic hormone (ADH) and hence urine flow. Although many other factors can also affect ADH secretion — e.g., emotion, drugs, alcohol, baroreceptor activity, or extracellular fluid volume (see text, Volume Receptors) — the osmoreceptor system is probably the major mechanism for regulating water balance.

C. Interplay of thirst and of the osmoreceptor system for release of ADH, in the maintenance of water balance as reflected in a normal plasma osmolality.

compose a sensitive and precise mechanism for maintaining water balance.

VOLUME RECEPTORS. Although the osmoreceptor system (Fig. 8-6B) is the main regulator of ADH secretion, there are other factors that modulate this rate, e.g., drugs, alcohol, catecholamines, and the volume of certain compartments. As to the last, it can be shown, for example, that experimental expansion of the intrathoracic blood volume — as by immersing the lower part of the body in water — will lead to a water diuresis by inhibiting the secretion of ADH. Conversely, breathing against positive pressure — which forces blood out of the thorax — stimulates the secretion of ADH. Such experiments have given rise to the concept of volume receptors, which may be located in the low-pressure portions of the circulation, as in the left atria or in the pulmonary veins. It is likely that the volume of extracellular fluid regularly modulates the osmoreceptor response, so that for any given osmotic stimulus the secretion of ADH is less when extracellular fluid is expanded than when it is contracted.

Thirst

Even though ADH is highly effective in regulating water balance, it alone does not suffice to maintain balance. For example, even in the face of maximal renal conservation of water, an obligatory loss of water (both renal and extrarenal; see Table 1-4) continues. This persistent loss will lead to dehydration — even in the face of maximal ADH — unless the loss is replaced by acquisition of water. How thirst governs that acquisition, and how it is integrated with ADH, is shown in Figure 8-6C. Hyperosmotic plasma stimulates not only the release of ADH but also thirst; and together — the first by renal conservation of water, the second by increased intake of water — they normalize the osmolality of plasma. The opposite chain of events sets in when the plasma is hyposmotic. Like the mechanism for ADH, that for thirst is prompt, sensitive, and precise.

Free Water

Free water refers to water that is free of solutes. In the kidney, free water is produced or "generated" in the ascending limbs of Henle and early distal tubules, where relatively more Na^+ and Cl^- than water are reabsorbed (see Fig. 8-1). Whether or not free water is excreted in the urine depends on ADH and the water permeability of the late distal tubules and collecting ducts. If the concentration of ADH in blood is low, much of the free water that was generated in the ascending limbs will not be reabsorbed, and hyposmotic urine will be excreted. Relative to the isosmotic plasma that was filtered, more water than solute will have been excreted, and in this sense the net result will be that free water has been removed or cleared from the plasma. When the concentration of ADH is high, all the generated free water, and more, will be reabsorbed and hyperosmotic urine will be excreted. The excretion of hyperosmotic urine reflects a net process in which relatively more solute than water was removed from isosmotic plasma. In this sense, no free water will have been removed or cleared from the plasma; in fact, a negative quantity of free water will have been cleared.

FREE-WATER CLEARANCE. The view that the excretion of hyposmotic or hyperosmotic urine represents the clearance of a positive and negative quantity of free water, respectively, from isosmotic plasma, led to the expression "free-water clearance" (C_{H_2O}). This is unfortunate, for unlike all other renal clearances, C_{H_2O} is *not* equal to $U_{H_2O} \cdot \dot{V}/P_{H_2O}$. However, the term is so well established in renal physiology that any attempt to change it is likely to cause more confusion than enlightenment. Hence, the term will be used in this book, but with the admonition that *it is not a classic renal clearance.*

Free-water clearance may be defined as the amount of distilled water that must be subtracted from or added to the urine in order to render that urine isosmotic with plasma. The formula for calculating this amount of distilled water is as follows:

$$C_{H_2O} = \dot{V} - C_{Osm} \tag{8-1}$$

where C_{Osm} = the osmolal clearance, or $U_{Osm} \cdot \dot{V}/P_{Osm}$.

When a hyposmotic urine of 100 mOsm/kg H_2O is formed, the urine flow is 10 ml per minute, and plasma osmolality is 300 mOsm/kg H_2O, then

$$C_{H_2O} = \frac{10 \text{ ml}}{\text{min}} - \left(\frac{100 \text{ mOsm}}{1,000 \text{ ml}} \cdot \frac{10 \text{ ml}}{\text{min}} \cdot \frac{1,000 \text{ ml}}{300 \text{ mOsm}} \right)$$

$$C_{H_2O} = 6.7 \text{ ml/min}$$

When a hyperosmotic urine of 1,000 mOsm/kg H_2O is formed, and the urine flow is 0.5 ml per minute, then

$$C_{H_2O} = \frac{0.5 \text{ ml}}{\text{min}} - \left(\frac{1,000 \text{ mOsm}}{1,000 \text{ ml}} \cdot \frac{0.5 \text{ ml}}{\text{min}} \cdot \frac{1,000 \text{ ml}}{300 \text{ mOsm}} \right)$$

$$C_{H_2O} = -1.2 \text{ ml/min}$$

That is, when hyposmotic urine is formed, the free-water clearance has a positive value, and when hyperosmotic urine is formed, this clearance has a negative value. Obviously, when the urine is isosmotic with plasma, C_{H_2O} will be zero.

In order to circumvent the awkward expression *negative free-water clearance,* the term $T^c_{H_2O}$ was coined. This refers to the net transport of free water in a reabsorptive direction when hyperosmotic urine is formed; the superscript "c" signifies that this net reabsorption occurs in the collecting ducts (Fig. 8-1A). $T^c_{H_2O}$ is equal to $-(C_{H_2O})$.

Summary

Water balance is maintained mainly through the regulation of thirst and of the secretion of antidiuretic hormone (ADH). When a subject is deprived of drinking water, the plasma becomes hyperosmotic, and this change stimulates thirst and increases the secretion of ADH from the posterior pituitary gland (Fig. 8-6C). Both effects tend to raise the total water content of the body — thirst by raising the intake of water, and ADH by increasing the water permeability of the late distal tubules and collecting ducts, which promotes renal conservation of water. Conversely, when a subject imbibes a large amount of water, the consequent dilution of the plasma inhibits both thirst and the secretion of ADH; and these changes tend to decrease the total water content of the body by decreasing the acquisition and increasing the excretion of water, respectively.

Concentrated (or hyperosmotic) urine is formed through passive reabsorption of water by means of the countercurrent mechanism. Countercurrent multiplication of the single effect of reabsorbing Na^+ and Cl^-, virtually without water, from ascending limbs of Henle results in progressive hyperosmolality of the medullary interstitium, the so-called corticopapillary osmotic gradient. Dissipation of the gradient by the medullary blood flow is minimized by the countercurrent configuration of the vasa recta, which enables them to function as countercurrent exchangers. In the presence of high concentrations of ADH and resultant high water permeability, water is reabsorbed passively in response to the osmotic gradient between late distal tubules and collecting ducts and the surrounding interstitium, and hyperosmotic urine is formed.

During formation of dilute urine, the countercurrent mechanism continues to function qualitatively in the same manner. But now, in the absence of ADH, water reabsorption from distal tubules and collecting ducts is minimized despite the existence of osmotic gradients. Consequently, hyposmotic urine is excreted.

Urea, the main end product of protein catabolism in mammals, serves a unique role in water conservation by this class of vertebrates. By "balancing itself," so to speak, in the renal medullary interstitium, urea can be excreted at a lesser cost of water than can other urinary solutes. The presence of urea in the countercurrent system also indirectly enhances the concentration of nonurea solutes in urine, possibly by "passive" countercurrent multiplication in the inner medulla.

The excretion of solute-free water is gauged in relation to the isosmotic plasma that is filtered. When urine is hyposmotic to plasma, relatively more water than solute must have been removed or cleared from the filtered plasma. Hence, under these circumstances the free-water clearance — a misnomer — has a positive sign. When urine is hyperosmotic to plasma, relatively less water than solute must have been removed (or cleared) from the filtered plasma; therefore, under these conditions C_{H_2O} is negative. Finally, when the urine is isosmotic with plasma, equivalent amounts of solute and water were cleared from the filtered plasma, and C_{H_2O} is zero.

Problem 8-1 Renal handling of salt, water, and urea in varying diuretic states. The following data were obtained on a healthy medical student, under three conditions: (a) while drinking ad libitum; (b) after 12 hours of thirsting; and (c) within 90 minutes after drinking 1 liter of tap water. Fill in the blanks, and be sure to specify units. Neglect corrections for plasma water and for Donnan distribution.

	$\dot{V}$ (ml/min)	U_{In} (mg/ml)	P_{In} (mg/ml)	GFR ( )	U/P Inulin	Proportion of Filtered Water (i.e., of GFR) Reabsorbed (%)
While drinking ad libitum	1.2	15.8	0.151			
After 12 hours of thirsting	0.75	25.2	0.155			
Within 90 minutes after drinking 1 liter water	15.0	1.23	0.154			

Problem 8-1 continued on page 182.

Problem 8-1 (Continued)

	P_{Na} (mEq/L)	Filtered Load of Na ( )	U_{Na} (mEq/L)	Urinary Na Excretion ( )	Proportion of Filtered Na Reabsorbed (%)
While drinking ad libitum	136		128		
After 12 hours of thirsting	144		192		
Within 90 minutes after drinking 1 liter water	134		10.2		

Problem 8-1 continued on page 183.

Problem 8-1 (Continued)

	U_{Osm} (mOsm/kg)	P_{Osm} (mOsm/kg)	C_{H_2O} ( )	$T^c_{H_2O}$ ( )	U_{UreaN}[a] (mg/100 ml)	P_{UreaN}[a] (mg/100 ml)	C_{Urea} ( )	Proportion of Filtered Urea Reabsorbed ( ) (%)
While drinking ad libitum	663	290			480	12		
After 12 hours of thirsting	1,000	300			720	15		
Within 90 minutes after drinking 1 liter water	100	287			48	10		

[a]Concentrations of urea are usually determined by measuring the amount of nitrogen in urea; hence, the expression *urea nitrogen*. The two nitrogen atoms constitute 28/60 of the urea molecule: $CO(NH_2)_2$. The clearance of urea (C_{Urea}) can be calculated without converting "Urea N" to "Urea," since the conversion factors for U_{UreaN} and P_{UreaN} cancel out.

Problem 8-2

Normally, in adult man, about 125 ml of plasma H_2O is filtered into Bowman's space each minute. Of this, about 124 ml per minute is reabsorbed. (a) In which parts of the nephron is the H_2O reabsorbed, and (b) what happens to the H_2O once it has been reabsorbed?

(c) In the same person, 660 ml of plasma enters the kidneys at an osmolality of 290 mOsm/kg H_2O, and 1 ml of urine leaves the kidneys at an osmolality of 700 mOsm/kg H_2O. What, then, is the osmolality of plasma that leaves the kidneys via the renal veins?

Appendix

The Cellular Action of ADH

Much has been learned in recent years about the means whereby ADH increases the water permeability of specialized epithelial membranes. The system is illustrated in Figure 8-7A for cells of the mammalian late distal tubule and collecting duct. ADH is a nonapeptide, which binds onto specific receptors located in the peritubular membrane. The interaction with the receptor stimulates the activation of an enzyme, adenylate cyclase, that catalyzes the formation of cyclic 3',5'-adenosine monophosphate (cyclic AMP) from adenosine triphosphate (ATP). Cyclic AMP serves as the intracellular mediator or messenger for ADH, and its concentration within the cell is controlled not only by its rate of formation from ATP but also by its rate of breakdown to adenosine 5'-monophosphate (5'-AMP) under the influence of the enzyme cyclic-AMP phosphodiesterase. Once formed, cyclic AMP induces changes in the luminal cell membrane that increase its permeability to water. These changes come about by a series of steps that are just being defined; they probably include the phosphorylation of specific membrane proteins under the influence of an enzyme, protein kinase, and somehow involve the function of microtubules and microfilaments.

It is not yet known just what the molecular changes are within the luminal membrane that alter its permeability to water. It appears likely that the changes involve fusion of the luminal membrane with cytoplasmic vesicles that are lined by membrane and that contain specialized proteins. The proteins are thought to be represented by clusters of intramembranous particles that can be visualized by the special technique of freeze-fracture electron microscopy (Fig. 8-7C), and that are probably the sites of increased water flow.

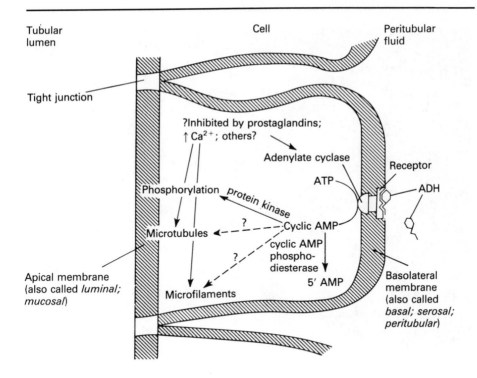

A

Fig. 8-7

A. Chain of events whereby antidiuretic hormone (ADH) is thought to increase
the permeability to water of cellular membranes in the late distal tubule and
collecting duct. Much of the schema is based on experiments that were conducted on other membranes that are also sensitive to ADH, most notably the
skin and urinary bladder of frogs and toads. Note that the receptors for ADH lie
in the serosal membrane, whereas the increased permeability is induced in the
mucosal membrane. The dashed arrows with question marks indicate that the
roles of microtubules and microfilaments in the action of ADH have not yet
been defined. Adapted from Dousa, T. P., and Valtin, H. *Kidney Int.* 10:46, 1976,
and reproduced from H. Valtin, *Renal Dysfunction: Mechanisms Involved in Fluid and
Solute Imbalance.* Boston: Little, Brown, 1979.

B, C. Freeze-fracture electron micrographs, showing surfaces within the frac-
ture of the luminal membrane from collecting ducts of a Brattleboro rat that
lacks ADH (B) and a Brattleboro rat that was treated with ADH (C). The arrows
point to some clusters of intramembranous particles that are thought to have
been incorporated in the membrane through fusion with cytoplasmic vesicles.
The clusters are probably the sites of increased water flow; note that there are
no clusters in (B), when ADH was absent. (The encircled arrowheads indicate
the shadowing direction.) From Harmanci, M. C., et al. *Am. J. Physiol.* 235 (Renal
Fluid Electrolyte Physiol. 4):F440, 1978. Analogous changes in response to ADH
have been demonstrated in anuran membranes (e.g., Chevalier, J., et al. *Cell Tissue Res.* 152:129, 1974; Kachadorian, W. A., et al. *Science* 190:67, 1975).

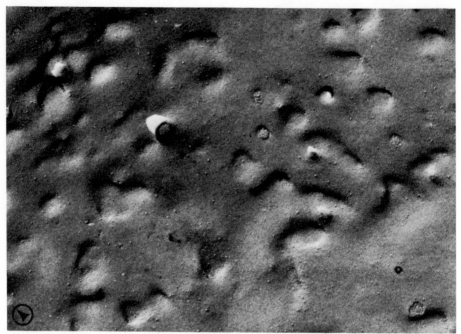

B

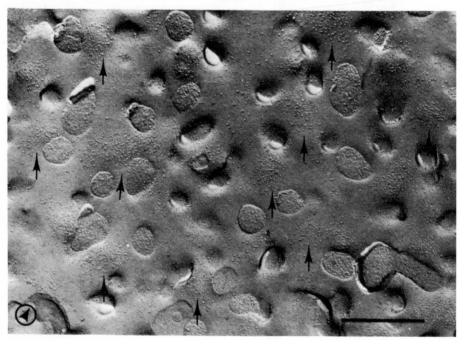

C

Selected References

General

Adolph, E. F., et al. *Physiology of Man in the Desert.* New York: Interscience, 1947.

Andersson, B. Regulation of water intake. *Physiol. Rev.* 58:582, 1978.

Andreoli, T. E., Grantham, J. J., and Rector, F. C., Jr. (Eds.). *Disturbances in Body Fluid Osmolality.* Bethesda: American Physiological Society, 1977.

Atherton, J. C., Hai, M.A., and Thomas, S. The time course of changes in renal tissue composition during water diuresis in the rat. *J. Physiol.* (Lond.) 197:429, 1968.

de Rouffignac, C., and Imbert, M. Données récentes sur les mécanismes de concentration et de dilution de l'urine. *J. Physiol.* (Paris) 71:181A, 1975.

Gamble, J. L. Physiological information gained from studies on the life raft ration. *Harvey Lect.* 42:247, 1947.

Gottschalk, C. W. Micropuncture studies of tubular function in the mammalian kidney. *Physiologist* 4:35, 1961.

Gottschalk, C. W., and Lassiter, W. E. Transport of Water: Renal Concentrating Mechanism. In G. Giebisch (Ed.), *Transport Organs,* vol. IVA. New York: Springer-Verlag, 1979.

Gottschalk, C. W., Lassiter, W. E., Mylle, M., Ullrich, K. J., Schmidt-Nielsen, B., O'Dell, R., and Pehling, G. Micropuncture study of composition of loop of Henle fluid in desert rodents. *Am. J. Physiol.* 204:532, 1963.

Gottschalk, C. W., and Mylle, M. Micropuncture study of the mammalian urinary concentrating mechanism: Evidence for the countercurrent hypothesis. *Am. J. Physiol.* 196:927, 1959.

Hays, R. M., and Levine, S. D. Pathophysiology of Water Metabolism. In B. M. Brenner and F. C. Rector, Jr. (Eds.), *The Kidney* (2nd ed.). Philadelphia: Saunders, 1981.

Jamison, R. L. Urine Concentration and Dilution. The Roles of Antidiuretic Hormone and Urea. In B. M. Brenner and F. C. Rector, Jr. (Eds.), *The Kidney* (2nd ed.). Philadelphia: Saunders, 1981.
A thorough and authoritative summary that contains, among other useful information, a table listing the permeability characteristics of the various parts of the nephron.

Jamison, R. L., and Kriz, W. *Urinary Concentrating Mechanisms. Structure and Function.* New York: Oxford University Press, 1982.

Jørgensen, C. B., and Skadhauge, E. (Eds.). *Osmotic and Volume Regulation.* Copenhagen: Munksgaard, 1978.

Knepper, M. A., Danielson, R. A., Saidel, G. M., and Post, R. S. Quantitative analysis of renal medullary anatomy in rats and rabbits. *Kidney Int.* 12:313, 1977.

Kuhn, W., and Ryffel, K. Herstellung konzentrierter Lösungen aus verdünnten durch blosse Membranwirkung. Ein Modellversuch zur Funktion der Niere. *Z. Physiol. Chem.* 276:145, 1942.

MacMillen, R. E., and Lee, A. K. Water metabolism of Australian hopping mice. *Comp. Biochem. Physiol.* 28:493, 1969.

Newburgh, J. D. The changes which alter renal osmotic work. *J. Clin. Invest.* 22:439, 1943.

Schmidt-Nielsen, K. *Desert Animals: Physiological Problems of Heat and Water.* London: Oxford University Press, 1964.
This book is now available in paperback form from Dover Publications, New York, 1979.

Schrier, R. W. (Ed.). Symposium on water metabolism. *Kidney Int.* 10:1, 1976.

Strauss, M. B. *Body Water in Man.* Boston: Little, Brown, 1957.

Ullrich, K. J., Kramer, K., and Boylan, J. W. Present knowledge of the countercurrent system in the mammalian kidney. *Prog. Cardiovasc. Dis.* 3:395, 1961.

Wolf, A. V. *Thirst: Physiology of the Urge to Drink and Problems of Water Lack.* Springfield, Ill.: Thomas, 1958.
Part II of this book contains several fascinating accounts of extreme acquisition and deprivation of water.

Countercurrent Multipliers and Exchangers

Berliner, R. W. The concentrating mechanism in the renal medulla. *Kidney Int.* 9:214, 1976.

Black, D. A. K. Renal rete mirabile. *Lancet* 2:1141, 1965.

de Rouffignac, C., and Morel, F. Micropuncture study of water, electrolytes, and urea movements along the loops of Henle in *Psammomys. J. Clin. Invest.* 48:474, 1969.

Jamison, R. L. Micropuncture study of segments of thin loop of Henle in the rat. *Am. J. Physiol.* 215:236, 1968.

Jamison, R. L. Micropuncture study of superficial and juxtamedullary nephrons in the rat. *Am. J. Physiol.* 218:46, 1970.

Kokko, J. P. Sodium chloride and water transport in the descending limb of Henle. *J. Clin. Invest.* 49:1838, 1970.

Kuhn, W., Ramel, A., Kuhn, H. J., and Marti, E. The filling mechanism of the swimbladder: Generation of high gas pressures through hairpin countercurrent multiplication. *Experientia* 19:497, 1963.

Marsh, D. J. Osmotic Concentration and Dilution of the Urine. In C. Rouiller and A. F. Muller (Eds.), *The Kidney,* vol. III. New York: Academic, 1971.

Marshall, E. K., Jr. The comparative physiology of the kidney in relation to theories of renal secretion. *Physiol. Rev.* 14:133, 1934.

Moore, L. C., Marsh, D. J., and Martin, C. M. Loop of Henle during the water-to-antidiuresis transition in Brattleboro rats. *Am. J. Physiol.* 239 (Renal Fluid Electrolyte Physiol. 8):F72, 1980.

Peter, K. *Untersuchungen über Bau und Entwickelung der Niere.* Jena: Fischer, 1909.

Scholander, P. F. Secretion of gases against high pressures in the swimbladder of deep sea fishes: II. The rete mirabile. *Biol. Bull.* 107:260, 1954.

Scholander, P. F. The wonderful net. *Sci. Am.* 196:96, 1957.

Schwartz, M. M., and Venkatachalam, M. A. Structural differences in thin limbs of Henle: Physiological implications. *Kidney Int.* 6:193, 1974.

Sperber, I. Studies on the mammalian kidney. *Zool. Bid. Uppsala* 22:249, 1944.

Stephenson, J. L. Countercurrent transport in the kidney. *Annu. Rev. Biophys. Bioeng.* 7:315, 1978.

Ullrich, K. J. Permeability Characteristics of the Mammaliam Nephron. In J. Orloff and R. W. Berliner (Eds.), *Handbook of Physiology,* section 8, Renal Physiology. Washington, D.C.: American Physiological Society, 1973.

Valtin, H. Structural and functional heterogeneity of mammalian nephrons. *Am. J. Physiol.* 233 (Renal Fluid Electrolyte Physiol. 2):F491, 1977.

Wirz, H. The Location of Antidiuretic Action in the Mammalian Kidney. In H. Heller (Ed.), *The Neurohypophysis.* London: Butterworth, 1957.

Wirz, H., Hargitay, B., and Kuhn, W. Lokalisation des Konzentrierungsprozesses in der Niere durch direkte Kryoskopie. *Helv. Physiol. Pharmacol. Acta* 9:196, 1951.

Role of Urea.
Passive Model

Andreoli, T. E., Berliner, R. W., Kokko, J. P., and Marsh, D. J. Questions and replies: Renal mechanisms for urinary concentrating and diluting processes. *Am. J. Physiol.* 235 (Renal Fluid Electrolyte Physiol. 4):F1, 1978.

Bonventre, J. V., Karnovsky, M. J., and Lechene, C. P. Renal papillary epithelial morphology in antidiuresis and water diuresis. *Am. J. Physiol.* 235 (Renal Fluid Electrolyte Physiol. 4):F69, 1978.

Bonventre, J. V., and Lechene, C. Renal medullary concentrating process: An integrative hypothesis. *Am. J. Physiol.* 239 (Renal Fluid Electrolyte Physiol. 8):F578, 1980.

Bonventre, J. V., Roman, R. J., and Lechene, C. Effect of urea concentration of pelvic fluid on renal concentrating ability. *Am. J. Physiol.* 239 (Renal Fluid Electrolyte Physiol. 8):F609, 1980.

Bray, G. W., and Preston, A. S. Effect of urea on urine concentration in the rat. *J. Clin. Invest.* 40:1952, 1961.

Burg, M. B., and Stephenson, J. L. Transport Characteristics of the Loop of Henle. In T. E. Andreoli, J. F. Hoffman, and D. D. Fanestil (Eds.), *Physiology of Membrane Disorders.* New York: Plenum, 1978. P. 661.

Crawford, J. D., Doyle, A. P., and Probst, J. H. Service of urea in renal water conservation. *Am. J. Physiol.* 196:545, 1959.

Gamble, J. L., McKhann, C. F., Butler, A. M., and Tuthill, E. An economy of water in renal function referable to urea. *Am. J. Physiol.* 109:139, 1934.

Gelbart, D. R., Battilana, C. A., Bhattacharya, J., Lacy, F. B., and Jamison, R. L. Transepithelial gradient and fractional delivery of chloride in thin loop of Henle. *Am. J. Physiol.* 235 (Renal Fluid Electrolyte Physiol. 4):F192, 1978.

Gunther, R. A., and Rabinowitz, L. Urea and renal concentrating ability in the rabbit. *Kidney Int.* 17:205, 1980.

Jamison, R. L., and Robertson, C. R. Recent formulations of the urinary concentrating mechanism: A status report. *Kidney Int.* 16:537, 1979.

Johnston, P. A., Battilana, C. A., Lacy, F. B., and Jamison, R. L. Evidence for a concentration gradient favoring outward movement of sodium from the thin loop of Henle. *J. Clin. Invest.* 59:234, 1977.

Kokko, J., and Rector, F. C., Jr. Countercurrent multiplication system without active transport in inner medulla. *Kidney Int.* 2:214, 1972.

Moore, L. C., and Marsh, D. J. How descending limb of Henle's loop permeability affects hypertonic urine formation. *Am. J. Physiol.* 239 (Renal Fluid Electrolyte Physiol. 8):F57, 1980.

Morgan, T., and Berliner, R. W. Permeability of the loop of Henle, vasa recta, and collecting duct to water, urea, and sodium. *Am. J. Physiol.* 215:108, 1968.

Schmidt-Nielsen, B. (Ed.). *Urea and the Kidney.* Amsterdam: Excerpta Medica, 1970.

Schmidt-Nielsen, B. Excretion in mammals: Role of the renal pelvis in the modification of the urinary concentration and composition. *Fed. Proc.* 36:2493, 1977.

Schmidt-Nielsen, B., and O'Dell, R. Structure and concentration mechanism in mammalian kidney. *Am. J. Physiol.* 200:1119, 1961.

Schütz, W., and Schnermann, J. Pelvic urine composition as a determinant of inner medullary solute concentration and urine osmolality. *Pflügers Arch. Ges. Physiol.* 334:154, 1972.

Stephenson, J. L. Concentration of urine in a central core model of the renal counterflow system. *Kidney Int.* 2:85, 1972.

Stephenson, J. L. Countercurrent transport in the kidney. *Annu. Rev. Biophys. Bioeng.* 7:315, 1978.

Stewart, J. Urea handling by the renal countercurrent system: Insights from computer simulation. *Pflügers Arch. Eur. J. Physiol.* 356:133, 1975.

Stewart, J., and Valtin, H. Computer simulation of osmotic gradient without active transport in renal inner medulla. *Kidney Int.* 2:264, 1972.

Stoner, L. C., and Roch-Ramel, F. The effects of pressure on the water permeability of the descending limb of Henle's loops of rabbits. *Pflügers Arch. Eur. J. Physiol.* 382:7, 1979.

Ullrich, K. J., Drenckhahn, F. O., and Jarausch, K. H. Untersuchungen zum Problem der Harnkonzentrierung und -verdünnung. Über das osmotische Verhalten von Nierenzellen und die begleitende Elektrolytanhäufung im Nierengewebe bei verschiedenen Diuresezuständen. *Pflügers Arch. Ges. Physiol.* 261:62, 1955.

Ullrich, K. J., and Jarausch, K. H. Untersuchungen zum Problem der Harkonzentrierung und Harnverdünnung. Über die Verteilung von Elektrolyten (Na, K, Ca, Mg, Cl, anorganischem Phosphat), Harnstoff, Aminosäuren und exogenem Kreatinin in Rinde und Mark der Hundeniere bei verschiedenen Diuresezuständen. *Pflügers Arch. Ges. Physiol.* 262:537, 1956.

Vogel, H. G., and Ullrich, K. J. (Eds.). *New Aspects of Renal Function.* Amsterdam: Excerpta Medica, 1978.
The special lecture in this symposium, as well as section IV, pertains to questions about the urinary concentrating process that remain largely unanswered.

Antidiuretic Hormone (ADH), Other Hormones, and Thirst

Bentley, P. J. *Endocrines and Osmoregulation.* New York: Springer-Verlag, 1971.

Berde, B. (Ed.). Neurohypophysial Hormones and Similar Polypeptides. In *Handbook of Experimental Pharmacology,* vol. XXIII. Berlin: Springer-Verlag, 1968.
A series of authoritative articles, with numerous, useful references. Topics covered include anatomy, chemistry, assays, physiology, pharmacology, and others.

Bie, P. Osmoreceptors, vasopressin, and control of renal water excretion. *Physiol. Rev.* 60:961, 1980.

Bisordi, J. E., Schlondorff, D., and Hays, R. M. Interaction of vasopressin and prostaglandins in the toad urinary bladder. *J. Clin. Invest.* 66:1200, 1980.

Blaschko, H. K. F., Gregory, R. A., Harris, G. W., and Kenner, G. W. (Organizers). Posterior pituitary hormones and neurophysiology: A discussion on polypeptide hormones. *Proc. R. Soc. Lond.* [Biol.] 170:3, 1968.

Brenner, B. M., and Stein, J. H. (Eds.). Hormonal Function and the Kidney. *Contemporary Issues in Nephrology,* vol. 4. New York: Churchill Livingstone, 1979.

Buggy, J., Hoffman, W. E., Phillips, M. I., Fisher, A. E., and Johnson, A. K. Osmosensitivity of rat third ventricle and interactions with angiotensin. *Am. J. Physiol.* 236 (Regulatory Integrative Comp. Physiol. 5):R75, 1979.

Carvounis, C. P., Carvounis, G., and Arbeit, L. A. Role of the endogenous kallikrein-kinin system in modulating vasopressin-stimulated water flow and urea permeability in the toad urinary bladder. *J. Clin. Invest.* 67:1792, 1981.

Charbardès, D., Gagnan-Brunette, M., Imbert-Teboul, M., Gontcharevskaia, O., Montégut, M., Clique, A., and Morel, F. Adenylate cyclase responsiveness to hormones in various portions of the human nephron. *J. Clin. Invest.* 65:439, 1980.

Dousa, T. P., and Valtin, H. Cellular actions of vasopressin in the mammalian kidney. *Kidney Int.* 10:46, 1976.

Dunn, F. L., Brennan, T. J., Nelson, A. E., and Robertson, G. L. The role of blood osmolality and volume in regulating vasopressin secretion in the rat. *J. Clin. Invest.* 52:3212, 1973.

Dunn, M. J. Renal Prostaglandins: Influences on Excretion of Sodium and Water, the Renin-Angiotensin System, Renal Blood Flow, and Hypertension. In B. M. Brenner and J. H. Stein (Eds.), Hormonal Function and the Kidney. *Contemporary Issues in Nephrology,* vol. 4. New York: Churchill Livingstone, 1979.

du Vigneaud, V. Hormones of the posterior pituitary gland: Oxytocin and vasopressin. *Harvey Lect.* 50:1, 1956.

Editorial. Prostaglandins in the kidney. *Lancet* 2:343, 1981.

Epstein, A. N., Kissileff, H. R., and Stellar, E. (Eds.). *The Neuropsychology of Thirst: New Findings and Advances in Concepts.* Washington, D.C.: Winston, 1973.

Epstein, M. Renal effects of head-out water immersion in man: Implications for an understanding of volume homeostasis. *Physiol. Rev.* 58:529, 1978.

Fitzsimons, J. T. Thirst. *Physiol. Rev.* 52:468, 1972.

Fitzsimons, J. T. *The Physiology of Thirst and Sodium Appetite.* Cambridge: Cambridge University Press, 1979.

Gauer, O. H., and Henry, J. P. Neurohormonal control of plasma volume. *Int. Rev. Physiol.* 9:145, 1976.

Gillespie, D. J., Sandberg, R. L., and Koike, T. I. Dual effect of left atrial receptors on excretion of sodium and water in the dog. *Am. J. Physiol.* 225:706, 1973.

Grantham, J. J. Action of antidiuretic hormone in the mammalian kidney. *Int. Rev. Physiol.* 6:247, 1974.

Grantham, J. J., and Orloff, J. Effect of prostaglandin E_1 on the permeability response of the isolated collecting tubule to vasopressin, adenosine 3',5'-monophosphate, and theophylline. *J. Clin. Invest.* 47:1154, 1968.

Grossman, A., Besser, G. M., Milles, J. J., and Baylis, P. H. Inhibition of vasopressin release in man by an opiate peptide. *Lancet* 2:1108, 1980.

Hall, D. A., and Varney, D. M. Effect of vasopressin on electrical potential difference and chloride transport in mouse medullary thick ascending limb of Henle's loop. *J. Clin. Invest.* 66:792, 1980.

Handler, J. S., and Orloff, J. The Mechanism of Action of Antidiuretic Hormone. In J. Orloff and R. W. Berliner (Eds.), *Handbook of Physiology,* section 8, Renal Physiology. Washington, D.C.: American Physiological Society, 1973.

Handler, J. S., and Orloff, J. Antidiuretic hormone. *Annu. Rev. Physiol.* 43:611, 1981.

Harmanci, M. D., Stern, P., Kachadorian, W. A., Valtin, H., and DiScala, V. A. Vasopressin and collecting duct intramembranous particle clusters: A dose-response relationship. *Am. J. Physiol.* 239 (Renal Fluid Electrolyte Physiol. 8):F560, 1981.

Hays, R. M. Antidiuretic hormone and water transfer. *Kidney Int.* 9:223, 1976.

Imbert-Teboul, M., Chabardès, D., Montégut, M., Clique, A., and Morel, F. Vasopressin-dependent adenylate cyclase activities in the rat kidney medulla: Evidence for two separate sites of action. *Endocrinology* 102:1254, 1978.

Imbert-Teboul, M., Chabardès, D., Montégut, M., Clique, A., and Morel, F. Impaired response to vasopressin of adenylate cyclase of the thick ascending limb of Henle's loop in Brattleboro rats with diabetes insipidus. *Renal Physiol.* 1:3, 1978.

Jackson, B. A., Edwards, R. M., Valtin, H., and Dousa, T. P. Cellular action of vasopressin in medullary tubules of mice with hereditary nephrogenic diabetes insipidus. *J. Clin. Invest.* 66:110, 1980.

Jard, S., Roy, C., Rajerison, R., Butlen, D., and Guillon, G. Comparative Studies with the ADH Receptors from Pig and Rat Kidney: Structure Activity Relationships and Receptor-Adenylate Cyclase Coupling. In M. Bergeron et al. (Eds.), *Prodeedings VII International Congress of Nephrology.* Basel: Karger, 1978.

Jewell, P. A., and Verney, E. B. An experimental attempt to determine the site of neurohypophysial osmoreceptors in the dog. *Philos. Trans. R. Soc. Lond.* Series B. [Biol.] 240:197, 1956–57.

Knobil, E., and Sawyer, W. H. (Eds.). The Pituitary Gland and Its Neuroendocrine Control, part 1. In *Handbook of Physiology,* vol. 4, section 7. Washington, D.C.: American Physiological Society, 1974.

Levine, S. D., Kachadorian, W. A., Levin, D. N., and Schlondorff, D. Effects of trifluoperazine on function and structure of toad urinary bladder. Role of calmodulin in vasopressin-stimulation of water permeability. *J. Clin. Invest.* 67:662, 1981.

Mogenson, G. J. Hypothalamic and Other Neural Mechanisms for the Control of Food and Water Intakes. In W. L. Veale and K. Lederis (Eds.), *Current Studies of Hypothalamic Function 1978,* vol. 2, *Metabolism and Behaviour.* Basel: Karger, 1978.

Morel, F., Chabardès, D., and Imbert-Teboul, M. Segmental Heterogeneity of the Nephron. In L. Takács (Ed.), *Proceedings of the XXVIII International Congress of Physiological Sciences.* Budapest: Akadémiai Kiadó, 1981.

North, W. G., LaRochelle, F. T., Jr., Morris, J. F., Sokol, H. W., and Valtin, H. Biosynthetic Specificity of Neurons Producing Neurohypophysial Principles. In K. Lederis and W. L. Veale (Eds.), *Current Studies of Hypothalamic Function 1978,* vol. 1, *Hormones.* Basel: Karger, 1978.

Orloff, J., Handler, J. S., and Bergstrom, S. Effect of prostaglandin (PGE_1) on the permeability response of toad bladder to vasopressin, theophylline and adenosine 3',5'-monophosphate. *Nature* 205:397, 1965.

Orloff, J., and Zusman, R. Role of prostaglandin E (PGE) in the modulation of the action of vasopressin on water flow in the urinary bladder of the toad and mammalian kidney. *J. Membr. Biol.* 40:297, 1978.

Peck, J. W., and Blass, E. M. Localization of thirst and antidiuretic osmoreceptors by intracranial injections in rats. *Am. J. Physiol.* 228:1501, 1975.

Robertson, G. L. The regulation of vasopressin function in health and disease. *Recent Prog. Horm. Res.* 33:333, 1977.

Robertson, G. L., and Athar, S. The interaction of blood osmolality and blood volume in regulating plasma vasopressin in man. *J. Clin. Endocrinol. Metab.* 42:613, 1976.

Rudinger, J. (Ed.). *Oxytocin, Vasopressin and Their Structural Analogues.* New York: Macmillan, 1964.

Sasaki, S., and Imai, M. Effects of vasopressin on water and NaCl transport across the in vitro perfused medullary thick ascending limb of Henle's loop of mouse, rat, and rabbit kidneys. *Pflügers Arch. Eur. J. Physiol.* 383:215, 1980.

Schafer, J. A., and Andreoli, T. E. Cellular constraints to diffusion. The effect of antidiuretic hormone on water flows in isolated mammalian collecting tubules. *J. Clin. Invest.* 51:1264, 1972.

Schnermann, J., Valtin, H., Thurau, K., Nagel, W., Horster, M., Fischbach, H., Wahl, M., and Liebau, G. Micropuncture studies on the influence of antidiuretic hormone on tubular fluid reabsorption in rats with hereditary hypothalamic diabetes insipidus. *Pflügers Arch. Ges. Physiol.* 306:103, 1969.

Schrier, R. W., Berl, T., and Anderson, R. J. Osmotic and nonosmotic control of vasopressin release. *Am. J. Physiol.* 236 (Renal Fluid Electrolyte Physiol. 5):F321, 1979.

Schwartz, I. L., and Schwartz, W. B. (Eds.). Symposium on antidiuretic hormones. *Am. J. Med.* 42:651, 1967.

Share, L., and Claybaugh, J. R. Regulation of body fluids. *Annu. Rev. Physiol.* 34:235, 1972.

Sieker, H. O., Gauer, O. H., and Henry, J. P. The effect of continuous negative pressure breathing on water and electrolyte excretion by the human kidney. *J. Clin. Invest.* 33:572, 1954.

Starling, E. H., and Verney, E. B. The secretion of urine as studied on the isolated kidney. *Proc. R. Soc. Lond.* Series B. [Biol.] 97:321, 1925.

Stokes, J. B. Integrated actions of renal medullary prostaglandins in the control of water excretion. *Am. J. Physiol.* 240 (Renal Fluid Electrolyte Physiol. 9):F471, 1981.

Valtin, H. Sequestration of urea and nonurea solutes in renal tissues of rats with hereditary hypothalamic diabetes insipidus: Effects of vasopressin and dehydration on the countercurrent mechanism. *J. Clin. Invest.* 45:337, 1966.

Verney, E. B. The antidiuretic hormone and the factors which determine its release. *Proc. R. Soc. Lond.* [Biol.] 135:25, 1947.

Wade, J. B., Kachadorian, W. A., and DiScala, V. A. Freeze-fracture electron microscopy: Relationship of membrane structural features to transport physiology. *Am. J. Physiol.* 232 (Renal Fluid Electrolyte Physiol. 1):F77, 1977.

Woodhall, P. B., and Tisher, C. C. Response of the distal tubule and cortical collecting duct to vasopressin in the rat. *J. Clin. Invest.* 52:3095, 1973.

9 : H^+ Balance

The Problem of Mammalian H^+ Balance

The pH of the blood of a normal person is alkaline, and it is maintained within the small range of about 7.37 to 7.42. A narrow range of pH is essential to normal metabolic function, probably because the activities of protein macromolecules such as enzymes, and elements required for blood clotting and muscle contraction, depend on an optimal pH. The extreme range of plasma pH that is compatible with life is approximately 6.8 to 8.0.

Despite the essential alkalinity, the mammalian body normally produces large amounts of acid, from two major sources. (1) Some 13,000 to 20,000 mMoles of CO_2 is produced daily as the result of oxidative metabolism; when processed, this CO_2 yields H^+ according to either or both of the following reactions:

$$CO_2 + H_2O \rightleftharpoons H_2CO_3 \rightleftharpoons H^+ + HCO_3^- \qquad (9\text{-}1)$$

and/or

$$\begin{array}{l} \quad\;\; HOH \rightleftharpoons H^+ \\ \quad\;\;\;\; \upharpoonleft\downharpoonright \\ CO_2 + OH^- \overset{C.A.}{\rightleftharpoons} HCO_3^- \end{array} \qquad (9\text{-}2)$$

Note that the final products are H^+ and HCO_3^-, whether the hydration of CO_2 is involved (Eq. 9-1) or the splitting of H_2O and subsequent hydroxylation of CO_2 (Eq. 9-2). There is evidence that carbonic anhydrase (C.A.) catalyzes reaction 9-2 but not 9-1. Because with either reaction the processing of CO_2 yields H^+, CO_2 is often referred to as a *volatile acid.* (2) In most western countries, where meat constitutes a large part of the diet, there is also a net daily production of some 40 to 60 mMoles of inorganic and organic acids that are not derived from CO_2. Sulfuric acid is produced from protein catabolism through the conversion of sulfur in the amino acid residues, cysteine, cystine, and methionine, as exemplified by the following reaction for methionine:

$$\underset{\text{methionine}}{2\, C_5H_{11}NO_2S} + 15\, O_2 \rightarrow 4\, H^+ + 2\, SO_4^{2-} + \underset{\text{urea}}{CO(NH_2)_2} + 7\, H_2O + 9\, CO_2 \qquad (9\text{-}3)$$

Formation of phosphoric acid during the catabolism of phospholipids makes a minor contribution. Because these acids, unlike CO_2, are not volatile or in equilibrium with a volatile component, they are known as *nonvolatile,* or *fixed,* acids. (When the diet consists mainly of vegetables and fruits, the net production of nonvolatile constituents consists of alkalis.)

In certain physiological and pathological states, the production of nonvolatile acids may rise as much as tenfold. Examples include the production of lactic acid during muscular exercise and states of hypoxia, and the production of aceto-acetic acid and β-hydroxybutyric acid during uncontrolled diabetes mellitus.

Thus, the problem of H^+ balance in most mammals is the defense of normal alkalinity in the face of a constant onslaught of acid.

In recent years, a number of medical experts have preferred a notation of *hydrogen ion concentration,* $[H^+]$, *rather than pH,* in analyzing acid-base disturbances. Both systems have advantages and disadvantages; one can easily switch from one to the other through the expression

$$pH \simeq - \log [H^+].$$
(9-4)

For the sake of clarity, we shall use only pH in this and the next chapter.

Buffering of Nonvolatile (Fixed) Acids

The very effective defense of alkalinity in a normal dog is illustrated in Figure 9-1. It compares the change in the pH of arterial blood plasma when 156 ml of a 1 N HCl solution was infused intravenously, with the drop in pH when the same amount of acid was gradually added to 11.4 liters of distilled water. This volume of distilled water is about equal to the total body water of the dog. In the dog, the pH dropped from 7.44 to 7.14, a state of severe acidosis but one compatible with survival. In contrast, the addition of just a few milliequivalents of H^+ to unbuffered distilled water lowered the pH sharply to a value that would have been fatal to the animal, and the final level was 1.84. This section deals with the mechanisms that permit such effective buffering in vivo.

First Line of Defense — Fast, Physicochemical Buffering

The following reaction is the prototype for physicochemical buffering:

Strong acid + Buffer salt $\rightleftharpoons$ Neutral salt + Weak acid   (9-5)

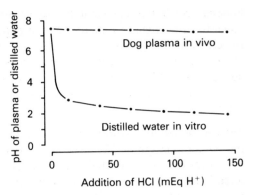

Fig. 9-1 : An experiment contrasting the effective buffering of HCl in a dog, with the lack of buffering when the same amount of acid is added to distilled water. The pH of the dog's arterial plasma decreased gradually from 7.44 to 7.14; that of unbuffered distilled water dropped precipitously to a level that would be fatal if it occurred in vivo. Redrawn from Pitts, R. F. *Harvey Lect.* **48**:172, 1953.

If hydrochloric acid is buffered by the bicarbonate buffer system, the reaction is:

$$H^+ + Cl^- + Na^+ + HCO_3^- \rightleftharpoons Na^+ + Cl^- + H_2CO_3 \qquad (9\text{-}6)$$

Insofar as physicochemical buffering reduces the amount of buffer salt and increases the amount of weak acid, this type of reaction only minimizes, but by no means prevents, a decrease in pH. This point can be illustrated by simple calculations, utilizing the derivation of the Henderson-Hasselbalch equation as it applies to the bicarbonate system:

$$pH = pK' + \log \frac{[HCO_3^-]}{[H_2CO_3]} \qquad (9\text{-}7)$$

The pK' (negative logarithm of the apparent dissociation constant) in Equation 9-7 is 3.5. Carbonic acid is in equilibrium with CO_2 (Eq. 9-1), and at the temperature and ionic concentration of the body fluids — and so long as carbonic anhydrase is present — there are approximately 400 molecules of dissolved CO_2 for every molecule of H_2CO_3. For that reason, a physiologically more meaningful form of Equation 9-7 is:

$$pH = pK' + \log \frac{[HCO_3^-]}{[\text{Dissolved } CO_2 + H_2CO_3]} \qquad (9\text{-}8)$$

In this equation, the pK' has a value of 6.1, reflecting the fact that the denominator is now some 400-fold higher than the one in

Equation 9-7. In the sense that the denominator of Equation 9-8 consists so overwhelmingly of CO_2 and not of H_2CO_3, the acid moiety of the bicarbonate buffer system is CO_2, even though it cannot donate H^+ (also called protons); in fact, some authorities speak of the "HCO_3^-/CO_2" buffer system rather than of the "HCO_3^-/H_2CO_3" system, and I shall use the former expression from now on.

The concentration of dissolved CO_2 in plasma is proportional to the partial pressure of CO_2 (P_{CO_2}) in the plasma, which is relatively easy to determine. The proportionality constant for plasma at 38°C, which converts P_{CO_2} in millimeters of mercury (mm Hg) to concentration of dissolved CO_2 expressed as millimoles per liter (mMoles/liter), is 0.03. Thus, ignoring the trace amounts that exist as H_2CO_3, the denominator in Equation 9-8 can be very closely approximated as $P_{CO_2} \cdot 0.03$, and this equation may be rewritten in a form that is most useful in physiological and clinical practice:

$$pH = 6.1 + \log \frac{[HCO_3^-]}{0.03 \cdot P_{CO_2}} \qquad (9\text{-}9)$$

In this equation, $[HCO_3^-]$ is expressed as mMoles/liter and P_{CO_2} in mm Hg. Substituting values for arterial plasma of man in normal H^+ balance:

$$pH = 6.1 + \log \frac{24 \text{ mMoles/L}}{0.03 \cdot 40 \text{ mm Hg}}$$

$$pH = 6.1 + \log \frac{24 \text{ mMoles/L}}{1.2 \text{ mMoles/L}} \qquad (9\text{-}10)$$

$$pH = 6.1 + \log 20$$

$$pH = 7.40$$

If 12 mMoles of HCl were added to each liter of extracellular fluid (which, except for a small Donnan effect, has the same ionic concentrations as plasma) — and if, for the moment, we say that all the acid is buffered by HCO_3^- (see below) — then physicochemical buffering would decrease the numerator and increase the denominator by 12 mMoles/liter each, according to the following reaction:

$$12\,H^+ + 12\,Cl^- + 24\,Na^+ + 24\,HCO_3^- \rightleftharpoons 12\,Na^+ + 12\,Cl^- + 12\,Na^+ + 12\,HCO_3^-$$
$$+ \ 12\,H_2CO_3$$
$$\Big\downarrow$$
$$12\,CO_2 + 12\,H_2O \qquad (9\text{-}11)$$

If this were to occur in a "closed system" — i.e., without a ventilatory system that can eliminate the newly generated CO_2 — the pH would drop to the fatal level of 6.06:

$$pH = 6.1 + \log \frac{12 \text{ mMoles/L}}{1.2 + 12 \text{ mMoles/L}}$$

$$pH = 6.1 + \log \frac{12 \text{ mMoles/L}}{13.2 \text{ mMoles/L}}$$

$$pH = 6.06$$

This dire consequence is prevented by the second line of defense, which, like physicochemical buffering, comes into play within seconds or minutes after the administration of HCl. [The above exposition represents a slight quantitative simplification in that it does not take into account two further factors: (1) By Equations 9-1 and 9-2, the concentration of HCO_3^- will be lowered as hyperventilation decreases the CO_2. (2) To the extent that the added HCl will be buffered not only by HCO_3^- but also by other buffers (see Utilization of the Various Buffers, below), the HCO_3^- concentration will be slightly higher and the CO_2 slightly lower than shown.]

Second Line of Defense — Fast, Respiratory Component

Because of the equilibrium in Equation 9-1, virtually all of the H_2CO_3 that was produced through physicochemical buffering is converted to CO_2 and H_2O (Eq. 9-11), and the CO_2 is excreted by the lungs. If all the extra CO_2 were excreted, returning the denominator to 1.2 mMoles/liter, the resulting pH would fall into the range that is compatible with survival.

$$pH = 6.1 + \log \frac{12 \text{ mMoles/L}}{1.2 \text{ mMoles/L}}$$

$$pH = 6.1 + \log 10$$

$$pH = 7.10$$

Respiratory compensation goes further, however. As a result of the lower pH of the blood, alveolar ventilation is increased, so that alveolar and hence arterial P_{CO_2} are decreased. Consequently the pH is returned toward, but not quite to, the normal value.

$$pH = 6.1 + \log \frac{12 \text{ mMoles/L}}{0.03 \cdot 23 \text{ mm Hg}}$$

$$pH = 6.1 + \log \frac{12 \text{ mMoles/L}}{0.69 \text{ mMoles/L}}$$

$$pH = 7.34$$

*Third Line of
Defense — Slow,
Renal Component*

Although respiratory compensation has, within minutes, restored the pH almost to normal, the stores of the main extracellular buffer have been depleted. This fact is reflected in the decrease of the HCO_3^- concentration from 24 to 12 mMoles/liter. Furthermore, some of the added H^+, although admittedly no longer in free solution, still remains within the body as weak acid. Both of these remaining abnormalities are corrected by the kidneys, which excrete H^+ and simultaneously replenish the depleted HCO_3^- stores. This process is a much slower one than the first two lines of defense, requiring hours to days rather than seconds or minutes. How the kidneys accomplish this task, which finally restores H^+ balance, is discussed in Chapter 10.

The above is a dramatic example that occurs only under artificial experimental conditions or in disease states. Nevertheless, these are the pathways by which the daily loads of nonvolatile acids are handled. The following quantitative comparison may put the normal, daily challenge from these fixed acids into perspective. An adult person weighing 70 kg has about 14 liters of extracellular fluid (about 20% of body weight; see Fig. 2-1). Hence the addition of 12 mMoles of HCl to each liter of extracellular fluid, as in the example described above, would be a total acid load to an adult human of 168 mMoles (12 mMoles/liter · 14 liters). Not only is the normal daily load of 40 to 60 mMoles of fixed acids merely about one-third of this amount, but also it is released relatively slowly over a 24-hour period, rather than in 1 to 2 hours, as in the above example. If, for the sake of illustration, about one-third of a total load of 48 mMoles were released after each meal, 16 mMoles (48 ÷ 3) would be added to 14 liters of extracellular fluid, i.e., an addition of about 1 mMole per liter of extracellular fluid. Since sulfuric acid is normally the major fixed acid (Eq. 9-3), the quantitative reaction would be as follows:

$$2\,H^+ + SO_4^{2-} + 24\,Na^+ + 24\,HCO_3^- \rightleftharpoons 2\,Na^+ + SO_4^{2-} + 22\,Na^+ + 22\,HCO_3^-$$

$$+\ 2\,H_2CO_3$$
$$\Updownarrow$$
$$2\,CO_2 + 2\,H_2O \qquad\qquad (9\text{-}12)$$

The resulting pH after physicochemical buffering would be:

$$pH = 6.1 + \log \frac{22\ \text{mMoles/L}}{3.2\ \text{mMoles/L}}$$

$$pH = 6.9$$

After elimination of the extra CO_2 through the lungs, the pH would be:

$$pH = 6.1 + \log \frac{22 \text{ mMoles/L}}{1.2 \text{ mMoles/L}}$$

$$pH = 7.36$$

This might cause only an undetectable increase in alveolar ventilation, thereby restoring the pH to near normal levels. However, what actually happens in a normal individual in the steady state is that the renal excretion of H$^+$ and reabsorption of HCO$_3^-$ (Third Line of Defense — see Chap. 10), which goes on continually, maintains the arterial plasma concentration of HCO$_3^-$ at about 24 mMoles/liter. Hence, the pH remains normal, as in Equation 9-10.

Buffering of the Volatile "Acid," CO$_2$

At the beginning of this chapter we cited the fact that some 13,000 to 20,000 mMoles of CO$_2$ is produced daily by an adult person, as the result of metabolic events. As shown in Equations 9-1 and 9-2, the processing of this CO$_2$ can generate H$^+$, and the production of CO$_2$ therefore potentially disturbs H$^+$ balance. Ultimately, elimination of all the CO$_2$ by the lungs prevents acidosis (Eq. 9-9); but before that elimination can occur, defense of alkalinity is threatened as the CO$_2$ is carried in the blood, from the cells where it is produced to the lungs where it is excreted. The extremely effective buffering in the blood is reflected in the fact that the difference in pH between venous blood, which goes to the lungs, and arterial blood, which leaves them, seldom exceeds 0.04 of a pH unit. This section deals with the mechanisms by which H$^+$ is buffered as CO$_2$ is transported in the blood.

Transport of CO$_2$ in Blood

The plasma P$_{CO_2}$ at the arterial end of tissue capillaries is about 40 mm Hg. Since the P$_{CO_2}$ is higher in tissue cells that produce CO$_2$, the gas will diffuse from the tissue cells into the capillary. The chain of events that then occurs is shown in Figure 9-2, and is as follows:

1. There is still no agreement whether CO$_2$ is processed mainly by hydration (Eq. 9-1) or by hydroxylation (Eq. 9-2). Because it is the latter reaction that is probably catalyzed by carbonic anhydrase (C.A.), I will use (in this chapter and the next) Equation 9-2 to show the processing of CO$_2$ within cells where C.A. is present; and I will use Equation 9-1 for extracellular fluids where C.A. is absent.

   Most cell membranes, including those of red blood cells (erythrocytes), are highly permeable to CO$_2$. Hence CO$_2$ diffuses not only into the plasma but also into the erythrocytes. Because there is much carbonic anhydrase in erythrocytes but none in plasma, CO$_2$ is processed much more rapidly within

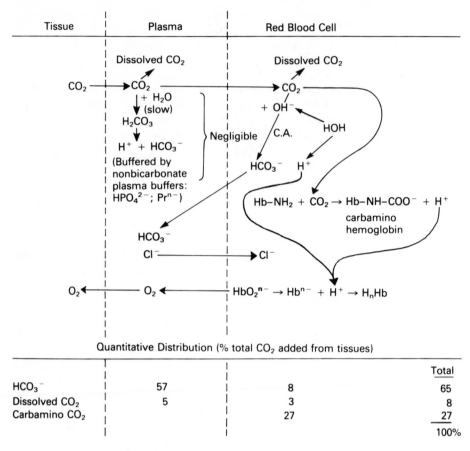

Tissue	Plasma	Red Blood Cell

Quantitative Distribution (% total CO_2 added from tissues)

	Plasma	Red Blood Cell	Total
HCO_3^-	57	8	65
Dissolved CO_2	5	3	8
Carbamino CO_2		27	27
			100%

Fig. 9-2 : Transport of CO_2 and buffering of H^+ by the blood. Adapted from Davenport, H. W. *The ABC of Acid-Base Chemistry* (6th ed.). Chicago: University of Chicago Press, 1974; and Masoro, E. J., and Siegel, P. D. *Acid-Base Regulation: Its Physiology, Pathophysiology and the Interpretation of Blood-Gas Analysis* (2nd ed.). Philadelphia: Saunders, 1977.

these cells than in the plasma. In fact, the processing is negligible in plasma; the little bit of H^+ that is formed from this reaction is buffered by the nonbicarbonate buffer anions of plasma, the proteins (Pr^{n-}) and phosphate (HPO_4^{2-}).

2. The rapid combination of CO_2 with OH^- within the erythrocytes yields HCO_3^-. Most of the newly formed HCO_3^- diffuses into the plasma, and Cl^- shifts into the erythrocytes. In this way, most of the CO_2 that is added to venous capillary blood is carried to the lungs as HCO_3^- in the plasma. A portion combines with hemoglobin to form carbamino hemoglobin, and an even smaller amount is carried as dissolved CO_2 within the erythrocytes.

The H$^+$ that is formed as water is split is buffered primarily by hemoglobin. The same is true of the H$^+$ that is released during the formation of carbamino hemoglobin.

3. In a normal, resting adult human, every liter of venous blood that goes to the lungs carries about 1.68 mMoles of extra CO_2 for excretion. The quantitative distribution of the various forms in which the added CO_2 is carried is shown at the bottom of Figure 9-2. About 65% of the 1.68 mMoles is carried as HCO_3^-, and the vast majority of this is carried in the plasma, even though virtually all of it was generated within the erythrocytes. The remainder is divided between dissolved CO_2 and carbamino CO_2. Of these, the major portion of dissolved CO_2 is carried in the plasma, whereas practically all the carbamino CO_2 is found in the erythrocytes.

Hemoglobin as a Buffer

As CO_2 is added to venous blood, the pH drops from about 7.40 in arterial blood to only about 7.37 in venous blood, rather than to about 7.32, which would be predicted. The mechanisms underlying this effect are shown in Figure 9-3.

The pK of oxygenated hemoglobin (HbO_2^{n-}) is lower than the pK of deoxygenated hemoglobin (Hb^{n-}; see Table 1-3); i.e., Hb^{n-} is

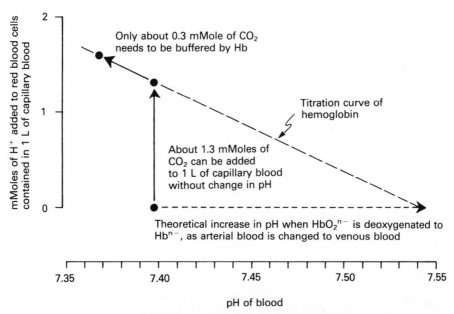

Fig. 9-3 : The special attributes of hemoglobin as a buffer. The pK of deoxygenated hemoglobin (Hb^{n-}) is higher than that of oxygenated hemoglobin (HbO_2^{n-}). Therefore, hemoglobin becomes a more effective buffer at precisely the moment when CO_2 and hence H$^+$ are added from the tissue cells to the blood.

less acidic than HbO_2^{n-}. As blood enters the arteriolar end of tissue capillaries, it gives up O_2 to the cells. The consequent reduction of HbO_2^{n-} to Hb^{n-} *would* cause a tremendous rise in pH were it not for the fact that CO_2, and hence H^+, is simultaneously added to the system. The net result of the change in pK of hemoglobin is that roughly 1.3 mMoles of CO_2 can be added to each liter of blood as it flows through the tissue capillaries, without changing the pH of that blood. Nearly 95% of the CO_2 that is added to each liter of venous blood, or about 1.6 mMoles of CO_2, is converted to H^+ (Fig. 9-2). Since 1.3 mMoles could be added without a change in pH, only about 0.3 mMole needs to be buffered by Hb^{n-}, and the drop in pH of venous blood is thus minimized.

Concept of Metabolic and Respiratory Disturbances

Primary Disturbances

Inspection of one form of the Henderson-Hasselbalch equation (Eq. 9-9) makes clear that an abnormality of plasma pH can result from a primary deviation of either the $[HCO_3^-]$ or the P_{CO_2}. Since the latter is regulated by the rate of alveolar ventilation, any disturbance in H^+ concentration that results from a primary change in P_{CO_2} is called respiratory. Thus, hypoventilation and retention of CO_2 lead to a reduction in pH that is called respiratory acidosis; hyperventilation and a fall in P_{CO_2} lead to a rise in pH that is called respiratory alkalosis. Changes in the concentration of HCO_3^- are brought about most commonly by the addition or loss of nonvolatile (fixed) acids or bases, which are derived mainly from metabolic processes. Hence, any abnormality of pH resulting primarily from a change in HCO_3^- is called metabolic. The endogenous production of aceto-acetic acid and β-OH butyric acid in uncontrolled diabetes mellitus leads to metabolic acidosis, while prolonged vomiting with loss of gastric HCl results in metabolic alkalosis.

Thus, there are four primary disturbances of H^+ balance (often called acid-base balance): (a) respiratory acidosis, (b) respiratory alkalosis, (c) metabolic acidosis, and (d) metabolic alkalosis.

Mixed Disturbances

Not infrequently, two primary disturbances, usually one respiratory and the other metabolic, occur simultaneously in the same individual. Such patients are said to have "mixed" acid-base disturbances. For example, a patient who manifests alveolar hypoventilation from emphysema may also have an obstructed duodenal ulcer leading to loss of HCl through vomiting. This patient would have a mixed disturbance of respiratory acidosis and metabolic alkalosis. Another patient may have both emphysema with retention of CO_2, and renal failure, which leads to the retention of fixed acids. This patient would have a mixed disturbance of respiratory acidosis and metabolic acidosis.

Since a mixed disturbance usually has a respiratory and a metabolic component, each of which may be acidosis or alkalosis, there are four major mixed disturbances: (a) respiratory acidosis plus metabolic acidosis, (b) respiratory acidosis plus metabolic alkalosis, (c) respiratory alkalosis plus metabolic acidosis, and (d) respiratory alkalosis plus metabolic alkalosis.

Compensatory
Responses

Most primary disturbances in H$^+$ balance tend to elicit a secondary response that partially corrects the pH. In the example cited earlier in this chapter, the addition of HCl led to a decrease in HCO_3^- and hence to metabolic acidosis. This disturbance was largely compensated for by the second line of defense, in which alveolar hyperventilation lowered the PCO_2 and thereby adjusted the pH to a near normal value.

This example illustrates two points: (a) that a compensatory response involves the system opposite to the one that caused the primary disturbance (e.g., *metabolic* alkalosis is compensated for by a *respiratory* response, and vice versa) and (b) that compensation shifts the pH *toward* but not to the normal value. Regarding the second point, in the example given earlier in this chapter, respiratory compensation moved the pH to 7.34 but not entirely into the normal range. The reason could be that ventilation may be controlled not only by pH but also by PCO_2. The latter declines as alveolar hyperventilation is induced, and the degree of hyperventilation will thus be set at a point where the stimulus to ventilation resulting from the decreased pH will be balanced by the inhibition to respiration resulting from the lowered arterial PCO_2.

Since primary disturbances may be either metabolic or respiratory in origin, and may cause either acidosis or alkalosis, there are four general types of compensatory responses: (1) Metabolic acidosis is compensated for within minutes by alveolar hyperventilation. (2) Metabolic alkalosis is accompanied by a respiratory compensation that decreases alveolar ventilation, although this response is less intense than during metabolic acidosis. (3) If the primary disturbance is respiratory acidosis, it is usually compensated for by increased renal excretion of H$^+$ and increased renal reabsorption of HCO_3^-. It takes days for this response to develop fully. The mechanisms by which it is accomplished are described in Chapter 10. (4) Finally, respiratory alkalosis is compensated for by a change in the metabolic component (the numerator) of Equation 9-9, namely, by decreased renal excretion of H^+ and decreased renal reabsorption of HCO_3^-; again, it takes days for this compensation to become fully effective.

Note that compensations for primary metabolic disturbances occur virtually immediately whereas those for primary respiratory disturbances materialize fully only after several days. The reason is that changes in alveolar ventilation almost instantly alter the level of PCO_2, while changes in renal function that alter the plasma $[HCO_3^-]$ take much longer. It is because of this difference in the time course of compensatory responses that primary respiratory disturbances — but not primary metabolic disturbances — are divided into acute (a few hours to approximately 2 days) and chronic (present for approximately 2 days or longer) phases. During acute respiratory acidosis or alkalosis, there will be a very slight rise or fall, respectively, of the plasma $[HCO_3^-]$ resulting from the chemical reactions shown in Equations 9-1 and 9-2; in chronic respiratory disturbances, the changes in plasma $[HCO_3^-]$ will be much greater because the kidneys have compensated by altering the reabsorptive rate for HCO_3^- (described further in Chap. 10).

The Important Buffers of Mammals

Thus far we have spoken almost exclusively about the bicarbonate and the hemoglobin buffer systems. In this section we shall emphasize that the body contains other important buffers, and that all these participate in the regulation of pH.

A buffer is a mixture of either a weak acid and its conjugate base, or a weak base and its conjugate acid. (Acid is here defined as a H^+ donor and base as a H^+ acceptor.) The buffers of physiological importance in mammals are all of the first type. They have been listed in Figure 9-4. These buffer systems are by no means limited to the plasma. They are found in all phases of the body fluids — plasma, interstitial fluid, intracellular fluid — and bone. The bicarbonate system predominates in plasma and interstitial fluid, while organic phosphates and proteins (especially hemoglobin) predominate in the intracellular spaces.

The Isohydric Principle

When several buffers exist in a common solution, as in a beaker, all the buffer pairs are in equilibrium with the same concentration of H^+. Expressed in the terminology of the Henderson-Hasselbalch equation, and for plasma — which is a common solution containing the bicarbonate, protein, and phosphate buffer systems — the isohydric principle can be stated as follows:

$$pH = pK_1' + \log \frac{[HCO_3^-]}{[CO_2]} = pK_2' + \log \frac{[HPO_4^{2-}]}{[H_2PO_4^-]} = pK_3' + \log \frac{[Prot^{n-}]}{[H_nProt]} \quad (9\text{-}13)$$

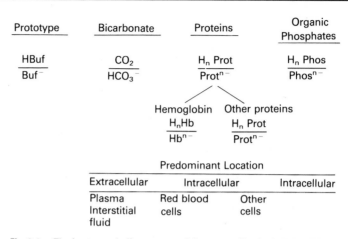

Prototype	Bicarbonate	Proteins	Organic Phosphates
$\dfrac{\text{HBuf}}{\text{Buf}^-}$	$\dfrac{CO_2}{HCO_3^-}$	$\dfrac{H_n\,Prot}{Prot^{n-}}$	$\dfrac{H_n\,Phos}{Phos^{n-}}$

Hemoglobin $\quad$ Other proteins

$\dfrac{H_nHb}{Hb^{n-}} \qquad \dfrac{H_n\,Prot}{Prot^{n-}}$

Predominant Location

Extracellular	Intracellular		Intracellular
Plasma Interstitial fluid	Red blood cells	Other cells	

Fig. 9-4 : The important buffer systems of the mammalian body fluid compartments. Note that CO_2 is denoted as the acid moiety of the bicarbonate buffer system, even though CO_2 is not a H$^+$ donor (see discussion of Eq. 9-8). The locations refer to quantitative predominance and are not exclusive except for hemoglobin in erythrocytes. The valence of phosphate is designated as indefinite because it is quantitatively an important chemical buffer mainly within the intracellular fluid, where its valence as organic phosphate is not known.

This principle has an important application in the analysis of acid-base disturbances, because one can infer the status of most of the body buffer pairs by determining the status of just one of them. In practice, one usually measures two of the three variables of the bicarbonate system, so that the third can easily be calculated (Eq. 9-9). For plasma, which is truly a homogeneous solution, knowledge of the bicarbonate system can thus be extended precisely to the phosphate and protein buffer pairs without actually measuring their concentrations.

Precise extension to the buffers in the other major fluid compartments is not possible because these compartments are not part of a homogeneous solution in which all the buffers are evenly distributed (Chap. 2). Largely because of the Gibbs-Donnan effect, and partly because of the metabolic production of acids, the pH is considerably lower (perhaps 7.00) within cells than in the plasma or interstitial fluid. Nevertheless, in many conditions of H$^+$ imbalance, the isohydric principle can be applied to infer qualitative changes in all or most of the body buffers from knowledge of the bicarbonate system alone. This is permissible because many acid-base disturbances represent relatively chronic situations in which the change in H$^+$ balance within one fluid compartment has been accompanied by qualitatively similar changes in the other compartments.

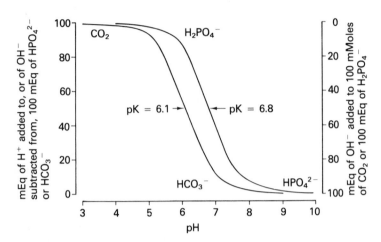

Fig. 9-5 : Titration curves for the bicarbonate and inorganic phosphate buffers in a closed system. Under these conditions, when the concentration of CO_2 cannot be kept low through diffusion to the outside, the bicarbonate system is a less effective buffer than phosphate. It is mainly because CO_2 can normally be eliminated by the lungs that the bicarbonate system is such an efficient physiological buffer. Modified from Pitts, R. F. *Physiology of the Kidney and Body Fluids* (3rd ed.). Chicago: Year Book, 1974.

Special Attributes of the Bicarbonate System

We have already reviewed the special properties of hemoglobin that render it extraordinarily suitable for buffering the H^+ that is formed when CO_2 is added to venous blood. In turn, the bicarbonate system has special attributes for buffering nonvolatile acids. Titration curves for the bicarbonate and inorganic phosphate buffers, which are found in plasma and interstitial fluid, are shown in Figure 9-5. Several points should be noted: (a) the pK is numerically equal to the pH existing when the weak acid and its conjugate base each compose 50% of the total concentration of that particular buffer; (b) the change in pH per quantum of H^+ or OH^- added is least in the linear portion of each titration curve; and (c) this linear portion of most effective chemical buffering extends roughly 1.0 pH unit to either side of the pK — from pH of about 5.1 to 7.1 for the bicarbonate system, and from about 5.8 to 7.8 for phosphate. In other words, in the range of plasma pH that is compatible with survival (about 6.8 to 8.0), each quantum of phosphate can buffer more H^+ than an equal quantum of bicarbonate. Nevertheless, bicarbonate plays a much more important physiological role as an extracellular buffer than does phosphate.

The reason for the seeming paradox is not only that the extracellular concentration of bicarbonate (about 24 mMoles/liter) is so much higher than that of phosphate (1 to 2 mMoles/liter; see

Table 1-2 and Fig. 2-2) but also, and more importantly, that bicarbonate has certain physiological properties that make it a uniquely effective buffer. The central property is that carbonic acid is in equilibrium with volatile CO_2, which can be rapidly excreted or retained by the lungs (see Second Line of Defense earlier in this chapter). Furthermore, both the acid moiety, CO_2, and the conjugate base, HCO_3^-, of the bicarbonate buffer system are more abundantly available from daily metabolic processes than are those of any other buffer system.

Utilization of the Various Buffers

ADDITION OF STRONG ACID. Earlier in this chapter when we described the buffering of nonvolatile (fixed) acids — i.e., of H$^+$ other than that generated by CO_2 (Eqs. 9-1 and 9-2) — we limited the analysis to the bicarbonate buffer system in plasma. This simplification was not seriously inaccurate, since an acid that is infused intravenously will initially have its impact on the plasma. The description, however, did not include the participation of the other buffer systems of the body. The total picture is presented in Figure 9-6, which indicates not only the time course for distribution of a fixed acid throughout the body fluid compartments but also the quantitative contribution of the major buffers. (The figure refers to the addition of an inorganic, or mineral, acid; details may be slightly different when the same amount of H$^+$ is added in the form of an organic acid, such as lactic acid.)

Figure 9-6 is based on experimental work in dogs that were given intravenous infusions of hydrochloric acid over periods of 1.5 to 3 hours. Within seconds to minutes, the acid is being handled by the various buffers of the blood. In the plasma, this process involves mainly the bicarbonate system, because its ionic concentration in plasma is so much greater than that of the proteins and inorganic phosphate (Table 1-2 and Fig. 2-2), and because CO_2, which is formed in the buffering reaction, is quickly eliminated via the lungs. The acid also quickly enters the erythrocytes, where it is buffered primarily by hemoglobin; bicarbonate, and to an even lesser extent organic phosphates, within erythrocytes contribute a little bit to the buffering. A small amount of the acid is buffered in the plasma, by bicarbonate that was derived from the erythrocytes through an exchange of Cl^- for HCO_3^-.

As soon as the HCl is infused into the plasma, it begins to enter the interstitial compartment. Although it takes about one-half hour for the acid to be evenly distributed between the plasma and interstitial fluid, the latter actually contributes more to the total buffering because its volume is about four times greater than that of plasma (see Fig. 2-1). Again, inorganic phosphate in the interstitium also participates, but to a negligible extent because its concentration in interstitial fluid is very low.

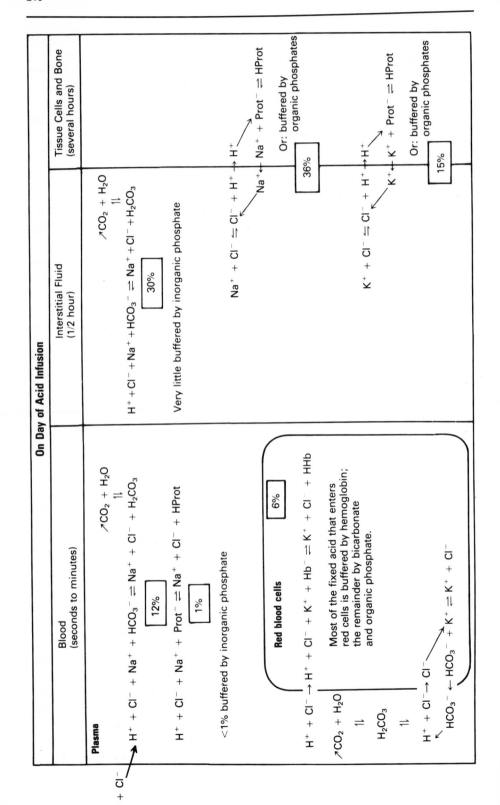

On Day of Acid Infusion

$H^+ + Cl^-$

Blood
(seconds to minutes)

Plasma

$$\nearrow CO_2 + H_2O$$
$$\rightleftharpoons$$
$$H^+ + Cl^- + Na^+ + HCO_3^- \rightleftharpoons Na^+ + Cl^- + H_2CO_3$$

12%

$$H^+ + Cl^- + Na^+ + Prot^- \rightleftharpoons Na^+ + Cl^- + HProt$$

1%

<1% buffered by inorganic phosphate

Red blood cells 6%

$$H^+ + Cl^- \rightarrow H^+ + Cl^- + K^+ + Hb^- \rightleftharpoons K^+ + Cl^- + HHb$$

Most of the fixed acid that enters red cells is buffered by hemoglobin; the remainder by bicarbonate and organic phosphate.

$$\nearrow CO_2 + H_2O$$
$$\rightleftharpoons$$
$$H_2CO_3$$
$$\rightleftharpoons$$
$$H^+ + Cl^- \rightarrow Cl^-$$
$$HCO_3^- \leftarrow HCO_3^- + K^+ \rightleftharpoons K^+ + Cl^-$$

Interstitial Fluid
(1/2 hour)

$$\nearrow CO_2 + H_2O$$
$$\rightleftharpoons$$
$$H^+ + Cl^- + Na^+ + HCO_3^- \rightleftharpoons Na^+ + Cl^- + H_2CO_3$$

30%

Very little buffered by inorganic phosphate

$$Na^+ + Cl^- \rightleftharpoons Cl^- + H^+ \rightleftharpoons H^+$$
$$Na^+ \leftarrow Na^+ + Prot^- \rightleftharpoons HProt$$

Or: buffered by organic phosphates

$$K^+ + Cl^- \rightleftharpoons Cl^- + H^+ \rightleftharpoons H^+$$
$$K^+ \leftarrow K^+ + Prot^- \rightleftharpoons HProt$$

Or: buffered by organic phosphates

Tissue Cells and Bone
(several hours)

36%

15%

24 Hours After Infusing Acid

About 25% of acid load has been excreted in the urine as titratable acid and NH_4^+ (see Chap. 10). Extracellular pH and ionic composition are nearly normal; therefore, 75% of the administered acid must be sequestered and buffered in tissue cells and bone.

2–6 Days After Infusing Acid

The remaining 75% of the administered acid is slowly released from tissue cells and bone, and excreted in the urine.

Fig. 9-6 : **Handling of the fixed inorganic acid, HCl, by intact dogs. For the sake of clarity, polyvalent anions such as proteins and hemoglobin have been drawn with a single negative sign. A slanted arrow next to CO_2 indicates that the CO_2 is quickly excreted through the lungs. The percentages enclosed in rectangles indicate the approximate proportion of the total acid load that is buffered by** each mechanism. Data from Swan, R. C., and Pitts, R. F. *J. Clin. Invest.* 34:205, 1955; Yoshimura, H., et al. *Jpn. J. Physiol.* 11:109, 1961; Pitts, R. F. *Physiology of the Kidney and Body Fluids* (3rd ed.). Chicago: Year Book, 1974; and Masoro, E. J., and Siegel, P. D. *Acid-Base Regulation: Its Physiology, Pathophysiology and the Interpretation of Blood-Gas Analysis* (2nd ed.). Philadelphia: Saunders, 1977.

Several hours elapse before the acid is evenly distributed throughout the intracellular compartment. Nevertheless, the contribution of the intracellular buffers is great. Utilization of these buffers — mainly proteins and organic phosphates — is accomplished by exchange of extracellular H^+ for either intracellular Na^+ or intracellular K^+. Some of the Na^+ probably comes from the apatite of bone, and the H^+ that is exchanged for this Na^+ enters into a chemical reaction with the apatite, finally being incorporated into HCO_3^-. The involvement of bone in buffering is probably much more important during chronic disturbances of acid-base balance (as in chronic renal failure) than during the relatively acute disturbance illustrated in Figure 9-6.

The relative quantitative contributions of the various buffers are indicated by the boxes in Figure 9-6, which give the percentage of the total acid load that is handled by each mechanism. It is clear that less than 15% is buffered in the plasma, and less than 20% by whole blood. To be emphasized is the fact that the largest proportion, or about one-half of the administered acid, is buffered in the intracellular compartment.

Although buffering of the acid has minimized changes in pH, restoration of external balance (for definition, see legend to Fig. 11-1) must await excretion of the acid load in the urine. This occurs during the ensuing several days. By the second day after the infusion, about 25% of the acid has been excreted, and both the pH and ionic composition of the extracellular fluids have returned to near normal values. It follows that 75% of the acid load must now reside within the cells and bone, where it is buffered. This remaining acid is slowly released into the extracellular fluids and excreted by the kidneys during the second to sixth days after the acid was given.

ADDITION OF STRONG ALKALI. When base is infused intravenously, or HCl is eliminated as by vomiting, the chain of events is similar to that discussed above, except that the reactions go in the opposite direction. There is a marked participation by the intracellular buffers, and the time course for the utilization of the various buffers is similar to that shown in Figure 9-6. Three differences should be noted, however: (a) respiratory compensation — i.e., alveolar hypoventilation due to an increase in pH — is less intense in metabolic alkalosis than in metabolic acidosis; (b) lactic acid moves out of skeletal muscle cells, to buffer the base in the extracellular fluid; and (c) the renal excretion of base, such as sodium bicarbonate, usually occurs more rapidly than does the renal excretion of H^+.

ADDITION OF THE VOLATILE "ACID," CO_2. If excess CO_2 is produced endogenously and there is no disorder of respiration, the surplus is quickly excreted through the lungs by the mechanisms shown in Figure 9-2. If, however, CO_2 is added from an external source, as by breathing a gas mixture containing 5% CO_2, or if CO_2 accumulates because of some disorder of respiration, there is a net addition of acid to the body, by the reactions shown in Equations 9-1 and 9-2. The chain of events that is set into motion under these circumstances is shown in Figure 9-7.

The first important point to recognize is that the H$^+$ produced when CO_2 is added cannot be buffered by the bicarbonate system. The reason is evident from Equation 9-14. When H$^+$ is buffered by HCO_3^- (as in Eqs. 9-11 and 9-12), carbonic acid is formed momentarily, and the final products are CO_2 and H_2O:

$$H^+ + HCO_3^- \rightleftharpoons H_2CO_3 \rightleftharpoons CO_2 + H_2O \qquad (9\text{-}14)$$

Since CO_2 and H_2O are the starting substrates when CO_2 is added to the body (Eqs. 9-1 and 9-2), reaction 9-14, under that circumstance, is being driven to the left, and it cannot simultaneously be driven to the right as would be required if the H$^+$ were to be buffered by HCO_3^-. Instead, the H$^+$ must be buffered by the nonbicarbonate buffers (proteins and phosphates), designated Buf$^-$ in the following reaction:

$$\left. \begin{array}{l} HOH \rightleftharpoons H^+ \\ \quad \updownarrow \quad \text{C.A.} \\ CO_2 + OH^- \rightleftharpoons HCO_3^- \end{array} \right\} \quad \begin{array}{l} + Na^+ \\ + Buf^- \end{array}$$

$$HBuf + Na^+ + HCO_3^- \qquad (9\text{-}15)$$

As is shown in Figure 9-4, the only buffer of quantitative importance in the extracellular fluid is the bicarbonate system. It follows, then, that very little of the H$^+$ that is generated when CO_2 is added to the body — in fact, less than 5% (Fig. 9-7) — can be buffered in the extracellular compartment, i.e., in the plasma and interstitial fluid.

A second important distinction between the addition of a fixed acid and the addition of the volatile "acid," CO_2, lies in the time required for the acid load to be distributed throughout the major fluid compartments. This process takes hours for a fixed acid (Fig. 9-6), whereas it occurs within minutes for CO_2 (Fig. 9-7), which diffuses so readily across both the vascular endothelium and the cell membrane.

Hemoglobin, of course, is the most abundant nonbicarbonate buffer in blood (Fig. 9-4). Consequently, a large proportion of the added volatile acid is buffered by the various mechanisms out-

At Onset of Hypoventilation

Blood (seconds to minutes)	Interstitial Fluid (minutes)	Tissue Cells and Bone (30–60 minutes)

Plasma

CO_2 →

$CO_2 + H_2O \rightleftharpoons H_2CO_3 \rightleftharpoons H^+ + HCO_3^-$

$H^+ + HCO_3^- + Na^+ + Prot^- \rightleftharpoons Na^+ + HCO_3^- + HProt$

[3%]

Red blood cells [29%]

$CO_2 \rightarrow CO_2$: Rapid conversion to HCO_3^- and H^+; formation of carbamino hemoglobin; buffering by hemoglobin; exchange of HCO_3^- for Cl^- — all as shown in Figure 9-2.

Interstitial Fluid

$CO_2 + H_2O \rightleftharpoons H_2CO_3 \rightleftharpoons H^+ + HCO_3^-$

$H^+ + HCO_3^- + 2\,Na^+ + HPO_4^{2-} \rightleftharpoons Na^+ + HCO_3^- + NaH_2PO_4$

[Negligible]

Several Hours

$Na^+ + HCO_3^- + HLac \rightleftharpoons H^+ + HCO_3^-$
$\rightleftharpoons Na^+ + Lac^-$

glucose or glycogen

$CO_2 + H_2O$

$Na^+ + HCO_3^- \rightleftharpoons HCO_3^- + H^+ \rightarrow H^+$
$Na^+ \rightarrow Na^+ + Prot^- \rightleftharpoons HProt$

$K^+ + HCO_3^- \rightleftharpoons HCO_3^- + H^+ \rightarrow H^+$
$K^+ \leftarrow K^+ + Prot^- \rightleftharpoons HProt$

Tissue Cells and Bone

$HOH \rightleftharpoons H^+$
$\underset{C.A.}{\rightleftharpoons} OH^- \rightleftharpoons HCO_3^-$

$CO_2 + OH^- \rightleftharpoons HCO_3^-$

$H^+ + HCO_3^- + K^+ + Prot^- \rightleftharpoons K^+ + HCO_3^- + HProt$

Or: buffered by organic phosphates

[?11%]

$\rightarrow Na^+ + Lac^-$ [6%]

$\rightarrow Na^+ + Prot^- \rightleftharpoons HProt$ Or: buffered by organic phosphates [37%]

$\rightarrow K^+ + K^+ + Prot^- \rightleftharpoons HProt$ Or: buffered by organic phosphates [14%]

2–5 Days After Onset of Hypoventilation

Renal excretion of H$^+$ and renal reabsorption of HCO$_3^-$ (see Chap. 10) restore plasma pH to nearly normal value.

Fig. 9-7 : Events that follow the retention of CO$_2$ (and hence the addition of H$^+$) due to prolonged alveolar hypoventilation. For the sake of clarity, polyvalent protein anions have been written with a single negative sign. The approximate proportion of the total acid load that is buffered by each mechanism is indicated by the percentages in the rectangles; the figure of 11% is uncertain. Data adapted from **Giebisch, G., et al.** *J. Clin. Invest.* **34:**231, 1955; **Pitts, R. F.** *Physiology of the Kidney and Body Fluids* (3rd ed.). Chicago: **Year Book, 1974;** and **Masoro, E. J., and Siegel, P. D.** *Acid-Base Regulation: Its Physiology, Pathophysiology and the Interpretation of Blood-Gas Analysis* (2nd ed.). Philadelphia: **Saunders, 1977.**

lined in Figure 9-2. Since CO_2 diffuses so easily across cell membranes, the reactions in erythrocytes occur within seconds to minutes after the onset of the disturbance. During this time, a relatively normal plasma pH will be preserved. However, since H^+ is simultaneously being formed in the interstitial compartment, where it initially cannot be buffered (since "only" HCO_3^- is available), there will then ensue a dramatic drop in plasma pH as the H^+ is distributed evenly throughout the plasma and interstitial fluid. It takes several hours before the intracellular nonhemoglobin buffers make a quantitatively significant contribution to handling the H^+ that was formed in the extracellular space. This is accomplished mainly by exchange of H^+ for Na^+ across cell membranes, by H^+ for K^+ exchange in very severe disturbances, and to a lesser extent by lactate moving out of cells. The H^+ that is formed within cells is buffered by the nonbicarbonate buffers in these cells.

Thus, since the H^+ generated when CO_2 is added cannot be buffered by the bicarbonate system, which exists mainly in the extracellular compartment, all but 3% of the added acid load is buffered either within cells (erythrocytes, tissue cells, and bone) or through buffers (lactate) derived from cells.

As was the case after the addition of strong acid, so here too the renal response is a relatively slow one requiring days before a new equilibrium state is reached. In this connection, a third difference between the addition of a fixed acid and the addition of volatile acid should be noted (alluded to earlier, in the last paragraph under Compensatory Responses). The events occurring on the day of adding strong acid (Fig. 9-6) include the rapid second line of defense, in which the excretion of CO_2 "adjusts" the denominator of the Henderson-Hasselbalch equation. Consequently, a near normal plasma pH is attained quickly. However, when the primary acid-base disturbance is respiratory (i.e., when the initial change is in the denominator of the Henderson-Hasselbalch equation; Eq. 9-9), the events occurring at the onset are limited to chemical buffering (Fig. 9-7), and compensatory "adjustment" of the numerator must await the much slower renal process. Hence, primary respiratory disturbances are accompanied by relatively marked deviations of pH during the first few days, and a near normal pH is attained only after a number of days.

DEFICIT OF THE VOLATILE "ACID," CO_2. The responses that set in when alveolar hyperventilation reduces CO_2, and hence H^+ (Eqs. 9-1 and 9-2), are analogous to those depicted in Figure 9-7, except that the reactions proceed in the opposite direction.

Summary

Every day, a person produces large quantities of acid. In an adult, this amounts to approximately 50 mMoles of nonvolatile acid derived from dietary proteins and phospholipids, and at least 13,000 mMoles of CO_2 [approximately 90% of which momentarily generates H$^+$ as the CO_2 is carried in the blood to the lungs where it is expired (Fig. 9-2)]. Despite these large loads of acid, the person maintains an alkaline plasma pH, which is crucial to survival.

The concept of CO_2 as an acid is complicated because CO_2 is not a proton-donor, nor does H_2CO_3 exist in appreciable amounts in the body fluids. Rather, most of the H$^+$ that results from the processing of metabolic CO_2 is derived from the dissociation of water (Eq. 9-2 and Fig. 9-2). As metabolic CO_2 enters the blood from tissue cells, this generation of H$^+$ poses a threat to H$^+$ balance. The decrease in pH is minimized by a special property of hemoglobin as a buffer, which makes nonoxygenated hemoglobin less acidic than oxygenated hemoglobin. Hence, as arterial capillary blood releases O_2, it can take up a great deal of H$^+$ without any change in pH (Fig. 9-3). Simultaneously, the CO_2 coming from the cells combines with the OH$^-$ of dissociated water to yield HCO_3^-, and it is mainly in this form that CO_2 is carried to the lungs for excretion.

Acids other than CO_2 do not have a volatile component; they are therefore known as nonvolatile, or "fixed," acids. Normally, such acids are derived from the catabolism primarily of proteins, and to a lesser extent of phospholipids. Acid-base balance in the presence of these acids is preserved by three lines of defense: (a) physicochemical buffering, which begins within seconds after introduction of the acid; (b) adjustments in alveolar ventilation, which occur within seconds or minutes; and (c) renal excretion of H$^+$ and renal reabsorption of HCO_3^-, which may take days to come to completion. The bicarbonate buffer system is especially effective in handling excesses or deficits of fixed acids because: (a) it involves an equilibrium with a volatile component, CO_2, which can be regulated by changes in alveolar ventilation; and (b) the substrates of this buffer system, namely, CO_2 and HCO_3^-, are readily available from metabolic processes.

Disturbances of H$^+$ balance may be either metabolic or respiratory in origin. The first will cause a deviation in the numerator of the Henderson-Hasselbalch equation (Eq. 9-9), which will tend to shift the pH in either an acid or an alkaline direction; the second will lead to a deviation in the denominator, which likewise may shift the pH in either direction. In most instances, a primary disturbance of one origin (i.e., metabolic or respiratory) is accompanied by a secondary, or compensatory, response of opposite origin (i.e., respiratory or metabolic, respectively), which restores the plasma pH toward normal. Compensations for primary metabolic disturbances are almost instantaneous, whereas those for primary respiratory disturbances become fully effective only after several days. When primary disturbances of metabolic and respiratory origin occur simultaneously in the same individual, the resulting state is known as a mixed disturbance.

A load of acid or alkali calls into play not only the buffers of the plasma but also those of interstitial fluid, cells, and bone. Roughly 50% of fixed acid is buffered within cells. In contrast, more than 95% of the H^+ resulting from an excess or deficit of CO_2 (Eqs. 9-1 and 9-2) is buffered intracellularly; this is so because this H^+ cannot be buffered by the bicarbonate system (Eqs. 9-14 and 9-15), which is overwhelmingly the predominant buffer of extracellular fluid, i.e., the plasma and interstitium.

The isohydric principle states that all buffer pairs in a common solution are in equilibrium with the same H^+ concentration. The various body fluid compartments do not represent a common solution. Nevertheless, the principle can be applied in most equilibrium states, to assess the approximate status of all buffers in the body. Most disturbances of H^+ balance result in a new equilibrium state (steady state), in which the changes in all body buffers are qualitatively similar. Hence, in relatively chronic acid-base disturbances, analysis of the bicarbonate buffer system in plasma may be extended to gain some knowledge about the other buffers.

Problem 9-1 The data below were obtained on each of four patients. Complete the analysis of the acid-base status of each patient by filling in the blank spaces.

Normal arterial values from Table 1-2: pH = 7.37 to 7.42; [HCO$_3^-$] = 23 to 25 mMoles/L; P$_{CO_2}$ = 37 to 43 mm Hg.

Cause of the Disturbance	Arterial Plasma			Type of Disturbance
	pH	P$_{CO_2}$ (mm Hg)	[HCO$_3^-$] (mM/L)	
Prolonged vomiting	7.55	44		
Ingestion of NH$_4$Cl[a]		28	10	
Hysterical hyperventilation	7.57		21	
Emphysema	7.33	68		

[a]The net effect of ingesting NH$_4$Cl is the addition of hydrochloric acid, by the following reaction:

2 NH$_4$Cl + CO$_2$ → 2 H$^+$ + 2 Cl$^-$ + H$_2$O + CO (NH$_2$)$_2$
                                             urea

Problem 9-2 Outline the sequential steps involved in the development of a steady state of: respiratory acidosis; metabolic alkalosis; and respiratory alkalosis.

What will be the pH of arterial plasma (i.e., acidotic, alkalotic, or unchanged) in the following mixed disturbances: respiratory acidosis plus metabolic acidosis; respiratory acidosis plus metabolic alkalosis; respiratory alkalosis plus metabolic acidosis; and respiratory alkalosis plus metabolic alkalosis?

Selected References *Note: Additional references — especially ones with more clinical connotations — are listed in: Valtin, H.* Renal Dysfunction: Mechanisms Involved in Fluid and Solute Imbalance. *Boston: Little, Brown, 1979. Chaps. 5, 6, and 12.*

General Bates, R. G. *Determination of pH. Theory and Practice.* New York: Wiley, 1964.

Christensen, H. N. *Body Fluids and the Acid-Base Balance.* Philadelphia: Saunders, 1964.

Cohen, J. J., and Kassirer, J. P. Acid-Base Metabolism. In M. H. Maxwell and C. R. Kleeman (Eds.), *Clinical Disorders of Fluid and Electrolyte Metabolism* (3rd ed.). New York: McGraw-Hill, 1980.

Cohen, J. J., and Kassirer, J. P. *Acid-Base.* Boston: Little, Brown, 1982.

Davenport, H. W. *The ABC of Acid-Base Chemistry* (6th ed.). Chicago: University of Chicago Press, 1974.

Davis, R. P. Logland: A Gibbsian view of acid-base balance. *Am. J. Med.* 42:159, 1967.

Dejours, P. (Ed.). Symposium on interaction of intra- and extracellular acid-base balance. *Respir. Physiol.* 33:1, 1978.

Fencl, V. Distribution of H^+ and HCO_3^- in Cerebral Fluids. In B. K. Siesjö and S. C. Sørensen (Eds.), *Ion Homeostasis of the Brain. The Regulation of Hydrogen and Potassium Ion Concentrations in Cerebral Intra- and Extracellular Fluids.* New York: Academic, 1971.

Henderson, L. J. *Blood: A Study in General Physiology.* New Haven: Yale University Press, 1928.

Hills, A. G. *Acid-Base Balance: Chemistry, Physiology, Pathophysiology.* Baltimore: Williams & Wilkins, 1973.

Huckabee, W. E. Henderson vs. Hasselbalch. *Clin. Res.* 9:116, 1961.

Lennon, E. J. Body Buffering Mechanisms. In E. D. Frohlich (Ed.), *Pathophysiology: Altered Regulatory Mechanisms in Disease.* Philadelphia: Lippincott, 1972.

Madias, N. E., Adrogué, H. J., Horowitz, G. L., Cohen, J. J., and Schwartz, W. B. A redefinition of normal acid-base equilibrium in man: Carbon dioxide tension as a key determinant of normal plasma bicarbonate concentration. *Kidney Int.* 16:612, 1979.

Masoro, E. J., and Siegel, P. D. *Acid-Base Regulation: Its Physiology, Pathophysiology and the Interpretation of Blood-Gas Analysis* (2nd ed.). Philadelphia: Saunders, 1977.
A concise and lucid exposition of the subject.

Nahas, G. G. (Ed.). Current concepts of acid-base measurement. *Ann. N.Y. Acad. Sci.* 133:1, 1966.
Two of the papers in this symposium, "Terminology of Acid-Base Disorders" and "Statement on Acid-Base Terminology," have also been reproduced in Ann. Intern. Med. *63:873, 1965.*

Pitts, R. F. *Physiology of the Kidney and Body Fluids* (3rd ed.). Chicago: Year Book, 1974.

Rector, F. C., Jr. (Ed.). Symposium on acid-base homeostasis. *Kidney Int.* 1:273, 1972.

Robin, E. D., Bromberg, P. A., and Cross, C. E. Some aspects of the evolution of vertebrate acid-base regulation. *Yale J. Biol. Med.* 41:448, 1969.

Rose, B. D. *Clinical Physiology of Acid-Base and Electrolyte Disorders.* New York: McGraw-Hill, 1977.

Schwartz, W. B., and Cohen, J. J. The nature of the renal response to chronic disorders of acid-base equilibrium. *Am. J. Med.* 64:417, 1978.

Schwartz, W. B., and Relman, A. S. Critique of the parameters used in evaluation of acid-base disorders. "Whole-blood buffer base" and "standard bicarbonate" compared with blood pH and plasma bicarbonate concentration. *N. Engl. J. Med.* 268:1382, 1963.

Siesjö, B. H. The regulation of cerebrospinal fluid pH. *Kidney Int.* 1:360, 1972.

Valtin, H. *Renal Dysfunction: Mechanisms Involved in Fluid and Solute Imbalance.* Boston: Little, Brown, 1979. Chaps. 5 and 6.

Waddell, W. J., and Bates, R. B. Intracellular pH. *Physiol. Rev.* 49:285, 1969.

Wiggins, P. M. Intracellular pH and the structure of cell water. *J. Theor. Biol.* 37:363, 1972.

Winters, R. W. (Ed.). *The Body Fluids in Pediatrics.* Boston: Little, Brown, 1973.

Winters, R. W., Engel, K., and Dell, R. B. *Acid-Base Physiology in Medicine: A Self-Instruction Program* (3rd ed.). Boston: Little, Brown, 1982.

Buffering

Bergstrom, W. H., and Wallace, W. M. Bone as a sodium and potassium reservoir. *J. Clin. Invest.* 33:867, 1954.

Boron, W. F. Intracellular pH transients in giant barnacle muscle fibers. *Am. J. Physiol.* 233 (Cell Physiol. 2):C61, 1977.

Burton, R. E. The roles of buffers in body fluid: Mathematical analysis. *Respir. Physiol.* 18:34, 1973.

German, B., and Wyman, J., Jr. The titration curves of oxygenated and reduced hemoglobin. *J. Biol. Chem.* 117:533, 1937.

Giebisch, G., Berger, L., and Pitts, R. F. The extrarenal response to acute acid-base disturbances of respiratory origin. *J. Clin. Invest.* 34:231, 1955.

Lemann, J., Jr., and Lennon, E. J. Role of diet, gastrointestinal tract and bone in acid-base homeostasis. *Kidney Int.* 1:275, 1972.

Lemann, J., Jr., Lennon, E. J., Goodman, A. D., Litzow, J. R., and Relman, A. S. The net balance of acid in subjects given large loads of acid or alkali. *J. Clin. Invest.* 44:507, 1965.

Lemann, J., Jr., Litzow, J. R., and Lennon, E. J. The effects of chronic acid loads in normal man: Further evidence for the participation of bone mineral in the defense against chronic metabolic acidosis. *J. Clin. Invest.* 45:1608, 1966.

Lennon, E. J., and Lemann, J., Jr. Defense of hydrogen ion concentration in chronic metabolic acidosis. *Ann. Intern. Med.* 65:265, 1966.

Pitts, R. F. Mechanisms for stabilizing the alkaline reserves of the body. *Harvey Lect.* 48:172, 1953.

Swan, R. C., Axelrod, D. R., Seip, M., and Pitts, R. F. Distribution of sodium bicarbonate infused into nephrectomized dogs. *J. Clin. Invest.* 34:1795, 1955.

Swan, R. C., and Pitts, R. F. Neutralization of infused acid by nephrectomized dogs. *J. Clin. Invest.* 34:205, 1955.

Tobin, R. B. Plasma, extracellular and muscle electrolyte responses to acute metabolic acidosis. *Am. J. Physiol.* 186:131, 1956.

Yoshimura, H., Fujimoto, M., Okumura, O., Sugimoto, J., and Kuwada, T. Three-step regulation of acid-base balance in body fluid after acid load. *Jpn. J. Physiol.* 11:109, 1961.

Primary and Mixed Disturbances

Brenner, B. M., and Stein, J. H. (Eds.). Acid-Base and Potassium Homeostasis. *Contemporary Issues in Nephrology,* vol. 2. New York: Churchill Livingstone, 1978.

Cahill, G. F., Jr. Ketosis. *Kidney Int.* 20:416, 1981.
The discussion is presented in "Nephrology Forum," which is a regular feature in this journal; it is the purpose of the fora "to relate the principles of basic science to clinical problems in nephrology."

Engel, K., Kildeberg, P., and Winters, R. W. Quantitative displacement of blood acid-base status in acute hypocapnia. *Scand. J. Clin. Lab. Invest.* 23:5, 1969.

Goodman, A. D., Lemann, J., Jr., Lennon, E. J., and Relman, A. S. Production, excretion, and net balance of fixed acid in patients with renal acidosis. *J. Clin. Invest.* 44:495, 1965.

Kassirer, J. P. Serious acid-base disorders. *N. Engl. J. Med.* 291:773, 1974.

Lemann, J., Jr., Lennon, E. J., Goodman, A. D., Litzow, J. R., and Relman, A. S. The net balance of acid in subjects given large loads of acid or alkali. *J. Clin. Invest.* 44:507, 1965.

Narins, R. G., and Emmett, M. Simple and mixed acid-base disorders: A practical approach. *Medicine* (Baltimore) 59:161, 1980.

Polak, A., Haynie, G. D., Hays, R. M., and Schwartz, W. B. Effects of chronic hypercapnia on electrolyte and acid-base equilibrium: I. Adaptation. *J. Clin. Invest.* 40:1223, 1961.

Tenney, S. M., and Lamb, T. W. Physiological Consequences of Hypoventilation and Hyperventilation. In W. O. Fenn and H. Rahn (Eds.), *Handbook of Physiology,* section 3, Respiration, vol. 2. Washington, D.C.: American Physiological Society, 1965.

Compensatory Responses

Brown, E. B., Jr. Physiological effects of hyperventilation. *Physiol. Rev.* 33:445, 1953.

Gennari, F. J., Goldstein, M. D., and Schwartz, W. B. The nature of the renal adaptation to chronic hypocapnia. *J. Clin. Invest.* 51:1722, 1972.

Madias, N. E., Adrogué, H. J., and Cohen, J. J. Maladaptive renal response to secondary hypercapnia in chronic metabolic alkalosis. *Am. J. Physiol.* 238 (Renal Fluid Electrolyte Physiol. 7):F283, 1980.

Nattie, E. E., and Romer, L. CSF HCO$_3^-$ regulation in isosmotic conditions: The role of brain Pco_2 and plasma HCO$_3^-$. *Respir. Physiol.* 33:177, 1978.

Nattie, E. E., and Tenney, S. M. Effect of potassium depletion on cerebrospinal fluid bicarbonate homeostasis. *Am. J. Physiol.* 231:579, 1976.

Pappenheimer, J. R. The ionic composition of cerebral extracellular fluid and its relation to control of breathing. *Harvey Lect.* 61:71, 1965.

Tuller, M. A., and Mehdi, F. Compensatory hypoventilation and hypercapnia in primary metabolic alkalosis. *Am. J. Med.* 50:281, 1971.

van Ypersele de Strihou, C., and Frans, A. The respiratory response to chronic metabolic alkalosis and acidosis in disease. *Clin. Sci. Mol. Med.* 45:439, 1973.

10 : Renal Excretion of H^+ and Conservation of HCO_3^-

Role of Kidneys in H^+ Balance

It is clear from Chapter 9 that the maintenance of a normal plasma pH depends on the preservation of a normal *ratio* between the weak acid and conjugate base components of each of the body buffers. By the isohydric principle (Eq. 9-13), these ratios can be determined precisely for all plasma buffers, from knowledge of the bicarbonate buffer system in plasma. Except for the slight correction necessitated by the Gibbs-Donnan effect, the plasma bicarbonate system will also reflect the ratio of all interstitial buffers; and as stated previously, in the steady state of most acid-base disturbances, any change in the plasma bicarbonate system will be accompanied by qualitatively similar changes of the intercellular buffers. It thus follows that regulating the ratio of the concentration of HCO_3^- to that of Pco_2 in plasma (Eq. 9-9) will tend to regulate the ratio of all other buffer pairs.

The weak acid component of the plasma bicarbonate buffer system is regulated as Pco_2 through alveolar ventilation (Eq. 9-9). Preservation of the conjugate base, HCO_3^-, is accomplished through the kidneys. This task involves two processes: (a) the reabsorption of virtually all the HCO_3^- that is filtered and (b) the reclamation of the HCO_3^- that was consumed in buffering fixed acids (Eq. 9-12). In the latter process, the H^+ ions of fixed acids that were incorporated into weak buffer acids are excreted by the kidneys. The combination of renal replenishment of HCO_3^- stores and renal excretion of the H^+ of fixed acids was described in Chapter 9 as the Third Line of Defense.

Reabsorption of Filtered HCO_3^-

Like Na^+ and other small solutes, HCO_3^- is freely filtered by the glomeruli. As is shown in Table 1-1, the daily filtered load of HCO_3^- in an adult human amounts to about 4,500 mEq. If even a very small portion of this were excreted in the urine, the normal stores of this important buffer would be quickly exhausted. This eventuality is prevented by avid tubular reabsorption of HCO_3^-, which normally amounts to more than 99.9% of the filtered load (Table 1-1).

In a series of classic studies conducted in the 1940s, R. F. Pitts and his colleagues showed conclusively that much of the acid that is excreted gets into the urine not by glomerular filtration but by tubular secretion. These workers reasoned that the source of this acid must be largely or exclusively carbon dioxide (Eq. 9-1), and they strengthened their thesis by demonstrating that inhibition of the enzyme carbonic anhydrase (C.A.; Eq. 9-2) greatly reduced or abolished the amount of acid that could be secreted. They suggested, furthermore, that acid was secreted in the form of H$^+$ ion in exchange for Na$^+$, rather than as molecular acid. A tremendous amount of subsequent experimental work by numerous investigators has proved the suggestions of Pitts to be largely correct. Figure 10-1 embodies these suggestions; although the schema varies in some details from that first drawn up by Pitts, the essence of his proposal has stood the test of time. Even now, some of the details are not fully settled.

Within tubular cells, water is split into H$^+$ and OH$^-$ (Fig. 10-1). [As stated in conjunction with Figure 9-2, this reaction rather than Equation 9-1 is chosen for the generation of H$^+$ because the hydroxylation of CO$_2$ (Eq. 9-2) is thought to be the reaction that is

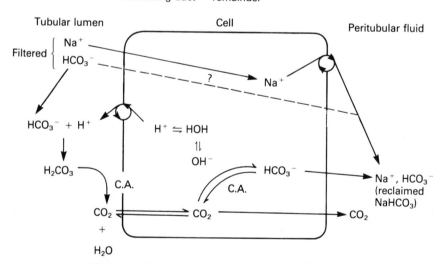

Proximal tubule 80–90%
Loop of Henle $\approx$ 2%
Distal tubule $\approx$ 8%
Collecting duct — remainder

Fig. 10-1 : Mechanism for the reabsorption of filtered HCO$_3$$^-$. C.A. stands for carbonic anhydrase; in the proximal tubule, but not in the distal tubule or collecting duct, tubular fluid is exposed to this enzyme, which is located in the luminal membrane. The percentages indicate the proportion of the filtered HCO$_3$$^-$ that is reabsorbed in each part of the nephron. In normal man producing a net amount of fixed acid, virtually all the filtered HCO$_3$$^-$ is conserved through reabsorption, either indirectly or directly.

catalyzed by carbonic anhydrase.] The H^+ is secreted into the tubular lumen; consideration of the transepithelial electrochemical potential difference (see, for example, Fig. 7-2) makes clear that this transport is almost certainly active all along the nephron, as denoted by the pump in the luminal membrane. In the tubular lumen, the secreted H^+ combines with filtered HCO_3^- to form H_2CO_3, which, within milliseconds, is converted to CO_2 and water under the influence of carbonic anhydrase. The arrow for the last step is deflected toward the cell to indicate that the carbonic anhydrase resides in the luminal cell membrane; tubular fluid is thus exposed to the enzyme even though carbonic anhydrase is not found in tubular fluid as such. The CO_2 that is formed within the lumen diffuses into the cell and peritubular fluid, although it is not in equilibrium with the latter space. The OH^- that results from the dissociation of water combines with CO_2 — again, under the influence of carbonic anhydrase — to form HCO_3^-, which diffuses into the peritubular fluid and blood. In addition, some filtered HCO_3^- is probably reabsorbed directly (indicated by the broken arrow with a question mark); disagreement persists on just how much HCO_3^- may be reabsorbed by this direct route. Finally, the filtered Na^+ is reabsorbed by mechanisms described in Chapter 7.

Note the net effects of the processes illustrated in Figure 10-1. For every filtered Na^+ that is reabsorbed, a HCO_3^- is returned to peritubular fluid and blood (as is indeed required for the preservation of electroneutrality) — possibly directly as HCO_3^- that was filtered, or indirectly as HCO_3^- derived from hydroxylated CO_2 or some other reaction (not shown); the indirect routes involve the disappearance of a filtered HCO_3^- through combination with secreted H^+. The mechanism shown in Figure 10-1 thus accomplishes the important task of *reclaiming virtually all of the filtered HCO_3^-* (Table 1-1). Note that it is not a mechanism for excreting H^+; to the extent that the CO_2 formed within the tubular lumen from secreted H^+ returns to the cell, ultimately to form more H^+ through hydroxylation, no net secretion of H^+ takes place.

The proportion of the total filtered HCO_3^- that disappears from tubular fluid in each of the major parts of the nephron is shown at the top of Figure 10-1. These values were derived by means of clearance ratios (see Answer to Problem 6-1, part 3), i.e., from knowledge of the concentrations of HCO_3^- and inulin in arterial plasma and tubular fluid. The concentration of HCO_3^- in the latter is often derived through measurement of the pH (Fig. 10-2) and P_{CO_2}, of tubular fluid and then application of the Henderson-Hasselbalch equation (Eq. 9-9). The results show that the vast majority of filtered HCO_3^- is reabsorbed in the proximal tubule, mainly in its early part as shown in Figure 7-3C.

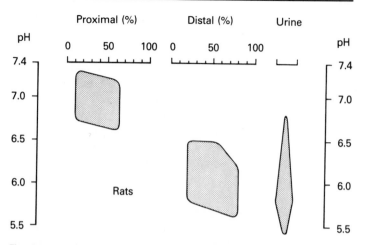

Fig. 10-2 : Changes in pH of tubular fluid in its course along the nephron. The enclosed areas cover the approximate range of values. Redrawn from Gottschalk, C. W., Lassiter, W. E., and Mylle, M. *Am. J. Physiol.* 198:581, 1960; and Vieira, F. L., and Malnic, G. *Am. J. Physiol.* 214:710, 1968.

FACTORS INFLUENCING THE RATE AT WHICH FILTERED HCO_3^- IS REABSORBED. The rate at which filtered HCO_3^- is returned to the blood can be affected by a number of factors, which often interact. Among the more important influences are the following: (1) the amount of HCO_3^- presented to the tubules; (2) the size of the extracellular fluid volume; (3) the arterial P_{CO_2}; (4) the concentration of Cl^- in the plasma; and (5) certain hormones.

1. Figure 10-3A shows a so-called titration curve for HCO_3^-, obtained in a fashion analogous to that described in Chapter 4 for glucose (Fig. 4-3). As the plasma HCO_3^- concentration is varied, so is the filtered load of this ion (GFR · $P_{HCO_3^-}$) and hence the amount of HCO_3^- that is presented to the tubules

Fig. 10-3

A. Titration curves for HCO_3^- in normal rats. Virtually all of the filtered HCO_3^- is reabsorbed unless the extracellular fluid volume is markedly expanded, in which case the reabsorptive rate is reduced despite a similar increase in the filtered load. The arrow indicates a normal arterial plasma HCO_3^- concentration (see Table 1-2). Adapted from Purkerson, M. L., et al. *J. Clin. Invest.* 48:1754, 1969.

B. Changes in the rate of HCO_3^- reabsorption in dogs as the arterial P_{CO_2} is either lowered through hyperventilation or raised through breathing gas mixtures containing increased concentrations of CO_2. Adapted from Rector, F. C., Jr., et al. *J. Clin. Invest.* 39:1706, 1960.

C. Influence of the plasma Cl^- concentration on the rate at which filtered HCO_3^- is reabsorbed. The data are from dogs in which the plasma Cl^- concentration was changed through the intravenous infusion of NaCl. From Pitts, R. F., and Lotspeich, W. D. *Am. J. Physiol.* 147:138, 1946.

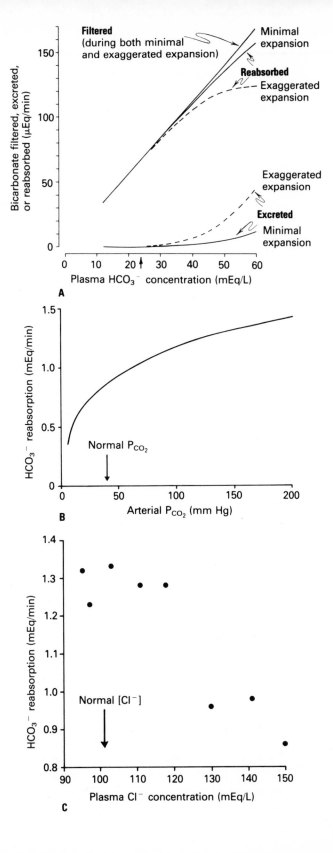

for reabsorption. Provided that other variables, such as the volume of extracellular fluid (see below), are held constant, the amount of HCO_3^- that is reabsorbed is almost the same as the load that is filtered into the tubules. The mechanism for this effect has not been clarified, save that the rate of HCO_3^- reabsorption appears to be closely linked to that of Na^+ reabsorption, especially in the early proximal tubule (Fig. 7-3C). It may thus be in part a consequence of the need to conserve Na^+ and maintain the extracellular fluid volume. The relationship shown in Figure 10-3A for minimal volume expansion protects H^+ balance and is reminiscent of the conservation of Na^+ (as discussed in Chap. 7, Challenges to Na^+ Balance), in that an increase in the filtered load of HCO_3^- (which could entail wastage of this important buffer) is immediately followed by increased reabsorption.

2. Also shown in Figure 10-3A is the effect of the extracellular fluid volume. When that volume is expanded markedly — as by infusing either $NaHCO_3$ or $NaCl$ — the reabsorption of filtered HCO_3^- is decreased, and the converse holds when the extracellular fluid volume is contracted. Although there appears to be a plateau for HCO_3^- reabsorption during exaggerated volume-expansion, a true Tm (see Chap. 4) for HCO_3^- does not exist. Again, the mechanisms by which extracellular fluid volume influences HCO_3^- reabsorption have not been fully clarified; the effect may be mediated mainly through changes in the plasma concentration of aldosterone (discussed below).

3. The influence of arterial P_{CO_2} is shown in Figure 10-3B. As P_{CO_2} is lowered (as by hyperventilation), the reabsorption of filtered HCO_3^- is decreased, and as P_{CO_2} is raised (as by alveolar hypoventilation), HCO_3^- reabsorption is increased. The effect is more marked during chronic than during acute alterations of the P_{CO_2}. The mechanisms that drive this response have not been conclusively identified. Some think that they involve the supply of more CO_2 substrate to the cell, but others consider this view too simplistic and have suggested that CO_2 may stimulate the secretory pump for H^+ or some other, related transport step. Whatever the mechanisms, it is clear from Equation 9-9 that the response will tend to correct the blood pH during a primary respiratory disturbance.

4. There is an inverse correlation between the plasma concentration of Cl^- and the rate at which filtered HCO_3^- is reabsorbed (Fig. 10-3C). This phenomenon may involve the well-known reciprocal relationship between the plasma concentrations of Cl^- and of HCO_3^-. In most situations, as the plasma Cl^- concentration falls, that of HCO_3^- rises, and vice versa; the same

is true when the initial event is a decrease or an increase in HCO$_3^-$. It is believed that the explanation for the reciprocal relationship involves the critical importance of maintaining extracellular fluid volume and hence Na$^+$ balance; that is, Na$^+$ reabsorption must be maintained, and, in order to preserve electroneutrality, either Cl$^-$ or HCO$_3^-$ must accompany the reabsorbed Na$^+$. In any case, given the reciprocal relationship, as plasma Cl$^-$ concentration rises, that of HCO$_3^-$ falls. Consequently, the filtered load of HCO$_3^-$ decreases, and that change, as discussed above in conjunction with Figure 10-3A, will lead to a decrease in the rate at which filtered HCO$_3^-$ is reabsorbed.

5. An increased plasma concentration of adrenal corticosteroids, as in Cushing's syndrome, leads to increased reabsorption of filtered HCO$_3^-$, and the converse occurs during adrenal cortical insufficiency (Addison's disease). Perhaps surprisingly, this effect is not mediated principally by influencing the renal handling of Na$^+$ or of K$^+$; it may involve an enhancement of H$^+$ transport by adrenal steroids.

Parathyroid hormone decreases the reabsorption of HCO$_3^-$; the mechanism is not known.

Replenishment of Depleted HCO$_3^-$ Stores

It was pointed out at the beginning of Chapter 9 that in persons whose diet is fairly high in protein there is a net daily production of nonvolatile (fixed) acids. These include sulfuric acid, resulting from protein catabolism, phosphoric acid, which is produced chiefly during the catabolism of phospholipids, and organic acids. These acids are buffered by the following types of reactions:

$$2\,H^+ + SO_4^{2-} + 2\,Na^+ + 2\,HCO_3^- \rightleftharpoons 2\,Na^+ + SO_4^{2-} + 2\,H_2O + 2\,CO_2 \nearrow \qquad (10\text{-}1)$$

$$2\,H^+ + HPO_4^{2-} + 2\,Na^+ + 2\,HCO_3^- \rightleftharpoons 2\,Na^+ + HPO_4^{2-} + 2\,H_2O + 2\,CO_2 \nearrow \qquad (10\text{-}2)$$

The CO$_2$ is eliminated via the lungs, as indicated by the diagonal arrows, and the two neutral salts, Na$_2$SO$_4$ and Na$_2$HPO$_4$, are filtered into Bowman's space. If these neutral salts were excreted in the urine, the body would soon become depleted of NaHCO$_3$, the main extracellular buffer that is utilized in neutralizing the fixed acids. The kidneys prevent such possible depletion of NaHCO$_3$, by two means: (a) the excretion of NH$_4^+$, which applies mainly to the handling of filtered Na$_2$SO$_4$; and (b) the excretion of titratable acid (T.A.), which pertains primarily to the filtered Na$_2$HPO$_4$. In both operations, HCO$_3^-$, newly formed within renal tubular cells, is absorbed into the peritubular blood along with Na$^+$ that was filtered.

Excretion of
Titratable Acid (T.A.)

As tubular fluid is acidified (Fig. 10-2) — both by the reabsorption of HCO_3^- and consequent decline of its concentration in tubular fluid (Eq. 9-9), and by the secretion of H^+ — the neutral salt Na_2HPO_4 is converted to the acid salt NaH_2PO_4 (for a depiction of this process, see Figure 10-6). The amount of strong base required to titrate the acid urine back to a pH of 7.40 (which is normally the pH of the glomerular filtrate) is *equal to the amount of titratable acid that was excreted in the urine.*

The probable schema for the formation of urinary T.A. is shown in Figure 10-4. The major reaction that generates the secreted H^+ is thought to be the dissociation of water; the OH^- that is simultaneously liberated combines with intracellular CO_2 under the catalysis of carbonic anhydrase, to form the HCO_3^- that is added to peritubular fluid and blood. Within the tubular lumen, the secreted H^+ combines with filtered $2 Na^+$, HPO_4^{2-} to form Na^+, $H_2PO_4^-$, which is excreted as T.A. in the urine. The second filtered Na^+ that is liberated in this reaction is reabsorbed to combine with the HCO_3^- that was newly formed within the cell. These reactions occur in all major parts of the nephron; in fact, they take place in the same cells as the schema depicted in Figure 10-1. But note that, whereas the net effect in Figure 10-1 is to recapture virtually all of the filtered HCO_3^-, the net effect in Figure 10-4 is to *replenish the blood with one HCO_3^- for every HCO_3^- that was consumed in buffering fixed H^+* (Eq. 10-2).

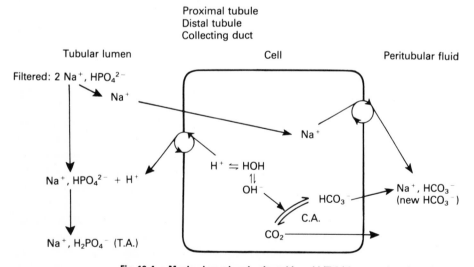

Fig. 10-4 : **Mechanism whereby titratable acid (T.A.) is created, and newly formed HCO_3^- is added to the blood along with a reabsorbed Na^+. In the proximal tubule, the CO_2 comes largely from the tubular lumen (see Fig. 10-1); in more distal parts of the nephron, it may come mainly from cellular metabolism. C.A. = carbonic anhydrase.**

FACTORS AFFECTING THE RATE OF T.A. EXCRETION. Two factors mainly influence the rate at which T.A. is excreted: the availability of urinary buffers and the pK of these buffers.

1. The effect of availability of urinary buffers is illustrated in Figure 10-5A, in which an increased supply of urinary buffer is reflected on the abscissa as increased excretion of phosphate. As more buffer is made available, more T.A. is excreted.

   The explanation involves a limiting concentration gradient for the transport of H$^+$ by renal cells. Besides HCO$_3^-$, inorganic phosphate is the main urinary buffer. At a pH of 7.4, at which it is filtered into Bowman's space, phosphate exists mainly as 2 Na$^+$,HPO$_4^{2-}$ (Fig. 10-6), and as the urine becomes more acid, it is converted to Na$^+$,H$_2$PO$_4^-$, which is the main urinary T.A. The minimal urinary pH is about 4.4, probably because collecting duct cells cannot transport H$^+$ against a concentration gradient exceeding about 1 : 1,000. When this minimal pH is attained (as it was in the experiment shown in Fig. 10-5A), virtually all the urinary phosphate is in the Na$^+$,H$_2$PO$_4^-$ form, and addition of even minute amounts of H$^+$ would then lead to a precipitous drop in pH (Fig. 10-6). Hence, under these conditions more H$^+$ can be excreted as T.A. only if more phosphate is filtered, i.e., only if the availability of more phosphate buffer in the tubular fluid enables the acceptance of more H$^+$ without a further drop in pH. This requirement was met by raising the plasma phosphate concentration and is reflected in the steadily increasing phosphate excretion in Figure 10-5A.

2. A buffer is most effective within ±1.0 pH unit of its pK (Fig. 9-5). Hence, given the normal pH of glomerular filtrate of about 7.4, phosphate with a pK of 6.8 can initially accept much more H$^+$ per unit drop in tubular fluid pH than can another buffer with a lower pK (Fig. 10-6). Furthermore, if the pK of the other buffer is close to the minimal urinary pH of 4.4, the total amount of H$^+$ that a quantum of that buffer can accept over the normal range of tubular fluid pH will be less than the amount accepted by the same quantum of phosphate. This fact is reflected in Figure 10-5B. Per millimole of buffer in the urine, more H$^+$ can be excreted as T.A. when phosphate is the main urinary buffer than when creatinine, with a pK of 4.97, is the main urinary buffer.

   This example illustrates the difference between *urinary acidification* and *H$^+$ excretion.* The ability to reduce the pH of urine, which is acidification, does not necessarily tell us much about the amount of H$^+$ being excreted. Note that the ordinate in Figure 10-6 shows the amount of H$^+$ excreted per

234

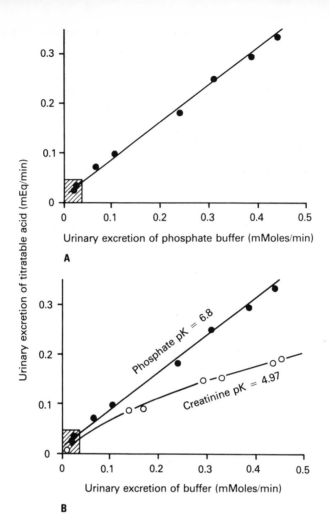

A

B

Fig. 10-5 : Two experiments in man, illustrating factors that influence the rate at which titratable acid (T.A.) is excreted in the urine. The experiments were done on the same person, who was either in a state of normal H^+ balance or in metabolic acidosis induced by ingesting NH_4Cl. This salt leads to acidosis through net addition of hydrochloric acid, as in the following reaction:

$$2\ NH_4Cl + CO_2 \rightleftharpoons 2\ HCl + H_2O + CO(NH_2)_2.$$
$$\text{urea}$$

A. In this experiment, the subject was in mild metabolic acidosis (plasma pH = 7.37; plasma HCO_3^- concentration = 14 mMoles/liter; urinary pH = 4.5). The points enclosed in the shaded rectangle represent excretion of endogenous phosphate; all other points were obtained during the intravenous infusion of inorganic phosphate at pH 7.40.

B. Differences in the amount of H^+ excreted as T.A., when phosphate is the main urinary buffer or when creatinine is the main buffer. The points for phosphate are those illustrated in (A); those for creatinine (open circles) are data obtained in the same subject (plasma pH = 7.38; plasma HCO_3^- concentration = 13 mMoles/liter; urinary pH = 5.1) when creatinine was infused intravenously instead of phosphate.

Both graphs slightly modified from Schiess, W. A., Ayer, J. L., Lotspeich, W. D., and Pitts, R. F. *J. Clin. Invest.* 27:57, 1948. It is of interest that the subject for these experiments was Dr. Pitts, whose work has contributed so much to our understanding of the renal regulation of acid-base balance.

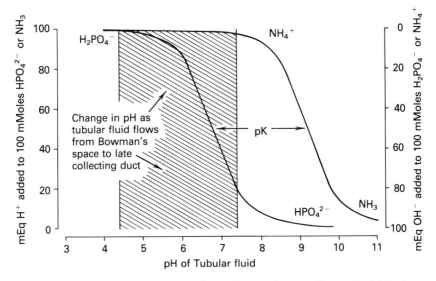

Fig. 10-6 : Titration of HPO_4^{2-} and NH_3 by H^+ as the pH of tubular fluid is de-creased from 7.4 in Bowman's space to 4.4 in the late collecting duct. With a pK of 9.2, the NH_3/NH_4^+ system is a relatively poor buffer in the pH range that ordi-narily exists in tubular fluid (shaded area). Nevertheless, a great deal of H^+ can be excreted as NH_4^+ because the supply of NH_3 from tubular cells is potentially plentiful (see Table 10-1). Adapted from Valtin, H. *Renal Dysfunction: Mechanisms Involved in Fluid and Solute Imbalance.* Boston: Little, Brown, 1979.

quantum of HPO_4^{2-} presented for titration. Therefore, if, say, 10 times more HPO_4^{2-} were to traverse the tubular system (as was done in the experiment shown in Fig. 10-5A by increasing the filtered load of phosphate), the amount of H^+ excreted could rise tenfold without any change in urinary pH.

Excretion of Ammonium — Nonionic Diffusion

If the formation of T.A. were the only mechanism for excreting H^+, the amount of H^+ that could be eliminated in the urine would be severely limited by the amount of phosphate that is filtered. As soon as the titration curve for phosphate would shift to the formation of H_3PO_4 from $Na^+,H_2PO_4^-$, urinary pH would fall below 4.4 (Fig. 10-6) and no more H^+ could be secreted by the renal tubular cells (see point 1 above). Yet, it can be shown that much more H^+ than that which appears as T.A. can be excreted in the urine even though the urine pH does not fall below the minimum value of 4.4. It was therefore apparent that an addi-tional mechanism existed for the excretion of H^+.

The observation that in acidosis there is a rise not only in urinary T.A. but also in urinary NH_4^+ raised the suspicion that NH_3 might be the additional acceptor for H^+, as by the following type of reaction:

$$H^+ + Cl^- + NH_3 \rightleftharpoons NH_4^+ + Cl^- \qquad (10\text{-}3)$$

Note that the H^+ is incorporated into the neutral salt NH_4Cl, so that this reaction would satisfy the requirement of excreting H^+ without a further decrease in urinary pH; in other words, neutral ammonium salts are not titratable acids.

The suspicion that the ammonia/ammonium system was involved was strengthened by the following findings: that the concentration of NH_3 is higher in renal venous blood than in renal arterial blood; that the delivery of NH_3 to the kidney from arterial blood is too low to account for the amount of NH_4^+ that is excreted in the urine; and that the concentration of NH_3 in arterial blood is unchanged in severe acidosis when urinary NH_4^+ excretion is greatly enhanced. The conclusion seemed inescapable that NH_3 must be produced within the kidney and that it is excreted as NH_4^+ in the urine after accepting a H^+.

The probable mechanism for the urinary excretion of NH_4^+ is illustrated in Figure 10-7. Here, too, the hydroxylation of CO_2 under the influence of carbonic anhydrase is thought to be the source of the HCO_3^- that is added to peritubular fluid and blood; and the H^+ that is simultaneously evolved from the splitting of water is secreted into the tubular lumen.

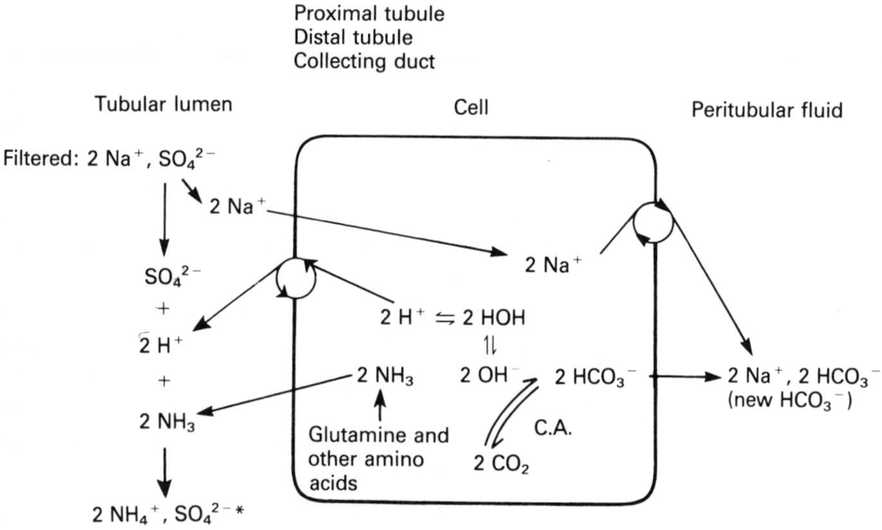

Fig. 10-7 : **Mechanism for the renal excretion of NH_4^+. Glutamine and other amino acid substrates come from the blood and enter the cell from the peritubular and luminal side. In the proximal tubule, the CO_2 comes largely from the tubular lumen (see Fig. 10-1); in more distal parts of the nephron, it may come mainly from cellular metabolism. C.A. = carbonic anhydrase.**

*The excretion of 2 NH_4^+, SO_4^{2-} is shown here, rather than that of NH_4^+, Cl^-, to indicate how the filtered Na_2SO_4 (which is derived from buffering of H_2SO_4; Eq. 10-1) is handled.

NH$_3$ is derived from glutamine and other amino acids in the blood, which are broken down within the renal tubular cells. This nonionized form is lipid-soluble and thus freely diffusible across virtually the entire cell membrane, which is composed largely of fat. NH$_3$ therefore diffuses passively down its concentration gradient into the tubular lumen. The pK of the NH$_3$/NH$_4^+$ buffer system is about 9.2 (Table 1-3). Therefore, at the pH of tubular fluid, H$^+$ avidly combines with NH$_3$ so that the system exists almost entirely in the NH$_4^+$ form (see Fig. 10-6). This ionized form, unlike NH$_3$, is not lipid-soluble and therefore traverses the cell membrane much less readily, since its transit is confined to the aqueous channels. Consequently, the NH$_4^+$ is trapped within the tubular lumen, and is then excreted in the form of neutral salts, such as NH$_4$Cl or (NH$_4$)$_2$SO$_4$. [For reasons explained in the legend to Figure 10-7, the excretion of 2 NH$_4^+$, SO$_4^{2-}$, rather than of NH$_4^+$, Cl$^-$, is shown; it should be realized, however, that NH$_4^+$ is excreted mainly as the chloride salt (see Answer to Problem 11-1 and its figure, as well as Fig. 10-9).] In the process, the HCO$_3^-$, which was newly formed within the tubular cell, is added to the blood along with the filtered Na$^+$ that is reabsorbed. As was the case with the excretion of T.A., the net result of the NH$_4^+$ mechanism is thus *the excretion of H$^+$, the replenishment of the body HCO$_3^-$ stores, and the reabsorption of filtered Na$^+$*. These reactions probably occur in all parts of the nephron.

NONIONIC DIFFUSION. The process by which the lipid-soluble, nonionized moiety of a buffer pair (e.g., NH$_3$) can readily diffuse across a cell membrane, while the lipid-insoluble, ionized member (e.g., NH$_4^+$) cannot, is known as nonionic diffusion or diffusion-trapping. Note that in the case of the urinary excretion of NH$_4^+$ this process aids the secretion of NH$_3$ and hence the excretion of H$^+$. The moment that NH$_3$ enters the tubular lumen, virtually all of it is converted to NH$_4^+$ (Figs. 10-6 and 10-7), so that a constant "sink" for the continued diffusion of NH$_3$ is maintained. This positive feedback, so to speak, is the more effective, the lower the urinary pH (Fig. 10-8); i.e., the secretion of NH$_3$ and, hence, the excretion of H$^+$ are most efficient in acidosis when more H$^+$ needs to be eliminated.

Nonionic diffusion is a common biological phenomenon that has important clinical applications in promoting the urinary excretion of weak acids and weak bases. An example of the utilization of this principle in the treatment of phenobarbital poisoning is given in Problem 10-1 and the corresponding Answer.

CONTROL OF RENAL NH$_3$ PRODUCTION AND EXCRETION. At least three factors influence the amount of NH$_3$ that is produced and secreted into the tubular lumen: the pH of the urine, the chronic-

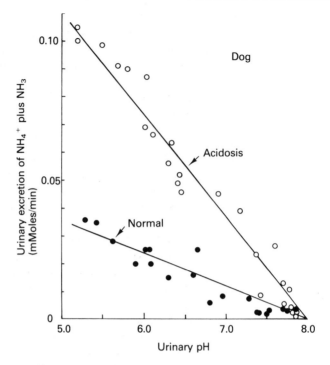

Fig. 10-8 : Influence of urinary pH and state of acid-base balance, on the urinary excretion of total ammonia (NH_4^+ plus NH_3). All the data were obtained
from one dog. At the beginning of each experiment the urinary pH was about
5.2, both in normal H^+ balance and after 48 hours of metabolic acidosis. The
urinary pH was then gradually increased in each instance by infusing $NaHCO_3$
intravenously. From Pitts, R. F. *Fed. Proc.* 7:418, 1948.

ity of acidosis, and the relative rates of flow of peritubular blood
and tubular fluid.

1. The influence of urinary pH was discussed above and is depicted in Figure 10-8. During both normal H^+ balance and
   states of metabolic acidosis, there is an inverse relationship
   between the urinary pH and the amount of total ammonia
   (i.e., NH_3 plus NH_4^+) that is excreted in the urine. The more
   acid the urine, the greater the proportion of total ammonia
   that exists in the ionized form (see Fig. 10-6); hence, the more
   acid the urine, the lower the urinary concentration of NH_3 and
   the greater the concentration difference promoting the passive diffusion of NH_3 from renal tubular cell into the tubular
   lumen. Since this NH_3 is immediately converted to NH_4^+
   within the tubular lumen, it cannot diffuse back into the cell,
   but is instead excreted.

2. The influence of the duration of acidosis is also illustrated in
   Figure 10-8, which shows that, *at any given urinary pH,* the

rate of total ammonia excretion is higher in acidosis (especially when present for hours or days) than during normal H$^+$ balance. It is important to note that this does not involve the explanation given in paragraph 1, since the difference can be detected at the same urinary pH. Rather, the explanation involves an increased renal production of NH$_3$, which is an important adaptive mechanism that enables increased excretion of H$^+$ during acidosis. Despite a great deal of work, it is not yet known precisely how this adaptation comes about.

3. When tubular fluid has the same pH as blood, which it usually does not (Fig. 10-2), the flow rates of these two solutions determine the rates of NH$_3$ diffusion into them. Since peritubular blood flow is much greater than the flow of tubular fluid, blood would carry off the NH$_3$ more rapidly and thereby maintain a more favorable sink for the further diffusion of NH$_3$. Normally, however, when tubular fluid is acid, about 75% of the NH$_3$ produced within renal cells diffuses into the tubular lumen, and about 25% into the blood. Under the admittedly unusual conditions, when the pH of the two fluids is equal, or when the pH is higher in tubular fluid than in blood, the majority of renal NH$_3$ diffuses into the blood; when the urinary pH is 8, virtually no NH$_3$ enters the tubular fluid (Fig. 10-8).

Relative Excretion Rates of Titratable Acid and Ammonium

Table 10-1 shows rates of H$^+$ excretion as NH$_4^+$ and as T.A., both in the normal situation and in two disease states that are characterized by disturbances of H$^+$ balance. It was pointed out in the beginning of Chapter 9 that in a normal person whose diet is relatively high in protein there is a net daily production of 40 to 60 mMoles of nonvolatile acids. In the steady (equilibrium) state, this amount of acid is excreted as H$^+$ combined with NH$_3$ or as T.A.; more H$^+$ is normally excreted as NH$_4^+$ than as T.A.

During uncontrolled diabetes mellitus, there is an overproduction of nonvolatile acids, mainly β-OH butyric acid. This leads to primary metabolic acidosis, which, as discussed earlier, increases the urinary excretion of NH$_4^+$ (Fig. 10-8). The pK of β-OH butyrate is slightly less than that of creatinine (Table 1-3); hence β-OH butyrate is ordinarily a less effective urinary buffer than are phosphate and creatinine (Figs. 10-5B and 10-6). During diabetic acidosis, however, the endogenous production and, hence, the filtered load of β-OH butyrate are so great that in this condition β-OH butyrate becomes the main urinary buffer, and T.A. appears primarily as β-OH butyric acid. Nevertheless, the data in Table 10-1 during diabetic acidosis show that the potential supply of NH$_3$ as a urinary buffer is enormous, and considerably greater than that of buffers that form titratable acids.

Table 10-1 : Relative excretion rates of ammonium and titratable acid (T.A.) in healthy persons and in two disease states that are accompanied by primary metabolic acidosis.

Condition	mEq of Urinary H^+ per Day
Health	
H^+ combined with NH_3	30 to 50
H^+ as T.A.	10 to 30
Diabetic acidosis	
H^+ combined with NH_3	300 to 500
H^+ as T.A.	75 to 250
Chronic renal disease	
H^+ combined with NH_3	0.5 to 15
H^+ as T.A.	2 to 20

From Pitts, R. F. *Science* 102:49;81, 1945. Published with permission.

During chronic renal disease, which is accompanied by a marked decrease in the amount of functioning renal tissue, there may be a reduction in both forms of fixed-acid excretion, depending largely on the protein content of the patient's diet. The reduction, however, is relatively much greater for NH_3 than for T.A. This is so because the rate of T.A. excretion depends largely on the urinary excretion of buffer (Fig. 10-5A), which may remain normal until renal disease advances very far; formation of NH_4^+, however, depends on the renal cellular production of NH_3, which is greatly curtailed as the amount of functioning renal tissue is reduced.

Summary

The kidneys play a major role in the regulation of H^+ balance by maintaining the normal body store (and hence concentration) of HCO_3^-, and by excreting the H^+ that is derived from the daily production of nonvolatile (fixed) acids. Preservation of the HCO_3^- store is accomplished through: (a) the reabsorption of virtually all the HCO_3^- that is filtered (Fig. 10-1); and (b) the formation of new HCO_3^- within renal cells and addition of this HCO_3^- to the blood (Figs. 10-4 and 10-7). Net excretion of H^+ also occurs via two mechanisms: (c) the excretion of titratable acid (T.A.; Fig. 10-4), which is quantified as the amount of strong base that must be added to acid urine in order to return the pH of that urine to7.4; and (d) the excretion of neutral NH_4^+ salts after H^+ has combined with secreted NH_3 (Fig. 10-7). The last process involves the principle of nonionic diffusion or diffusion-trapping.

In the text of this chapter, each of these processes was described separately, both for the sake of clarity and to account for the various aspects of H^+ balance quantitatively. It must be realized, however, that the major mechanisms take place simultaneously

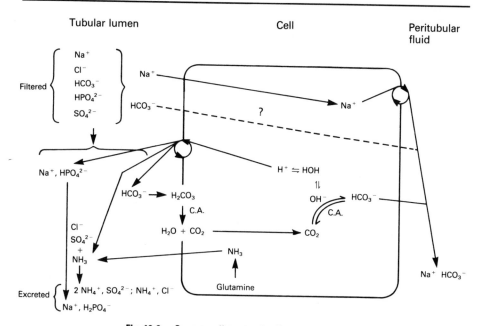

Fig. 10-9 : Summary diagram, showing the various means by which the kidneys help maintain H^+ balance. Although each mechanism occurs in virtually all parts of the nephron, some processes predominate in one part (e.g., titration of filtered HCO_3^- in the proximal tubule) while others predominate in another part (e.g., titration of NH_3 in the collecting duct). The diagram is a simplification, which does not show some unresolved questions; it is likely, for example, that the hydroxylation of CO_2 is not the only source for secreted H^+, and that carbonic anhydrase has a function in the peritubular membrane (possibly to enhance HCO_3^- transport) as well as in the luminal membrane and cytoplasm.

in the same cells, that the secreted H^+ comes from a common cellular pool, and that the kidney does not distinguish a H^+ that is destined to combine with filtered HCO_3^- from one that will combine with HPO_4^{2-} or NH_3; nor will it distinguish a reabsorbed HCO_3^- that was generated within the cell from one that was initially filtered, or a reabsorbed Na^+ that came from $NaHCO_3$ from one that came from the chloride, phosphate, sulfate, or some other filtered salt. In order to emphasize these points, the processes are summarized in Figure 10-9, where they are shown as occurring in a single tubular cell.

The rate at which filtered HCO_3^- is reabsorbed is affected by: the filtered load of HCO_3^-, expansion or contraction of the extracellular fluid, the arterial P_{CO_2}, the concentration of Cl^- in the plasma, and certain hormones, notably adrenal corticosteroids and parathyroid hormone. The rate of T.A. excretion is influenced principally by: the availability of buffers within the tubular fluid, and the pK of those buffers. And the rate of urinary NH_4^+ excretion is governed by: the pH of the urine, the chronicity of acidosis, and the relative rates of flow of peritubular blood as compared to tubular fluid, especially when the urinary pH is equal to or higher than the pH of plasma.

Normally, about three-fourths of the daily endogenous load of nonvolatile acid is excreted as NH_4^+, and the remainder as T.A. The potential supply of NH_3 as a H^+ acceptor is very large, rising as much as tenfold in states such as diabetic acidosis. Since NH_3 is generated within renal cells, however, this adaptive mechanism may be greatly curtailed in chronic renal disease, when the total amount of functioning renal tissue is reduced.

Problem 10-1

UTILIZATION OF THE PRINCIPLE OF NONIONIC DIFFUSION IN THE TREATMENT OF PHENOBARBITAL POISONING. A 23-year-old woman is admitted to the emergency ward in coma and with a history of having ingested a large amount of phenobarbital. Her respirations are shallow, and her systemic blood pressure is somewhat low. The patient is several times incontinent of urine, which probably means that urine production is adequate despite the mild hypotension.

After instituting measures to re-establish normal respiration and to support the systemic circulation, the attending physician begins efforts to hasten the excretion of phenobarbital. Although much of the drug is metabolized in the liver, as much as 30% of the total dose may be excreted unchanged by the kidney. The compound, having a molecular weight of 232 daltons, enters the tubular system mainly through filtration, and it is then passively reabsorbed. Many physicians would choose to treat this patient by means of dialysis, either with an artificial kidney or through peritoneal dialysis. When the urine flow is adequate, however, as in this patient, forced diuresis and alkalinization of the urine is an acceptable alternative mode of therapy.

The attending physician therefore begins to infuse mannitol and $NaHCO_3$ intravenously. Mannitol, with a molecular weight of 182 daltons (Table 1-5), is freely filtered but very poorly or not at all reabsorbed. Hence, by contributing to the osmolality of tubular fluid, mannitol inhibits the passive reabsorption of water and initiates a diuresis. By this means, mannitol decreases the passive reabsorption of phenobarbital, analogous to the reduction of passive urea reabsorption when the urine flow is increased (Fig. 4-4). The infusion of $NaHCO_3$ will alkalinize the urine, shift the titration of the weak acid phenobarbital (pK of 7.2) toward the ionized form (Fig. 10-6), and thereby diminish the passive reabsorption of phenobarbital through the process of nonionic diffusion.

It is determined that the concentration of total phenobarbital (i.e., the nonionized plus the ionized form) in this patient is 10 mg per 100 ml of plasma. About 40% of phenobarbital is bound to plasma proteins. On admission, the plasma pH is 7.3 (primary respiratory acidosis due to depression of the respiratory center) and urinary pH is 5.2; after correction of the alveolar hypoventilation through assisted respiration, and infusion of NaHCO$_3$, the plasma pH is 7.7 and the urinary pH is 8.2. The pK of the phenobarbital system is 7.2. Given these facts, complete the table below.

	Total Unbound Phenobarbital in Plasma (mg/100 ml)	Ratio of Unbound Phenobarbital: [Ionized] / [Nonionized]	Plasma Concentration of Unbound Phenobarbital	
			Ionized	Nonionized (mg/100 ml)
Plasma, pH 7.3				
Plasma, pH 7.7				
Urine, pH 5.2	—		—	—
Urine, pH 8.2	—		—	—

Problem 10-2   Is NH$_4$Cl a titratable acid (T.A.)? Defend your answer, utilizing Figure 10-6.

Problem 10-3   Theoretically, to what extent could urine be acidified just by reabsorbing filtered HCO$_3^-$, without excretion of T.A.? *Hint:* Apply the Henderson-Hasselbalch equation (Eq. 9-9), using a pK' of 6.1 and a P$_{CO_2}$ for urine of 40 mm Hg.

Selected References

General

Arruda, J. A. L., and Kurtzman, N. A. Acid-Base Physiology and Pathophysiology. In S. Klahr and S. G. Massry (Eds.), *Contemporary Nephrology*, vol. 1. New York: Plenum, 1981.

Baruch, S. (Ed.). Symposium on renal metabolism. *Med. Clin. North Am.* 59:505, 1975.
This symposium was held in honor of Dr. Robert F. Pitts, whose work elucidated many of the mechanisms by which the kidney regulates H$^+$ balance. In a beautifully written and learned Dedication that introduces this volume, Dr. Erich E. Windhager describes the qualities that made Dr. Pitts a greatly admired teacher and investigator.

Brenner, B. M., and Stein, J. H. (Eds.). Acid-Base and Potassium Homeostasis. *Contemporary Issues in Nephrology*, vol. 2. New York: Churchill Livingstone, 1978.

Cohen, J. J., and Kassirer, J. P. *Acid-Base.* Boston: Little, Brown, 1982.

Gennari, F. J., and Cohen, J. J. Role of the kidney in potassium homeostasis: Lessons from acid-base disturbances. *Kidney Int.* 8:1, 1975.

Karlmark, B., and Danielson, B. G. Titratable acid, P$_{CO_2}$, bicarbonate and ammonium ions along the rat proximal tubule. *Acta Physiol. Scand.* 91:243, 1974.

Levine, D. Z. Difficulties in the micropuncture evaluation of proximal renal bicarbonate reabsorption: An overview for the general reader. *Can. J. Physiol. Pharmacol.* 56:354, 1978.

Malnic, G., and Giebisch, G. Cellular Aspects of Renal Tubular Acidification. In G. Giebisch (Ed.), *Transport Organs,* vol. IVA. New York: Springer-Verlag, 1979.

Malnic, G., and Steinmetz, P. R. Transport processes in urinary acidification. *Kidney Int.* 9:172, 1976.

Masoro, E. J., and Siegel, P. D. *Acid-Base Regulation: Its Physiology, Pathophysiology and the Interpretation of Blood-Gas Analysis* (2nd ed.). Philadelphia: Saunders, 1977.

Pitts, R. F. Mechanisms for stabilizing the alkaline reserves of the body. *Harvey Lect.* 48:172, 1953.

Rector, F. C., Jr. (Ed.). Symposium on acid-base homeostasis. *Kidney Int.* 1:273, 1972.

Schulz, I., Sachs, G., Forte, J. G., and Ullrich, K. J. (Eds.). *Hydrogen Ion Transport in Epithelia.* Developments in Bioenergetics and Biomembranes, vol. 4. Amsterdam: Elsevier/North Holland, 1980.

Simpson, D. P. Control of hydrogen ion homeostasis and renal acidosis. *Medicine* (Baltimore) 50:503, 1971.

Simpson, D. P., and Hager, S. R. pH and bicarbonate effects on mitochondrial anion accumulation. Proposed mechanism for changes in renal metabolite levels in acute acid-base disturbances. *J. Clin. Invest.* 63:704, 1979.

Steinmetz, P. R. Excretion of acid by the kidney: Functional organization and cellular aspects of acidification. *N. Engl. J. Med.* 278:1102, 1968.

Steinmetz, P. R. Cellular mechanisms of urinary acidification. *Physiol. Rev.* 54:890, 1974.

Tannen, R. L. Control of acid excretion by the kidney. *Annu. Rev. Med.* 31:35, 1980.

Warnock, D. G., and Rector, F. C., Jr. Renal Acidification Mechanisms. In B. M. Brenner and F. C. Rector, Jr. (Eds.), *The Kidney* (2nd ed.). Philadelphia: Saunders, 1981.

H⁺ Secretion

Al-Awqati, Q. H^+ transport in urinary epithelia. *Am. J. Physiol.* 235 (Renal Fluid Electrolyte Physiol. 4):F77, 1978.

Aronson, P. S. Identifying secondary active solute transport in epithelia. *Am. J. Physiol.* 240 (Renal Fluid Electrolyte Physiol. 9):F1, 1981.

Brodsky, W. A. (Ed.). Anion and proton transport. *Ann. N.Y. Acad. Sci.* 341:1, 1980.
Part II of this symposium deals especially with the kidney and related epithelia, but the rest of the volume contains a great deal of useful and interesting information.

Cohen, L. H., and Steinmetz, P. R. Control of active proton transport in turtle urinary bladder by cell pH. *J. Gen. Physiol.* 76:381, 1980.

DeSousa, R. C., Harrington, J. T., Ricanati, E. S., Shelkrot, J. W., and

Schwartz, W. B. Renal regulation of acid-base equilibrium during chronic administration of mineral acid. *J. Clin. Invest.* 53:465, 1974.

Gottschalk, C. W., Lassiter, W. E., and Mylle, M. Localization of urine acidification in the mammalian kidney. *Am. J. Physiol.* 198:581, 1960.

Green, H. H., Steinmetz, P. R., and Frazier, H. S. Evidence for proton transport by turtle bladder in presence of ambient bicarbonate. *Am. J. Physiol.* 218:845, 1970.

Hulter, H. N., Licht, J. H., Bonner, E. L., Jr., Glynn, R. D., and Sebastian, A. Effects of glucocorticoid steroids on renal and systemic acid-base metabolism. *Am. J. Physiol.* 239 (Renal Fluid Electrolyte Physiol. 8):F30, 1980.

Malnic, G., Mello-Aires, M., and Giebisch, G. Micropuncture study of renal tubular hydrogen ion transport during alterations of acid-base equilibrium in the rat. *Am. J. Physiol.* 222:147, 1972.

Murer, H., Hopfer, U., and Kinne, R. Sodium/proton antiport in brush-border-membrane vesicles isolated from rat small intestine and kidney. *Biochem. J.* 154:597, 1976.

Schwartz, J. H., Finn, J. T., Vaughan, G., and Steinmetz, P. R. Distribution of metabolic CO$_2$ and the transported ion species in acidification by turtle bladder. *Am. J. Physiol.* 226:283, 1974.

Tam, S.-C., Goldstein, M. B., Stinebaugh, B. J., Chen, C.-B., Gougoux, A., and Halperin, M. L. Studies on the regulation of hydrogen ion secretion in the collecting duct in vivo: Evaluation of factors that influence the urine minus blood P$_{CO_2}$ difference. *Kidney Int.* 20:636, 1981.

Terao, N., and Tannen, R. L. Characterization of acidification by the isolated perfused rat kidney: Evidence for adaptation by the distal nephron to a high bicarbonate diet. *Kidney Int.* 20:36, 1981.

Ullrich, K. J., Rumrich, G., and Baumann, K. Renal proximal tubular buffer-(glycodiazine) transport. Inhomogeneity of local transport rate, dependence on sodium, effect of inhibitors and chronic adaptation. *Pflügers Arch. Eur. J. Physiol.* 357:149, 1975.

Vieira, F. L., and Malnic, G. Hydrogen ion secretion by rat renal cortical tubules as studied by an antimony microelectrode. *Am. J. Physiol.* 214:710, 1968.

Warnock, D. G., and Rector, F. C., Jr. Proton secretion by the kidney. *Annu. Rev. Physiol.* 41:197, 1979.

Ziegler, T. W., Fanestil, D. D., and Ludens, J. H. Influence of transepithelial potential difference on acidification in the toad urinary bladder. *Kidney Int.* 10:279, 1976.

Conservation of Filtered HCO$_3^+$

Boylan, J. W., Antkowiak, D. E., and Calkins, J. Maximum rates of bicarbonate reabsorption by the dogfish kidney. *Bull. Mount Desert Island Biol. Lab.* 13:17, 1973.

Burg, M. B., and Green, N. Bicarbonate transport by isolated perfused rabbit proximal convoluted tubules. *Am. J. Physiol.* 233 (Renal Fluid Electrolyte Physiol. 2):F307, 1977.

Cogan, M. G., Maddox, D. A., Warnock, D. G., Lin, E. T., and Rector, F. C., Jr. Effect of acetazolamide on bicarbonate reabsorption in the proximal tubule of the rat. *Am. J. Physiol.* 237 (Renal Fluid Electrolyte Physiol. 6):F447, 1979.

Cohen, L. HCO_3-Cl exchange transport in the adaptive response to alkalosis by turtle bladder. *Am. J. Physiol.* 239 (Renal Fluid Electrolyte Physiol. 8):F167, 1980.

DuBose, T. D., Jr., Pucacco, L. R., and Carter, N. W. Determination of disequilibrium pH in the rat kidney in vivo: Evidence for hydrogen secretion. *Am. J. Physiol.* 240 (Renal Fluid Electrolyte Physiol. 9):F138, 1981.

DuBose, T. D., Jr., Pucacco, L. R., Seldin, D. W., Carter, N. W., and Kokko, J. P. Microelectrode determination of pH and Pco_2 in rat proximal tubule after benzolamide: Evidence for hydrogen ion secretion. *Kidney Int.* 15:624, 1979.

Fuller, G. R., MacLeod, M. B., and Pitts, R. F. Influence of administration of potassium salts on the renal tubular reabsorption of bicarbonate. *Am. J. Physiol.* 182:111, 1955.

Gennari, F. J., Caflisch, C. R., Johns, C., Maddox, D. A., and Cohen, J. J. Pco_2 measurements in surface proximal tubules and peritubular capillaries of the rat kidney. *Am. J. Physiol.* 242 (Renal Fluid Electrolyte Physiol. 11):F78, 1982.

Gennari, F. J., Johns, C., and Caflisch, C. R. Effect of benzolamide on pH in the proximal tubules and peritubular capillaries of the rat kidney. *Pflügers Arch. Eur. J. Physiol.* 387:69, 1980.

Giebisch, G., MacLeod, M. B., and Pitts, R. F. Effect of adrenal steroids on renal tubular reabsorption of bicarbonate. *Am. J. Physiol.* 183:377, 1955.

Kassirer, J. P., and Schwartz, W. B. Correction of metabolic alkalosis in man without repair of K^+ deficiency: A re-evaluation of the role of potassium. *Am. J. Med.* 40:19, 1966.

Kurtzman, N. A. Regulation of renal bicarbonate reabsorption by extracellular volume. *J. Clin. Invest.* 49:586, 1970.

Levine, D. Z. Effect of acute hypercapnia on proximal tubular water and bicarbonate reabsorption. *Am. J. Physiol.* 221:1164, 1971.

Maren, T. H. Chemistry of the renal reabsorption of bicarbonate. *Can. J. Physiol. Pharmacol.* 52:1041, 1974.

McKinney, T. D., and Burg, M. B. Bicarbonate and fluid reabsorption by renal proximal straight tubules. *Kidney Int.* 12:1, 1977.

McKinney, T. D., and Burg, M. B. Bicarbonate transport by rabbit cortical collecting tubules. Effect of acid and alkali loads in vivo on transport in vitro. *J. Clin. Invest.* 60:766, 1977.

Mello-Aires, M., and Malnic, G. Peritubular pH and Pco_2 in renal tubular acidification. *Am. J. Physiol.* 228:1766, 1975.

Pitts, R. F., and Lotspeich, W. D. Bicarbonate and the renal regulation of acid base balance. *Am. J. Physiol.* 147:138, 1946.

Purkerson, M. L., Lubowitz, H., White, R. W., and Bricker, N. S. On the influence of extracellular fluid volume expansion on bicarbonate reabsorption in the rat. *J. Clin. Invest.* 48:1754, 1969.

Rector, F. C., Jr., Carter, N. W., and Seldin, D. W. The mechanism of bicarbonate reabsorption in the proximal and distal tubules of the kidney. *J. Clin. Invest.* 44:278, 1965.

Schwartz, G. J., Weinstein, A. M., Steele, R. E., Stephenson, J. L., and

Burg, M. B. Carbon dioxide permeability of rabbit proximal convoluted tubules. *Am. J. Physiol.* 240 (Renal Fluid Electrolyte Physiol. 9):F231, 1981.

Slaughter, B. D., Osiecki, H. S., Cross, R. B., Budtz-Olsen, O., and Jedrzejczyk, H. The regulation of bicarbonate reabsorption: The role of arterial pH, P_{CO_2} and plasma bicarbonate concentration. *Pflügers Arch. Eur. J. Physiol.* 349:29, 1974.

Sohtell, M., and Karlmark, B. In vivo micropuncture P_{CO_2} measurements. *Pflügers Arch. Eur. J. Physiol.* 363:179, 1976.

Walser, M., and Mudge, G. H. Renal Excretory Mechanisms. In C. L. Comar and F. Bronner (Eds.), *Mineral Metabolism.* New York: Academic, 1960.

Titratable Acid and Ammonia

Balagura-Baruch, S. Renal Metabolism and Transfer of Ammonia. In C. Rouiller and A. F. Muller (Eds.), *The Kidney,* vol. III. New York: Academic, 1971.

Burch, H. B., Chan, A. W. K., Alvey, T. R., and Lowry, O. H. Localization of glutamine accumulation and tubular reabsorption in rat nephron. *Kidney Int.* 14:406, 1978.

Cheema-Dhadli, S., and Halperin, M. L. Role of the mitochondrial anion transporters in the regulation of ammoniagenesis in renal cortex mitochondria of the rabbit and rat. *Eur. J. Biochem.* 99:483, 1979.

Curthoys, N. P., and Shapiro, R. A. Effect of metabolic acidosis and of phosphate on the presence of glutamine within the matrix space of rat renal mitochondria during glutamine transport. *J. Biol. Chem.* 253:63, 1978.

Goldstein, L. Ammonia production and excretion in the mammalian kidney. *Int. Rev. Physiol.* 11:283, 1976.

Goldstein, L. Adaptation of renal ammonia production to metabolic acidosis: A study in metabolic regulation. *Physiologist* 23 (1):19, 1980.

Kamm, D. E., and Strope, G. L. The effects of acidosis and alkalosis on the metabolism of glutamine and glutamate in renal cortex slices. *J. Clin. Invest.* 51:1251, 1972.

Lemieux, G., Vinay, P., Baverel, G., Briere, R., and Gougoux, A. Relationship between lactate and glutamine metabolism in vitro by the kidney: Differences between dog and rat and importance of alanine synthesis in the dog. *Kidney Int.* 16:451, 1979.

Malnic, G., Mello-Aires, M., deMello, G. B., and Giebisch, G. Acidification of phosphate buffer in cortical tubules of rat kidney. *Pflügers Arch. Eur. J. Physiol.* 331:275, 1972.

Nash, T. P., Jr., and Benedict, S. R. The ammonia content of the blood, and its bearing on the mechanism of acid neutralization in the animal organism. *J. Biol. Chem.* 48:463, 1921.

Pitts, R. F. The renal regulation of acid base balance with special reference to the mechanism for acidifying the urine. *Science* 102:81, 1945.

Pitts, R. F. Control of renal production of ammonia. *Kidney Int.* 1:297, 1972.

Pitts, R. F. Production and Excretion of Ammonia in Relation to Acid-Base Regulation. In J. Orloff and R. W. Berliner (Eds.), *Handbook of Physi-*

ology, section 8, Renal Physiology. Washington, D.C.: American Physiological Society, 1973.

Pitts, R. F., and Alexander, R. S. The nature of the renal tubular mechanism for acidifying the urine. *Am. J. Physiol.* 144:239, 1945.

Ross, B., and Guder, W. G. (Eds.). *Biochemical Aspects of Renal Function.* Oxford: Pergamon, 1980. Chap. 2.

Sajo, I. M., Goldstein, M. B., Sonnenberg, H., Stinebaugh, B. J., Wilson, D. R., and Halperin, M. L. Sites of ammonia addition to tubular fluid in rats with chronic metabolic acidosis. *Kidney Int.* 20:353, 1981.

Tannen, R. L. Ammonia metabolism. *Am. J. Physiol.* 235 (Renal Fluid Electrolyte Physiol. 4):F265, 1978.

Tannen, R. L., and Ross, B. D. Ammoniagenesis by the isolated perfused rat kidney: The critical role of urinary acidification. *Clin. Sci. Mol. Med.* 56:353, 1979.

Ullrich, K. J., and Papavassiliou, F. Bicarbonate reabsorption in the papillary collecting duct of rats. *Pflügers Arch. Eur. J. Physiol.* 389:271, 1981.

Carbonic Anhydrase   Karlmark, B., Ågerup, B., and Wistrand, P. J. Renal proximal tubular acidification. Role of brush-border and cytoplasmic carbonic anhydrase. *Acta Physiol. Scand.* 106:145, 1979.

Lönnerholm, G., and Ridderstråle, Y. Intracellular distribution of carbonic anhydrase in the rat kidney. *Kidney Int.* 17:162, 1980.

Maren, T. H. Carbonic anhydrase: Chemistry, physiology, and inhibition. *Physiol. Rev.* 47:595, 1967.

Maren, T. H. Carbon dioxide equilibria in the kidney: The problems of elevated carbon dioxide tension, delayed dehydration, and disequilibrium pH. *Kidney Int.* 14:395, 1978.

Maren, T. H. Current status of membrane-bound carbonic anhydrase. *Ann. N.Y. Acad. Sci.* 341:246, 1980.

Norby, L. H., Bethencourt, D., and Schwartz, J. H. Dual effect of carbonic anhydrase inhibitors on H^+ transport by the turtle bladder. *Am. J. Physiol.* 240 (Renal Fluid Electrolyte Physiol. 9):F400, 1981.

Tinker, J. P., Coulson, R., and Weiner, I. M. Dextran-bound inhibitors of carbonic anhydrase. *J. Pharmacol. Exp. Ther.* 218:600, 1981.

Wistrand, P. J., and Kinne, R. Carbonic anhydrase activity of isolated brush border and basal-lateral membranes of renal tubular cells. *Pflügers Arch. Eur. J. Physiol.* 370:121, 1977.

Nonionic Diffusion   Hill, J. B. Salicylate intoxication. *N. Engl. J. Med.* 288:1110, 1973.

Levy, G., Lampman, T., Kamath, B. L., and Garrettson, L. K. Decreased serum salicylate concentrations in children with rheumatic fever treated with antacid. *N. Engl. J. Med.* 293:323, 1975.

Milne, M. D., Scribner, B. H., and Crawford, M. A. Non-ionic diffusion and the excretion of weak acids and bases. *Am. J. Med.* 24:709, 1958.

Waddell, W. J., and Butler, T. C. The distribution and excretion of phenobarbital. *J. Clin. Invest.* 36:1217, 1957.

11 : Renal Handling of K^+: K^+ Balance

The status of K^+ in the body and the dynamics of K^+ balance are shown in Figure 11-1. Note the following points: (1) The concentration of K^+ is high within cells and low in extracellular fluid. This difference is thought to be maintained by active transport of K^+ into cells, which is coupled to active extrusion of Na^+ from cells in a variable ratio (Figs. 2-6, 11-3, and 11-4); that is, there is not necessarily a one-to-one exchange of K^+ for Na^+. (2) Less than 5% of total body K^+ (Table 1-3) resides in the extracellular compartment. (3) Dietary intake of K^+ in a healthy adult human varies from approximately 50 to 150 mEq per day. (4) Most of this daily intake is excreted by the kidneys, which are the primary regulators of external K^+ balance.

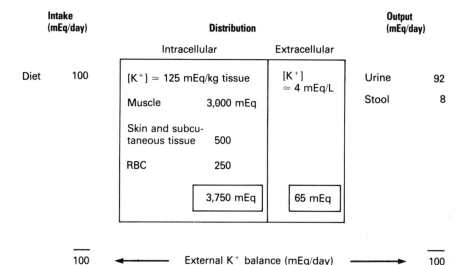

Fig. 11-1 : **The status of potassium in the body and the dynamics of K^+ balance in a healthy adult person. The distribution of K^+ is superimposed on the relative sizes of the intracellular and extracellular compartments (see Fig. 2-7). Detailed description in the text.** *External balance* **refers to the entire body; net shifts between the intracellular and extracellular compartments (see Fig. 11-5B) are described as** *internal balance.* **[K^+] = concentration of potassium. Adapted from Black, D. A. K., in Maxwell, M. H., and Kleeman, C. R. (Eds.),** *Clinical Disorders of Fluid and Electrolyte Metabolism* **(2nd ed.). New York: McGraw-Hill, 1972, and reproduced from Valtin, H.** *Renal Dysfunction: Mechanisms Involved in Fluid and Solute Imbalance.* **Boston: Little, Brown, 1979.**

Normal concentration of K^+, both within cells and in the extracellular fluid, is essential to some very basic processes, such as cell growth, the operation of enzymes, neuromuscular function including that of the myocardium, and H^+ balance. Possibly for this reason, and because the kidney is the major organ that excretes K^+, potassium balance frequently comes into play in the analysis of clinical problems in nephrology: H^+ imbalance; nephrogenic defects of urinary concentration; diuretic therapy; acute renal failure; and hypertension, among others.

Net Transport of K^+ in Various Parts of the Nephron

Several times in this text, we have mentioned heterogeneity of nephrons (for example, see Chap. 7, Reabsorptive Events Along Proximal Tubules). The recognition that a given major component of the nephron, such as the distal tubule, can be subdivided into at least four segments that are structurally and functionally distinct is assuming increasing importance, especially for the transport of K^+; in addition, there are often major differences between a given segment of an outer cortical nephron as opposed to the same segment belonging to a juxtamedullary nephron. However, for the sake of clarity in the ensuing discussion, I shall distinguish only an early from a late distal tubule, and a cortical from an outer or inner medullary collecting duct (for orientation of these parts, see Fig. 1-2).

Results of micropuncture studies are summarized in Figure 11-2; additional conclusions, on portions of the nephron that are not accessible to micropuncture, have been inferred from experiments on isolated, perfused tubules (Fig. 7-5). Normally (Fig. 11-2A), the fraction of filtered K^+ that is excreted in the urine is considerably less than 1.0, i.e., there is net reabsorption of the filtered K^+ so that only about 10 to 20% of the filtered load is excreted. It is clear from the graph, however, that net reabsorption does not occur in all parts of the nephron. The fraction of filtered K^+ that remains at various sites declines in the proximal tubule, from about 0.7 at 20% of proximal length — about the first accessible site of micropuncture — to about 0.3 at 70%, the last accessible site. Only about 0.08, or 8% of the filtered K^+

Fig. 11-2 : Net transport of K^+ in various parts of the nephron, as revealed by micropuncture studies in rats on different diets. A negative slope of the points reflects reabsorption; a positive slope, secretion. When the points for ureteral urine lie below the interrupted horizontal lines at 1.0, there has been net reabsorption of K^+ by the entire kidney; when the urine points lie above these lines, net secretion has occurred. The site of micropuncture was determined at the end of each experiment by microdissection of the nephron. Enclosure in brackets denotes concentration. The rationale for using the concentration ratios given on the ordinate, in order to calculate the fraction of the filtered K^+ that is found at the various sites, is explained in footnote b to Problem 4-1 (p. 78). Redrawn from Malnic, G., Klose, R. M., and Giebisch, G. *Am. J. Physiol.* 206:674, 1964.

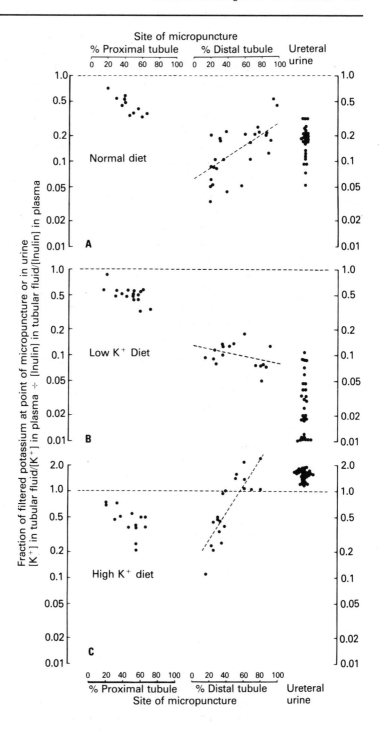

remains at the first 20% of the distal tubule. Therefore, net reabsorption must have taken place in the intervening segments, and most or all of this probably occurred in the nonaccessible portion of the proximal tubule and in the thick ascending limb of Henle. As fluid courses through the distal tubule, there is net secretion, for the fraction of filtered K^+ rises from a mean of about 0.08 to about 0.3. Often, events in the collecting duct can be roughly inferred from the difference between urine and fluid collected from the late portion of the distal tubule. The fact that the mean fraction in the urine is lower than the mean in the late distal tubule reflects significant net reabsorption of K^+ in the collecting duct, probably in the outer and inner medullary portions. Thus, as pointed out by G. Giebisch, urinary excretion of K^+ is regulated by several sequential steps: net reabsorption in the proximal tubule and ascending limb of Henle, net secretion in the late distal tubule and cortical collecting duct, a small, variable component of either net reabsorption or net secretion in the outer medullary collecting duct, and reabsorption in the inner medullary collecting duct.

As is shown in Figure 11-2B, however, net movement of K^+ in the distal tubule is not always in a secretory direction. When the intake of K^+ is low, avid conservation of K^+ occurs, so that only 1 to 10% of the filtered load is excreted in the urine. Under these circumstances, net secretion of K^+ in the distal tubule is abolished, and there may even be moderate net reabsorption. Note that net movement in the other parts of the nephron has changed very little, except for more marked reabsorption by inner medullary collecting ducts. This suggests that modulations in net movement of K^+ in the distal tubule largely determine changes in the urinary excretion of K^+; in other words, the regulation of K^+ balance occurs mainly in the distal tubule. This point is further emphasized by the results depicted in Figure 11-2C.

Net tubular secretion of K^+ by the *entire* kidney under certain conditions was simultaneously and independently demonstrated by R. W. Berliner and G. H. Mudge and their respective associates. This process is reflected in Figure 11-2C by 1.2 to 2.0 times the filtered amount of K^+ appearing in the urine when the animals were placed on a high-K^+, low-Na^+ diet. Even under these conditions, there was net reabsorption in the proximal tubule, to about the same extent as in the conditions shown in Figure 11-2A and B. Thus, even when more than the filtered load is excreted, at least 80% of the filtered K^+ is first reabsorbed in the proximal tubule and possibly in the ascending limb of Henle, which process is then followed by marked net secretion in the distal tubule. When the body is challenged with particularly large loads of K^+, as much as 3½ times more K^+ may be excreted than was filtered; under these conditions, marked secretion of K$^+$ into the cortical collecting duct (as well as into the late distal tubule) probably contributes importantly to the regulation of K$^+$ balance.

In summary, net transport of K$^+$ by the entire kidney varies with the conditions. Normally, about 10 to 20% of the filtered load is excreted, and on a low K$^+$ intake, the excreted fraction is even lower. But when the intake of K$^+$ is high, more than the filtered amount of K$^+$ may be excreted. Under all these conditions, at least 80% of the filtered load is first reabsorbed. Thus, it is primarily through changes of net transport in the distal tubule and cortical collecting duct that the excretion of K$^+$ is regulated.

Mechanisms of K$^+$ Transport

Reabsorption

PROXIMAL TUBULE. Movement of K$^+$ across the proximal tubular epithelium is illustrated in Figure 11-3, which is an extension of Figure 7-2. As was pointed out in connection with the latter figure, the transepithelial electrical potential difference (P.D.)

Proximal Tubule

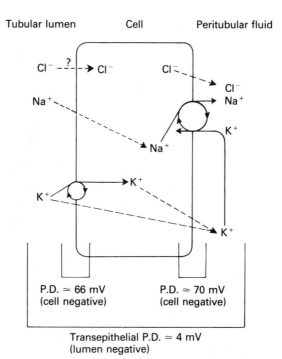

Tubular lumen   Cell   Peritubular fluid

P.D. $\simeq$ 66 mV (cell negative)

P.D. $\simeq$ 70 mV (cell negative)

Transepithelial P.D. $\simeq$ 4 mV (lumen negative)

Fig. 11-3 : Movement of K$^+$ across proximal tubular cells. This diagram is an extension of Figure 7-2 and shows, in addition, proximal net reabsorption of K$^+$. Broken arrows signify passive transport; solid arrows, active transport via a metabolic pump.

changes from lumen negative in the early proximal convolution to lumen positive in the later portion (see also Fig. 7-3C). The concentration of K^+ within tubular fluid also changes, from equal to that in peritubular plasma to slightly higher. For these reasons, and because intracellular concentrations of K^+ are not yet known precisely, the mode of K^+ reabsorption in the proximal tubule has not been fully defined. Under normal conditions, most K^+ is probably reabsorbed passively, both across the cell (especially where the P.D. is lumen positive) and through lateral intercellular channels (see Fig. 7-3C; this route is not shown in Fig. 11-3). There is little doubt, however, that there is also a component of active K^+ reabsorption in the proximal tubule, especially in those parts where the P.D. is lumen negative. Since it is the entry of K^+ from lumen into cell that must, under some circumstances and at some sites, proceed against an electrochemical potential gradient, the pump is located in the luminal membrane. The intracellular K^+ concentration is not yet known precisely; it is probably sufficiently higher than that in peritubular fluid to permit passive movement of K^+ from cell into peritubular fluid, despite the electrical P.D. across the peritubular membrane, which tends to hold K^+ within the cell.

It was pointed out in Chapter 2 and at the beginning of this chapter that the characteristically high intracellular K^+ concentration is maintained in part by active transport. This fact is indicated in Figure 11-3 by the attachment of K^+ to the peritubular pump for Na^+. Although there appears to be a reciprocal relationship between the movement of Na^+ and of K^+ across the membrane of most cells in the body (see Fig. 2-6), the mechanism is not a simple one-to-one exchange whereby an ion of Na^+ is carried in one direction at the same time that an ion of K^+ is transported in the opposite direction. For example, H^+ as well as Na^+ may move in a direction opposite to that of K^+ (see Fig. 11-5B). But whatever the exchange, its location in the peritubular membrane (also called basolateral, basal, or serosal; see Fig. 8-7A) emphasizes the point that this membrane of renal tubular cells — in contrast to the luminal membrane — may be viewed as sharing the characteristics of most cell membranes in the body.

DISTAL TUBULE. Although the distal tubule normally secretes K^+, under certain conditions (Fig. 11-2B) it may reabsorb this ion. If this occurs, the reabsorption must be active, as indicated by the luminal pump in Figure 11-4.

Secretion

Net secretion of K^+ takes place predominantly in the late distal tubule but also in the cortical collecting duct. Because there are some differences between the two — for example, the cortical

Late Distal Tubule

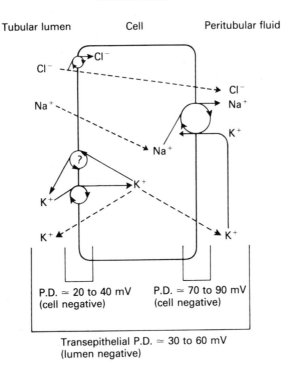

Transepithelial P.D. $\simeq$ 30 to 60 mV
(lumen negative)

Fig. 11-4 : Movement of K$^+$ across late distal tubular cells. This figure is an extension of Figure 7-6. The active component of secretion across the luminal membrane is not yet proved. The situation is similar in cortical collecting ducts except that active secretion (in addition to passive) is certain, and there is no net reabsorption.

collecting duct does not reabsorb K$^+$ in the net, while the distal tubule may — only events in the distal tubule are portrayed in Figure 11-4. Knowing the transepithelial P.D. for late distal tubule and the K$^+$ concentration in peritubular plasma, and then inserting these values into the Nernst equation, one can predict the K$^+$ concentration within tubular fluid that would result, at equilibrium, from passive distribution of K$^+$. Under most experimental conditions, the K$^+$ concentration that is measured in late distal tubular fluid has been found to be lower than the theoretical prediction. This means not only that net K$^+$ secretion can be accounted for on the basis of passive diffusion but also that this passive movement is partially counteracted by active reabsorption. Note a semantic paradox in the above conclusion: We speak of passive secretion of K$^+$ from peritubular plasma to lumen even though we know that uptake of K$^+$ from peritubular fluid into the cell is an active step (Fig. 11-4). The resolution to the paradox is that the ability to *account* for net movement on the basis of passive diffusion does not preclude the interposition of an active step. But beyond that, secretion of K^+ may in part be active, not only across the peritubular membrane but also across the luminal membrane. The secretory pump in the latter membrane has been labeled with a question mark in Figure 11-4, for while active secretion across the luminal membrane exists in the cortical collecting duct, the evidence is not yet conclusive for the late distal tubule.

In summary: In the late distal tubule, secretion of K^+ from cell into tubular lumen is largely passive, although it probably has an active component; the net secretory process is partly modified by active reabsorption. In the cortical collecting duct, secretion is both passive and active, and there appears to be no reabsorption.

The magnitude of distal secretion is determined by several variables: (a) the difference between the K^+ concentration in the tubular cell and that within the tubular lumen, which difference is regulated largely by the activity of the peritubular pump (Fig. 11-4); (b) the flow rate of tubular fluid, which, acting as a sink, ultimately operates through (a) above; and (c) the magnitude of the P.D. across the luminal membrane. That is, other influences being equal, the rate of K^+ secretion will be greater, the higher the intracellular K^+ concentration, the higher the flow rate keeping K^+ concentration low within tubular fluid, and the lower the electrical P.D. which, being cell negative (Fig. 11-4), tends to hold K^+ within the cell.

Factors Influencing Rate of K^+ Excretion

It has been known for many years that certain physiological or pathological conditions are associated with characteristic changes in the urinary excretion of K^+. Some of the major conditions and the associated changes have been listed in Table 11-1. Alterations in urinary K^+ excretion result primarily or solely from changes in the rate or the direction of net K^+ transport in the distal tubule and cortical collecting duct, or both. It is therefore not surprising that the possible mechanisms listed in Table 11-1 involve mainly the factors listed in the preceding paragraph, which influence the rate of K^+ secretion.

INTAKE OF K^+. It was shown in Figure 11-2 that lowering or raising the dietary intake of K^+ could result in enhancement of net reabsorption or a shift to net secretion, respectively, by the entire kidney. These adaptations were paralleled by changes in the rate of net K^+ secretion in the late distal tubule. The mechanism involves primarily changes in the peritubular uptake of K^+. For example, when the intake of K^+ is increased, there is enhanced movement of K^+ into the cell, not only at the peritubular mem-

Table 11-1 : Conditions that influence the rate of urinary K^+ excretion, and possible mechanisms through which each condition mainly exerts its influence.

Condition	Change in K^+ Excretion	Possible Mechanisms*
K^+ intake		
High	Increased	Increased distal secretion resulting from: Increased peritubular uptake of K^+, leading to increased intracellular K^+ concentration ?Increased aldosterone
Low	Decreased	Decrease in distal tubular net secretion and possibly shift to net reabsorption, probably resulting from changes opposite to those listed above Increased net reabsorption by inner medullary collecting ducts
Adrenal mineralo-corticoids		
Excess	Increased	Increased secretion by cortical collecting ducts, probably resulting from: Increased peritubular uptake of K^+ Increased luminal permeability to K^+ Decreased P.D. across luminal membrane
Deficiency	Decreased	Decreased secretion by cortical collecting ducts, probably due to opposite changes
H^+ balance		
Alkalosis	Increased	Increased secretion by late distal tubules and cortical collecting ducts due to increased peritubular uptake of K^+ and consequent increased intracellular K^+ concentration
Acute acidosis	Decreased	Decreased secretion by late distal tubules and cortical collecting ducts, probably resulting from the opposite effects
Na^+ intake		
High	Increased	Increased secretion by late distal tubules and cortical collecting ducts due to: Increased delivery of Na^+ to distal sites, possibly augmenting peritubular uptake of K^+ Increased flow rate of tubular fluid ?Decreased K^+ concentration in distal tubular fluid ?Decreased P.D. across luminal membrane
Low	Decreased	Increased reabsorption of K^+ in outer and inner medullary collecting ducts Decreased secretion by late distal tubules and cortical collecting ducts due to changes opposite to those listed above
Diuretics		
Chlorothiazide	Increased ⎫	Increased secretion by late distal tubules and cortical collecting ducts resulting from increased delivery of Na^+ and water to distal sites and from the other effects listed above under high Na^+ intake
Furosemide	Increased ⎪	
Ethacrynic acid	Increased ⎬	
Mannitol	Increased ⎭	
Triamterene	Decreased	Decreased secretion by late distal tubules but probably mainly by cortical collecting ducts, due to: ?Increased electrical P.D. across luminal membrane retarding movement of K^+ from cell into lumen
Spironolactone	Decreased	Decreased secretion by cortical collecting ducts resulting from competitive inhibition of aldosterone

*For some conditions, the main mechanisms that have been identified are listed; for others, reasonable speculations are mentioned. The lists are not necessarily exhaustive.

brane of distal cells (Fig. 11-4) but also at the surface of most body cells. With adaptation to prolonged high intake of K^+, the increased peritubular uptake of K^+ involves an enhancement of Na-K-activated ATPase in the basolateral membrane, and it probably also entails an increase in the plasma level of aldosterone. The converse chain of events during K^+ deprivation presumably leads to decreased distal secretion and possibly even to reabsorption; in addition, there is increased net reabsorption of K^+ in inner medullary collecting ducts under these conditions.

ADRENAL MINERALOCORTICOIDS. In keeping with the major sites of action of mineralocorticoids (see Chap. 7, Challenges to Na^+ Balance. Changes in Na^+ Intake), these steroids stimulate secretion of K^+, and hence its urinary excretion, mainly in the cortical collecting ducts, and possibly in those of the outer medulla as well. The effect is mediated by at least three changes: increased peritubular uptake of K^+, increased permeability of the luminal membrane to K^+, and decreased electrical P.D. across the luminal membrane. The opposite effects probably account for decreased excretion of K^+ in adrenal insufficiency.

H^+ BALANCE. Alkalosis, whether it be metabolic or respiratory in origin, is usually associated with increased urinary excretion of K^+, and *acute* acidosis of either metabolic or respiratory origin is accompanied by decreased K^+ excretion. (Chronic states of acidosis are often accompanied by increased K^+ excretion, perhaps because of increased delivery of Na^+ to distal parts of the nephron; see below.) Figure 11-5A shows that modulations in secretion of K^+ by late distal tubules and cortical collecting ducts are responsible for changes in K^+ excretion. Under control conditions, the fraction of the filtered K^+ rises along the course of the distal tubule (Fig. 11-2A). This fraction is about 0.1 at 20% of the length — the earliest portion accessible to micropuncture — and about 0.3 toward the end of the distal tubule. When acute respiratory acidosis is induced in rats by raising the concentration of CO_2 in the inspired air to 15%, the rate of distal tubular K^+ secretion is decreased, as reflected in the lesser slope. A similar inhibitory effect on secretion is seen in acute metabolic acidosis induced by an intravenous infusion of NH_4Cl. On the other hand, when states of alkalosis are induced, either through hyperventilation (respiratory) or through an intravenous infusion of $NaHCO_3$ (metabolic), the rate of distal tubular K^+ secretion is greatly enhanced. The cluster of the points at 20% of distal tubular length again emphasizes the fact that the handling of K^+ up to the early distal tubule is identical under the various conditions of H^+ balance.

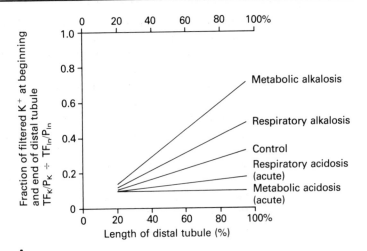

A

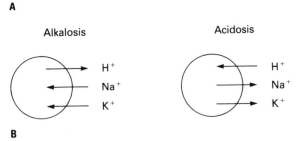

B

Fig. 11-5

A. Effect of changes in H$^+$ balance on the rate of distal tubular K$^+$ secretion in rats. The means for inducing the various states of alkalosis and acidosis are described in the text. The rationale for calculating the fraction of filtered K$^+$ by means of the so-called [TF/P] K/In is described in footnote b to Problem 4-1 (p. 78). Redrawn from Giebisch, G. Renal Potassium Excretion. In Rouiller, C., and Muller, A. F. (Eds.). *The Kidney,* vol. III. New York: Academic, 1971.

B. Reciprocal movement of H$^+$, Na$^+$, and K$^+$ during disturbances of H$^+$ balance. The circles represent body cells surrounded by extracellular fluid. In epithelial cells, such as those lining renal tubules, these shifts take place across the peritubular membrane. From Valtin, H. *Renal Dysfunction: Mechanisms Involved in Fluid and Solute Imbalance.* Boston: Little, Brown, 1979.

The mechanism for the modulation of K$^+$ secretion is primarily a change in the peritubular uptake of K$^+$ and hence a shift in the intracellular K$^+$ concentration. The change in peritubular uptake can be ascribed, in turn, to reciprocal movement of H$^+$ and K$^+$ at the peritubular membrane of cells lining the late distal tubules and cortical collecting ducts. The schema depicted in Figure 11-5B is thought to occur in virtually all cells, not just those lining the distal nephron. During alkalosis, the low extracellular concentration of H$^+$ promotes movement of H$^+$ out of cells, and reciprocally, K$^+$, as well as Na$^+$, moves into the cells. The converse occurs during acidosis. (Note that at times, Na^+ and K^+ can traverse the cell membrane in the same direction; they do not exclusively move in opposite directions, as shown in Fig. 11-3 and 11-4.) The explanation for these shifts is not fully understood. It might involve the intracellular buffering of H^+ as depicted in the lower right-hand quadrant of Figure 9-6, or some consequence of a change in intracellular pH, such as changes in the ionization of certain intracellular compounds or a change in electrical P.D. But whatever the explanation, the shifts shown in Figure 11-5B are known to involve renal tubular cells, and the consequent changes in K^+ concentration within cells of late distal tubules and cortical collecting ducts are the main causes for the alterations of K^+ secretion during disturbances of H^+ balance.

INTAKE OF Na^+. In most instances there is a direct correlation between the increased urinary excretion of Na^+ that follows a high intake of Na^+, and the urinary excretion of K^+. The converse also holds when the intake of Na^+, and hence the urinary excretion of Na^+, is reduced. It is important to realize, however, that there are notable exceptions, when changes in the urinary excretion of these two ions do not parallel one another. One example is the so-called escape from adrenal mineralocorticoids; when these hormones are administered for a prolonged period, Na^+ excretion returns to control values while K^+ excretion remains elevated.

There are several mechanisms whereby Na^+ influences the rate of K^+ excretion, and not all of them have been fully clarified. With a high intake of Na^+, the increased excretion of K^+ is mainly due to increased secretion in late distal tubules and cortical collecting ducts. One critical element causing the enhanced secretion is increased delivery of Na^+ to these tubular sites, which may launch a chain of events whereby increased passive entry of Na^+ into distal cells stimulates the pump in the peritubular membrane and reciprocally increases peritubular uptake of K^+ (Fig. 11-4). Another important element is increased flow rate of fluid past the distal secreting sites; this effect probably increases the "sink" for K^+ diffusion into the lumen, even though the intratubular concentration of K^+ is not invariably decreased as flow is augmented. Finally, it is possible that a decrease in the magnitude of the electrical P.D. across the luminal membrane promotes secretion of K^+ through a lesser tendency to "hold" K^+ within the electrically negative cell (Fig. 11-4).

Perhaps surprisingly, the influences that decrease urinary excretion of K^+ during a low Na^+ intake are not simply the reverse of those listed in the preceding paragraph. Although decreased secretion of K^+ may play a role, the most important element is enhanced reabsorption of K^+, certainly in the inner medullary collecting ducts and probably in those of the outer medulla as well.

DIURETICS. The diuretics constitute a group of pharmacological agents that increase the urinary excretion of NaCl and water by inhibiting the reabsorption of Na^+ or of Cl^- — or both — in various parts of the nephron. The most effective, and hence most commonly used, diuretics (the first four listed in Table 11-1) also tend to increase the urinary excretion of K^+; with prolonged use of the diuretic, this increased excretion can lead to serious K^+ depletion. The mechanisms entail greater secretion of K^+ by the late distal tubules and cortical collecting ducts, which results from inhibition of Na^+ and Cl^- reabsorption proximal to these sites and hence increased delivery of Na^+ to these sites. Thus, the various factors listed in Table 11-1 under high Na^+ intake are responsible for increasing K^+ secretion during use of the common diuretics.

Several, less frequently used, diuretics decrease K^+ excretion. They are rarely prescribed by themselves, but more commonly as adjuvants with the more effective diuretics. They fall into two classes: the so-called K^+-sparing diuretics, of which triamterene is an example, and the antagonists of the adrenal mineralocorticoids, exemplified by spironolactone. Both decrease secretion of K^+, predominantly or solely in cortical collecting ducts, but by different mechanisms. Triamterene may do so by increasing the electrical P.D. across the luminal membrane; spironolactone by competitive binding to the nuclear receptor for aldosterone, and hence through the mechanisms listed in Table 11-1 for deficiency of adrenal mineralocorticoids.

Summary

Maintenance of a normal intracellular K^+ concentration is essential to many cellular functions. The kidney is the major organ through which K^+ is excreted; changes in the renal handling of K^+ are therefore primarily responsible for maintaining K^+ balance.

K^+ undergoes bidirectional net transport in its course through the nephron. At least 80% of the filtered load of K^+ is reabsorbed in the proximal tubules and ascending limbs of Henle under all circumstances. In late distal tubules, there is normally net secretion of K^+, and this might be converted into net reabsorption in certain conditions such as K^+ deprivation. Cortical collecting ducts secrete K^+, those in the outer medulla may either reabsorb or secrete it, and inner medullary collecting ducts reabsorb K^+. For the entire kidney, there may be either avid net reabsorption of K^+ or marked net secretion. The rate of urinary K^+ excretion can thus vary widely, and this rate is governed primarily by changes in the magnitude of net secretion in the late distal tubules and collecting ducts.

Reabsorption of K^+ in the proximal tubule occurs by a combination of passive and active transport processes. If net K^+ reabsorption takes place in the distal tubule, its mode of transport must be active. Net secretion of K^+ across the luminal cell membrane of late distal tubules and cortical collecting ducts is largely passive, although an active component exists with certainty in the cortical collecting duct and probably in the late distal tubule as well. The magnitude of secretion is governed by three major influences: (a) the gradient for K^+ concentration between tubular cell and tubular lumen, which is determined mainly by the peritubular uptake of K^+ and the consequent intracellular K^+ concentration; (b) the flow rate of Na^+ and water through the late distal tubules and cortical collecting ducts; and (c) the magnitude of the electrical P.D. across the luminal membrane of secreting cells.

Many factors — among them the dietary intake of K^+ and Na^+, adrenal mineralocorticoids, H^+ balance, and the use of diuretics — can alter the rate of urinary K^+ excretion. These alterations are brought about mainly by changing the rate of secretion in the late distal tubules or cortical collecting ducts, or both — changes that are mediated in turn by influencing one or more of the three elements listed above. Two notable exceptions are low intake of K^+ or of Na^+, when increased reabsorption of K^+ by medullary collecting ducts constitutes a major adjustment.

Problem 11-1

Now that you have become an expert on renal function, you can answer these questions:

What are the urinary pH and osmolality of a healthy adult human whose diet is normal and contains protein? What are the major solutes in such urine, and what is the approximate concentration of each solute?

Selected References

General

Berliner, R. W. Renal mechanisms for potassium excretion. *Harvey Lect.* 55:141, 1961.

Berliner, R. W., and Kennedy, T. J., Jr. Renal tubular secretion of potassium in the normal dog. *Proc. Soc. Exp. Biol. Med.* 67:542, 1948.

Brenner, B. M., and Berliner, R. W. Transport of Potassium. In J. Orloff and R. W. Berliner (Eds.), *Handbook of Physiology,* section 8, Renal Physiology. Washington, D.C.: American Physiological Society, 1973.

DeFronzo, R. A., Lee, R., Jones, A., and Bia, M. Effect of insulinopenia and adrenal hormone deficiency on acute potassium tolerance. *Kidney Int.* 17:586, 1980.

Giebisch, G. Renal Potassium Transport. In G. Giebisch (Ed.), *Transport Organs,* vol. IVA. New York: Springer-Verlag, 1979.

Giebisch, G., Malnic, G., and Berliner, R. W. Renal Transport and Control of Potassium Excretion. In B. M. Brenner and F. C. Rector, Jr. (Eds.), *The Kidney* (2nd ed.). Philadelphia: Saunders, 1981.

Kernan, R. P. *Cell K.* Washington, D.C.: Butterworth, 1965.

Leaf, A., and Santos, R. F. Physiologic mechanisms in potassium deficiency. *N. Engl. J. Med.* 264:335, 1961.

Mudge, G. H., Foulks, J., and Gilman, A. The renal excretion of potassium. *Proc. Soc. Exp. Biol. Med.* 67:545, 1948.

O'Connor, G., and Kunau, R. T. Renal Transport of Hydrogen and Potassium. In B. M. Brenner and J. H. Stein (Eds.), *Contemporary Issues in Nephrology,* vol. 2. New York: Churchill Livingstone, 1978.

Tannen, R. L. (Ed.). Symposium on potassium homeostasis. *Kidney Int.* 11:389, 1977.

Wright, F. S. Potassium transport by the renal tubule. *Int. Rev. Physiol.* 6:79, 1974.

K$^+$ Transport in Various Parts of the Nephron

Battilana, C. A., Dobyan, D. C., Lacy, F. B., Bhattacharya, J., Johnston, P. A., and Jamison, R. L. Effect of chronic potassium loading on potassium secretion by the pars recta or descending limb of the juxtamedullary nephron in the rat. *J. Clin. Invest.* 62:1093, 1978.

Bengele, H. H., McNamara, E. R., and Alexander, E. A. Potassium secretion along the inner medullary collecting duct. *Am. J. Physiol.* 236 (Renal Fluid Electrolyte Physiol. 5):F278, 1979.

Bennett, C. M., Brenner, B. M., and Berliner, R. W. Micropuncture study of nephron function in the rhesus monkey. *J. Clin. Invest.* 47:203, 1968.

Crayen, M., and Thoenes, W. Architektur und cytologische Charakterisierung des distalen Tubulus der Rattenniere. *Fortschr. Zool.* 23:279, 1975.

Giebisch, G., Boulpaep, E. L., and Whittembury, G. Electrolyte transport in kidney tubule cells. *Philos. Trans. R. Soc. Lond.* Series B. [Biol.] 262:175, 1971.

Giebisch, G., Malnic, G., Klose, R. M., and Windhager, E. E. Effect of ionic substitutions on distal potential differences in rat kidney. *Am. J. Physiol.* 211:560, 1966.

Grantham, J. J., Burg, M. B., and Orloff, J. The nature of transtubular Na and K transport in isolated rabbit renal collecting tubules. *J. Clin. Invest.* 49:1815, 1970.

Gross, J. B., Imai, M., and Kokko, J. P. A functional comparison of the cortical collecting tubule and the distal convoluted tubule. *J. Clin. Invest.* 55:1284, 1975.

Jamison, R. L., Work, J., and Schafer, J. A. New pathways for potassium transport in the kidney. *Am. J. Physiol.* 242 (Renal Fluid Electrolyte Physiol. 11):F297, 1982.

LeGrimellec, C., Poujeol, P., and de Rouffignac, C. ^{3}H-inulin and electrolyte concentrations in Bowman's capsule in rat kidney. Comparison with artificial ultrafiltration. *Pflügers Arch. Eur. J. Physiol.* 354:117, 1975.

Malnic, G., Klose, R. M., and Giebisch, G. Micropuncture study of renal potassium excretion in the rat. *Am. J. Physiol.* 206:674, 1964.

Malnic, G., Klose, R. M., and Giebisch, G. Micropuncture study of distal tubular potassium and sodium transport in rat nephron. *Am. J. Physiol.* 211:529, 1966.

Reineck, H. J., Osgood, R. W., and Stein, J. H. Net potassium addition beyond the superficial distal tubule of the rat. *Am. J. Physiol.* 235 (Renal Fluid Electrolyte Physiol. 4):F104, 1978.

Schafer, J. A. Response of the collecting duct to the demands of homeostasis. *Physiologist* 22 (No. 5):44, 1979.

Schwartz, G. J., and Burg, M. B. Mineralocorticoid effects on cation transport by cortical collecting tubules in vitro. *Am. J. Physiol.* 235 (Renal Fluid Electrolyte Physiol. 4):F576, 1978.

Sonnenberg, H. Medullary collecting-duct function in antidiuretic and in salt- or water-diuretic rats. *Am. J. Physiol.* 226:501, 1974.

Stokes, J. B. Consequences of potassium recycling in the renal medulla. *J. Clin. Invest.* 70:219, 1982.

Watson, J. F. Potassium reabsorption in the proximal tubule of the dog nephron. *J. Clin. Invest.* 45:1341, 1966.

Wiederholt, M., Sullivan, W. J., Giebisch, G., Curran, P. F., and Solomon, A. K. Potassium and sodium transport across single distal tubules of *Amphiuma. J. Gen. Physiol.* 57:495, 1971.

Wright, F. S. Increasing magnitude of electrical potential along the renal distal tubule. *Am. J. Physiol.* 220:624, 1971.

Wright, F. S., and Giebisch, G. Renal potassium transport: Contributions of individual nephron segments and populations. *Am. J. Physiol.* 235 (Renal Fluid Electrolyte Physiol. 4):F515, 1978.

Mechanisms of
K$^+$ Transport

Duarte, C. G., Chomety, F., and Giebisch, G. Effect of amiloride, ouabain, and furosemide on distal tubular function in the rat. *Am. J. Physiol.* 221:632, 1971.

Fujimoto, M., Kubota, T., and Kotera, K. Electrochemical profile of K and Cl ions across the proximal tubule of bullfrog kidneys. A study using double-barreled ion-sensitive microelectrodes. *Contrib. Nephrol.* 6:114, 1977.

Giebisch, G. Effect of Diuretics on Renal Tubular Potassium Transport. In W. Siegenthaler, R. Beckerhoff, and W. Vetter (Eds.), *Diuretics in Research and Clinics.* Stuttgart: Thieme, 1977.

Giebisch, G. (Chairman). Symposium on problems of epithelial potassium transport: Special consideration of the nephron. *Fed. Proc.* 40:2395, 1981.
This collection of papers includes reports on models other than the kidney, such as the colon and the midgut of insects.

Good, D. W., and Wright, F. S. Luminal influences on potassium secretion: Transepithelial voltage. *Am. J. Physiol.* 239 (Renal Fluid Electrolyte Physiol. 8):F289, 1980.

Khuri, R. N., Wiederholt, M., Strieder, N., and Giebisch, G. Effects of flow rate and potassium intake on distal tubular potassium transfer. *Am. J. Physiol.* 228:1249, 1975.

Kunau, R. T., Jr., Webb, H. L., and Borman, S. C. Characteristics of the relationship between the flow rate of tubular fluid and potassium transport in the distal tubule of the rat. *J. Clin. Invest.* 54:1488, 1974.

Macknight, A. D. C. Epithelial transport of potassium. *Kidney Int.* 11:391, 1977.

Malnic, G., Klose, R. M., and Giebisch, G. Microperfusion study of distal tubular potassium and sodium transfer in rat kidney. *Am. J. Physiol.* 211:548, 1966.

Mello-Aires, M., Giebisch, G., and Malnic, G. Kinetics of potassium transport across single distal tubules of rat kidney. *J. Physiol.* (Lond.) 232:47, 1973.

O'Neil, R. G., and Helman, S. I. Transport characteristics of renal collecting tubules: Influences of DOCA and diet. *Am. J. Physiol.* 233 (Renal Fluid Electrolyte Physiol. 2):F544, 1977.

Silva, P., Brown, R. S., and Epstein, F. H. Adaptation to potassium. *Kidney Int.* 11:466, 1977.

Silva, P., Ross, B. D., Charney, A. N., Besarab, A., and Epstein, F. H. Potassium transport by the isolated perfused kidney. *J. Clin. Invest.* 56:862, 1975.

Wright, F. S. Sites and mechanisms of potassium transport along the renal tubule. *Kidney Int.* 11:415, 1977.

Regulation of
K⁺ Excretion

Adler, S., and Fraley, D. S. Potassium and intracellular pH. *Kidney Int.* 11:433, 1977.

Boudry, J. F., Stoner, L. C., and Burg, M. B. Effect of acid lumen pH on potassium transport in renal cortical collecting tubules. *Am. J. Physiol.* 230:239, 1976.

Cooke, R. E., Segar, W. E., Cheek, D. B., Coville, F. E., and Darrow, D. C. The extrarenal correction of alkalosis associated with potassium deficiency. *J. Clin. Invest.* 31:798, 1952.

Cortney, M. A. Renal tubular transfer of water and electrolytes in adrenalectomized rats. *Am. J. Physiol.* 216:589, 1969.

Foulkes, E. C. On the mechanism of chlorothiazide-induced kaliuresis in the rabbit. *J. Pharmacol. Exp. Ther.* 150:406, 1965.

Gardner, L. I., MacLachlan, E. A., and Berman, H. Effect of potassium deficiency on carbon dioxide, cation, and phosphate content of muscle. *J. Gen. Physiol.* 36:153, 1952.

Gatzy, J. T. The effect of K⁺-sparing diuretics on ion transport across the excised toad bladder. *J. Pharmacol. Exp. Ther.* 176:580, 1971.

Gennari, F. J., and Cohen, J. J. Role of the kidney in potassium homeostasis: Lessons from acid-base disturbances. *Kidney Int.* 8:1, 1975.

Giebisch, G. Effects of Diuretics on Renal Transport of Potassium. In M. Martinez-Maldonado (Ed.), *Methods in Pharmacology*, vol. 4A, *Renal Pharmacology.* New York: Plenum, 1976.

Gross, J. B., and Kokko, J. P. Effects of aldosterone and potassium-sparing diuretics on electrical potential differences across the distal nephron. *J. Clin. Invest.* 59:82, 1977.

Hayslett, J. P., and Binder, H. J. Mechanism of potassium adaptation. *Am. J. Physiol.* 243 (Renal Fluid Electrolyte Physiol. 12):F103, 1982.

Irvine, R. O. H., Saunders, S. J., Milne, M. D., and Crawford, M. A. Gradients of potassium and hydrogen ion in potassium-deficient voluntary muscle. *Clin. Sci. Mol. Med.* 20:1, 1961.

Kashgarian, M., Taylor, C. R., Binder, H. J., and Hayslett, J. P. Amplification of cell membrane surface in potassium adaptation. *Lab. Invest.* 42:581, 1980.

Khuri, R. N., Wiederholt, M., Strieder, N., and Giebisch, G. Effects of flow rate and potassium intake on distal tubular potassium transfer. *Am. J. Physiol.* 228:1249, 1975.

Linas, S. L., Peterson, L. N., Anderson, R. J., Aisenbrey, G. A., Simon, F. R., and Berl, T. Mechanism of renal potassium conservation in the rat. *Kidney Int.* 15:601, 1979.

Malnic, G., Mello-Aires, M., and Giebisch, G. Potassium transport across renal distal tubules during acid-base disturbances. *Am. J. Physiol.* 221:1192, 1971.

Miller, R. B., Tyson, I., and Relman, A. S. pH of isolated resting skeletal muscle and its relation to potassium content. *Am. J. Physiol.* 204:1048, 1963.

Mudge, G. H., Foulks, J., and Gilman, A. Renal secretion of potassium in the dog during cellular dehydration. *Am. J. Physiol.* 161:159, 1950.

Muntwyler, E., and Griffin, G. E. Effect of potassium on electrolytes of rat plasma and muscle. *J. Biol. Chem.* 193:563, 1951.

Peterson, L. N., and Wright, F. S. Effect of sodium intake on renal potassium excretion. *Am. J. Physiol.* 233 (Renal Fluid Electrolyte Physiol. 2):F225, 1977.

Rabinowitz, L. Aldosterone and renal potassium excretion. *Renal Physiol.* 2:229, 1979.

Rabinowitz, L., Gunther, R. A., and Sarason, R. L. Renal sodium and potassium excretion in sheep given amiloride. *Am. J. Vet. Res.* 40:688, 1979.

Rastegar, A., Biemesderfer, D., Kashgarian, M., and Hayslett, J. P. Changes in membrane surfaces of collecting duct cells in potassium adaptation. *Kidney Int.* 18:293, 1980.

Sastrasinh, S., and Tannen, R. L. Mechanism by which enhanced ammonia production reduces urinary potassium excretion. *Kidney Int.* 20:326, 1981.

Seely, J. F., and Dirks, J. H. Site of action of diuretic drugs. *Kidney Int.* 11:1, 1977.

Silva, P., Hayslett, J. P., and Epstein, F. H. The role of Na-K-ATPase in potassium adaptation. *J. Clin. Invest.* 52:2665, 1973.

Sonnenberg, H. Effect of adrenalectomy on medullary collecting-duct function in rats before and during blood volume expansion. *Pflügers Arch. Eur. J. Physiol.* 368:55, 1977.

Stanton, B. A., and Giebisch, G. H. Regulation of Potassium Homeostasis. In R. A. Corradino (Ed.), *Functional Regulation at the Cellular Levels.* Amsterdam: Elsevier/North Holland, 1982.

Stanton, B., Biemesderfer, D., Wade, J. B., and Giebisch, G. Structural and functional study of the rat distal nephron: Effects of K^+ adaptation and depletion. *Kidney Int.* 19:36, 1981.

Stoner, L. C., Burg, M. B., and Orloff, J. Ion transport in cortical collecting tubule; effect of amiloride. *Am. J. Physiol.* 227:453, 1974.

Toussaint, C., and Vereerstraeten, P. Effects of blood pH changes on potassium excretion in the dog. *Am. J. Physiol.* 202:768, 1962.

Answers to Problems

Problem 1-1

Except for some minor differences (see Chap. 4, Quantifying Reabsorption), the concentration of Na^+ is the same in the plasma that is filtered into Bowman's space as it is in the plasma before it is filtered. Furthermore, since 92% of plasma is made up of water, we equate the amount of water filtered with the amount of plasma that is filtered. Hence, the so-called filtered load of Na^+ — i.e., the rate at which Na^+ is filtered through the glomerular capillaries into Bowman's space — is 180 L/day $\times$ 139 mEq/L, or 25,020 mEq per day.

If the urine flow is 1.1 ml per minute and the concentration of Na^+ in that urine is 95 mEq/liter (i.e., 0.095 mEq/ml), then the rate of urinary excretion of Na^+ is 1.1 ml/min $\times$ 0.095 mEq/ml, or 0.1045 mEq per minute. There are 60 $\times$ 24, or 1,440, min in each day; hence the urinary excretion of Na^+ in this example is 0.1045 mEq/min $\times$ 1,440 min, or 150 mEq per day.

Since 25,020 mEq per day was filtered into the tubules, and only 150 mEq per day was excreted, 24,870 mEq per day must have been reabsorbed; that is, 24,870/25,020 $\times$ 100, or 99.4% of the filtered load of Na^+ was reabsorbed.

Problem 1-2

A solution of 0.9% NaCl contains 0.9 g of NaCl per 100 ml, or 9 g of NaCl per liter. Since the atomic weight of Na^+ is 23 and that of Cl^- is 35, 1 mole (or gram molecule) of NaCl weighs 58 g and 1 mMole of NaCl weighs 58 mg. Therefore, 9,000 mg of NaCl (which is contained in 1 liter of the solution) represents 155 mMoles of NaCl. At this concentration, the 155 mMoles of NaCl is completely dissociated into the ionic constituents of Na^+ and Cl^-; the solution therefore contains 155 mEq (or mMoles) of Na^+ and 155 mEq of Cl^-, and these are the values that one obtains when analyzing a solution of 0.9% NaCl in a flame photometer.

The osmolality of a solution is a function solely of the *number of discrete particles* that it contains; that is, it is a function of its colligative properties, which depend on the interaction between the solute and the solvent molecules. Because of this interaction, the osmolality is less than the sum of 155 mMoles of Na^+ and

155 mMoles of Cl^-. Rather, it is 282 mOsm/kg H_2O when measured in an osmometer, as by determining the depression of the freezing point. Dividing the measured osmolality by the millimoles in solution yields the so-called osmotic coefficient (in this case, 282/310, or 0.91).

A 5% solution of glucose contains 50 g of glucose per liter. Since the molecular weight of glucose is 180, 50 g of glucose represents 278 mMoles of glucose. Nonelectrolytes also have colligative properties, and for a 278-mMolar solution of glucose, the osmotic coefficient is approximately 0.99; hence, the addition of 5 g of glucose to each 100 ml of 0.9% NaCl adds about 275 mMoles to each liter, and the new solution would have an osmolality of approximately 557 mOsm/kg H_2O.

One molecule of $CaCl_2$ contains one ion of calcium with a valence of two, and two ions of chloride, each with a valence of one. Therefore, 1 mMole of $CaCl_2$ contains 2 mEq of calcium and 2 mEq of chloride.

Since 1 mMole of $CaCl_2$ contains 1 mMole of calcium and 2 mMoles of chloride, it would contribute 3 mOsm to a solution if the osmotic coefficient were 1.0.

Problem 2-1

Plasma Volume

Equation 2-2:

$$\frac{\text{Volume of}}{\text{compartment}} = \frac{\text{Amount of substance given} - \text{Amount of substance lost}}{\text{Concentration of substance in the compartment}}$$

$$= \frac{10 \text{ mg} - 0}{0.4 \text{ mg/100 ml}}$$

$$= \frac{10 \text{ mg}}{1} \cdot \frac{100 \text{ ml}}{0.4 \text{ mg}}$$

$$= \frac{1000}{0.4}, \text{ or 2,500 ml, or 2.5 L}$$

Whole Blood Volume

$$\frac{\text{Plasma volume}}{55\%} = \frac{\text{Whole blood volume}}{100\%}$$

$$\frac{2,500 \text{ ml}}{55} = \frac{\text{Whole blood volume}}{100}$$

$$\text{Whole blood volume} = \frac{2,500 \cdot 100}{55} = 4,545 \text{ ml, or 4.5 L}$$

Problem 2-2

Total Body Water

Again, one uses Equation 2-2:

$$TBW = \frac{99.8 \text{ g} - (99.8 \cdot 0.004)}{0.2 \text{ g/100 ml}}$$

$$= \frac{99.4 \text{ g}}{0.2 \text{ g/100 ml}}$$

$$= \frac{99.4 \text{ g}}{1} \cdot \frac{100 \text{ ml}}{0.2 \text{ g}}$$

$$= 49,700 \text{ ml, or } 49.7 \text{ L}$$

Extracellular Fluid Volume

$$ECW = \frac{100 \text{ } \mu Ci - (100 \cdot 0.04)}{0.0064 \text{ } \mu Ci/ml}$$

$$= \frac{96 \text{ } \mu Ci}{0.0064 \text{ } \mu Ci/ml}$$

$$= \frac{96 \text{ } \mu Ci}{1} \cdot \frac{ml}{0.0064 \text{ } \mu Ci}$$

$$= 15,000 \text{ ml, or } 15 \text{ L}$$

N.B. To the extent that the distribution of sulfate between plasma and interstitial fluid is governed by the Gibbs-Donnan equilibrium, the concentration of radiosulfate will be slightly greater in the interstitium than in plasma. Since interstitial fluid constitutes about three-quarters of the extracellular compartment, the above calculation will slightly overestimate the amount of ECW.

Intracellular Volume

From Table 2-1:

$$ICW = TBW - ECW$$

$$= 49.7 - 15.0$$

$$= 34.7 \text{ L}$$

Problem 2-3

The answers are shown in Figure 2-A. In clinical parlance, the new steady state following a loss of fluid is known as volume contraction and a gain of fluid as volume expansion. The change in volume, as well as the adjectives *isosmotic, hyperosmotic,*

Healthy state

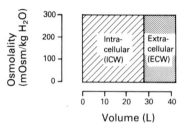

Types of volume contraction

Isosmotic   Hyperosmotic   Hyposmotic

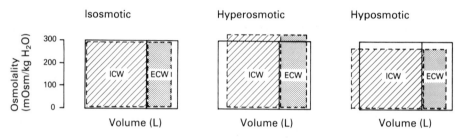

Types of volume expansion

Isosmotic   Hyperosmotic   Hyposmotic

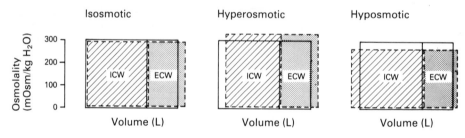

Fig. 2-A : Types of contraction and expansion of the body fluid compartments. The plasma and the interstitial fluid are here portrayed as a single extracellular compartment. In each diagram, the healthy state is drawn in solid lines and the new steady state in dashed lines. This type of portrayal, known as a *Darrow-Yannet diagram,* was introduced by these two workers in a classic contribution on this subject (*J. Clin. Invest.* 14:266, 1935). From H. Valtin, *Renal Dysfunction: Mechanisms Involved in Fluid and Solute Imbalance.* Boston: Little, Brown, 1979.

and *hyposmotic,* refers to the *extracellular* fluid in the new steady state.

(a) *Loss of isosmotic fluid.* Initially the fluid is lost from the plasma, and this loss is largely replenished from the interstitial space because of a change in Starling forces. Therefore, the entire extracellular compartment contracts, but since the loss is isosmotic, there will be no major change in the osmolality of extracellular fluid, and hence no shift of H_2O in or out of the intracellular space. The final result will be a reduction in the volume of the extracellular fluid, but no change in its osmolality; that is, isosmotic contraction will have occurred.

(b) *Loss of "pure" H_2O.* In persons lost in the desert or patients with fever (as well as in normal individuals — Table 1-4), much H_2O is lost even when they are not sweating. This loss, which occurs by evaporation from the skin and breath, is called *insensible H_2O loss* because it is not perceived, as is sweat. This evaporative H_2O comes first from the plasma, which thereby becomes hyperosmotic with respect to the other body fluids, and this change in turn causes a shift of H_2O from the interstitial into the plasma compartment. The consequent rise in the osmolality of the interstitial fluid causes H_2O to flow out of the intracellular compartment. That is, in hyperosmotic contraction, the volume of all the major fluid compartments is decreased.

(c) *Loss of NaCl.* Patients with adrenal insufficiency actually lose some H_2O initially, but then they retain H_2O even though loss of NaCl continues. The net result is therefore loss of NaCl in excess of H_2O, and this decrement results in decreased osmolality of extracellular fluid. Consequently, H_2O will shift from the extracellular into the intracellular space, and the new steady state will show contraction of the extracellular compartment and expansion of the intracellular space, with both having an osmolality that is less than normal.

(d) *Gain of isosmotic fluid.* Edema fluid is essentially a solution of NaCl that has the same osmolality as plasma. The analysis of this situation is therefore similar to the one given for Figure 2-4 except that in generalized edema the fluid is added to the body through failure of the kidneys to excrete it, not through intravenous infusion. Generalized edema is the classic example of isosmotic expansion, which represents a selective enlargement of the extracellular compartment, without change in osmolality.

(e) *Gain of NaCl.* As with loss of NaCl, so with a gain thereof the subject initially retains H_2O; but thereafter, the net result is addition of NaCl in excess of H_2O. Consequently, the osmolality of plasma rises, and there is then a shift of H_2O from the intracellular into the extracellular compartment until the two equilibrate at a higher osmolality. Therefore, in the new steady state of hyperosmotic expansion, the extracellular compartment is expanded, the intracellular is contracted, and the osmolality of both is greater than normal.

(f) *Gain of "pure" H_2O.* In the syndrome of inappropriate ADH secretion (SIADH), a sustained normal or high plasma concentration of the antidiuretic hormone (ADH or vasopressin) causes the kidneys to retain H_2O (see Chap. 8). This H_2O at first enters the plasma, causing its osmolality to decline. This change, in turn, causes a shift of H_2O into the interstitial space, and as the osmolality of that space decreases, there is a further shift of H_2O into the intracellular compartment. Thus, a gain of "pure" H_2O is shared by all the major body fluid compartments, which equilibrate at an osmolality that is below the normal value.

Problem 3-1 Sample calculations illustrating the independence of the inulin clearance from the plasma concentration of inulin and from the rate of urine flow in a dog.

Urine Flow (ml/min)	Inulin Concentration		Inulin Clearance (ml/min)
	Plasma (mg/ml)	Urine (mg/ml)	
1.2	0.9	45	60.0
1.3	1.4	68	63.1
1.0	2.3	141	61.3
1.4	3.8	168	61.9
1.2	5.7	294	61.9
1.3	0.5	23	59.8
2.1	0.6	17	59.5
3.1	0.4	8	62.0
5.7	0.5	5	57.0
6.6	0.5	4.6	60.7

Modified from Shannon, J. A. *Am. J. Physiol.* 112:405, 1935.

Problem 3-2 Sample calculations illustrating the identity of the inulin and creatinine clearances in a dog under physiological conditions.

Urine Flow (ml/min)	Inulin			Creatinine		
	Plasma (mg/100 ml)	Urine (mg/100 ml)	Clearance (ml/min)	Plasma (mg/100 ml)	Urine (mg/100 ml)	Clearance (ml/min)
1.0	104	5,076	48.8	13.7	673	49.1
1.1	106	4,601	47.7	14.7	630	47.1
0.9	108	6,017	50.1	16.0	890	50.1
1.0	109	5,137	47.1	16.6	792	47.7

Modified from Shannon, J. A. *Am. J. Physiol.* 112:405, 1935.

**Table 3-A : Attainment of a steady state for inulin during a
stable intravenous infusion of inulin in a healthy adult human.**

Elapsed Time (min)	Rate of Inulin Infusion (mg/min)	GFR (ml/min)	P_{In} (mg/ml)	Urinary Excretion of Inulin (mg/min)
1	72	120	0.005	0.6
5	72	120	0.02	2.4
10	72	120	0.05	6.0
50	72	120	0.24	28.8
100	72	120	0.47	56.4
110	72	120	0.6	72.0
120	72	120	0.6	72.0

Problem 3-3

1. The urinary excretion of inulin at each time interval is given in Table 3-A. The values were derived by calculating the filtered load of inulin ($P_{In} \cdot$ GFR), which is equal to the urinary excretion of inulin, since this compound is neither reabsorbed nor secreted by the tubules.

There is danger of a circular argument here: Inulin was given in order to measure the GFR, yet we have utilized the GFR in order to calculate the urinary excretion of inulin. In practice, one measures the urinary excretion as $U_{In} \cdot \dot{V}$ and determines the GFR as $U_{In} \cdot \dot{V}/P_{In}$ (just as in Fig. 3-4), *once a steady state is reached.* What we are doing here is utilizing, retrospectively, that steady-state value of GFR in order to illustrate how the steady state is attained and to re-emphasize some points about the renal handling of inulin.

2. So long as the rate of inulin infusion exceeds its urinary excretion, inulin will continue to accumulate in the body, and the plasma concentration of inulin will rise; this is known as a positive balance for inulin. It will stop rising once the input of inulin by infusion equals its output via the urine, for at that point inulin will stop accumulating in the body.

3. By definition, the steady state is reached when input equals output (at 110 minutes in Table 3-A). Note another feature of the steady state: The plasma concentration of inulin is stable during this state, and it levels out at that point where the product of the plasma concentration and the GFR (i.e., the rate at which inulin is filtered into Bowman's space) is equal to the rate of infusion of inulin.

4. The value of 120 ml per minute for a normal GFR in this problem was chosen to be different from the value in Figure 3-4 in order to emphasize that there is a wide range of normality: 85 to 125 ml per minute for women, and 97 to 140 ml per minute for men.

Problem 4-1 Renal handling of inorganic phosphate in dogs.

Urine Flow (ml/min)	Phosphate Phosphorus[a]			Creatinine			Phosphate Phosphorus[a]			Clearance Ratio: Phosphate Clearance/Creatinine Clearance
	Plasma (mg/100 ml)	Urine (mg/100 ml)	Clearance (ml/min)	Plasma (mg/100 ml)	Urine (mg/100 ml)	Clearance (ml/min)	Filtered (mg/min)	Excreted (mg/min)	Reabsorbed (mg/min)	
6.8	1.25	0.07	0.4	33.9	427	85.7	1.07	0.005	1.07	0.005
9.2	2.75	0.46	1.5	31.2	283	83.4	2.29	0.04	2.25	0.018
9.7	3.70	2.95	7.7	32.5	274	81.8	3.03	0.29	2.74	0.094
8.7	4.64	9.10	17.1	33.3	321	83.9	3.89	0.79	3.10	0.203
6.7	9.34	69.0	49.5	34.5	423	82.1	7.67	4.62	3.05	0.603
8.2	13.0	95.7	60.4	34.5	352	83.7	10.88	7.85	3.03	0.722
10.0	31.7	208	65.6	38.7	293	75.7	24.00	20.80	3.20	0.867

[a]The values were measured as phosphate phosphorus; they have been converted from milligrams to millimoles of inorganic phosphate in Table 4-1 and Figure 4-1. Slightly modified from Pitts, R. F., and Alexander, R. S. *Am. J. Physiol.* 142:648, 1944. Used with permission of the American Physiological Society.

These calculations emphasize that the concept of clearance is by no means restricted to inulin or creatinine. As explained in footnote b to this problem (p. 78), the clearance ratio is a useful calculation in renal physiology. In this instance, it tells us that at a plasma phosphate phosphorus concentration of 1.25 mg per 100 ml, 0.005 or 0.5% of the phosphate that was filtered was excreted; i.e., 99.5% of the filtered phosphate was reabsorbed. In contrast, at a plasma phosphate phosphorus concentration of 31.7 mg per 100 ml, 86.7% of the filtered phosphate was excreted, and 13.3% was reabsorbed.

Problem 4-2 Handling of urea by the kidneys of an adult human at varying rates of urine flow.

V̇ (ml/min)	Urine Concentration Inulin (mg/ml)	Urea (mM/L)	Plasma Concentration Inulin (mg/ml)	Urea (mM/L)	GFR (ml/min)	Urea Filtered (mM/min)	Excreted (mM/min)	Reabsorbed (mM/min)	Urea Excreted* (% of filtered load)	Reabsorbed* (% of filtered load)
0.4	144	300	0.5	5	115	0.58	0.12	0.46	21	79
0.8	75	263	0.5	5	120	0.60	0.21	0.39	35	65
1.0	60	240	0.5	5	120	0.60	0.24	0.36	40	60
3.1	20	119	0.5	5	124	0.62	0.37	0.25	60	40
10.2	5.8	37	0.5	5	118	0.59	0.38	0.21	64	36

*Note that these values can be calculated in two ways. (1) From line 1, the % of filtered urea excreted equals (0.12/0.58) · 100 or 20.7%, and the % of filtered urea reabsorbed equals (0.46/0.58) · 100 or 79.3%. (2) Alternatively, as explained in footnote b to Problem 4-1 (p. 78), one can utilize the clearance ratio to derive the same answers without having to measure urine flow and without first calculating the actual amounts filtered, excreted, and reabsorbed. Using this ratio (U/P urea ÷ U/P inulin), the fraction of filtered urea excreted equals 300/5 ÷ 144/0.5 or 0.208 (20.8%), and the fraction reabsorbed equals 1.000 − 0.208 or 0.792 (79.2%).

Lesson: The answer to this problem emphasizes the dependence of passive urea reabsorption upon the renal handling of water (see Fig. 4-4). The chemical concentration gradient favoring urea reabsorption in the terminal portions of the collecting ducts is reflected by the U/P ratio for urea (i.e., the ratio of the urinary concentration of urea to the plasma concentration of urea); note that the higher this ratio, the greater the rate of urea reabsorption.

Problem 5-1 Determination of renal plasma flow (RPF), renal blood flow (RBF), and filtration fraction (FF), using PAH and inulin in dogs. The extraction ratio of PAH (E_{PAH}) changes during the postnatal period, when these data were obtained.

Age (days)	Urine Flow (μl per min per g of kidney)[c]	U_{PAH} (mg/100 ml)	Pa_{PAH}[a] (mg/100 ml)	Pv_{PAH}[a] (mg/100 ml)	E_{PAH}	RPF (μl per min per g of kidney)[c]	RBF[b] (μl per min per g of kidney)[c]	C_{in} (μl per min per g of kidney)[c]	FF
2	3.8	104	2.60	2.16	0.17	898	1,633	130	0.14
21	2.7	283	1.70	1.08	0.36	1,232	2,240	270	0.22
40	5.2	664	3.00	1.23	0.59	1,951	3,547	630	0.32
60	3.2	672	1.20	0.34	0.72	2,501	4,547	790	0.32
74	2.3	3,516	3.10	0.52	0.83	3,134	5,698	1,200	0.38

[a] Pa_{PAH} and Pv_{PAH} = concentration of PAH in arterial and renal venous plasma, respectively.
[b] Assume that the hematocrit = 0.45.
[c] Values have been expressed per gram of kidney in order to correct for any changes that might be due to growth of the kidney during the postnatal period.
Abstracted from Horster, M., and Valtin, H. *J. Clin. Invest.* 50:779, 1971.

Lessons: (1) Since the extraction ratio for PAH is so low at the early postnatal stages, there is a large difference between the effective renal plasma flow (ERPF; given by the clearance of PAH) and the true renal plasma flow (RPF), which utilizes the Fick principle (p. 92). (2) The filtration fraction (FF) must be calculated using RPF; it cannot be determined accurately using ERPF. (3) In dogs, the mature value for GFR (C_{in}) and RPF, when expressed per unit of time and per gram of kidney, is reached by approximately 3 to 3½ months of age.

Table 6-A : Results obtained on micropuncture samples.

Flow Rate of Tubular Fluid ($\dot{v}$) (nl/min)	Concentrations in Tubular Fluid (TF)		Concentrations in Arterial Plasma (P)	
	Na$^+$ (mEq/L)	Inulin (mg/100 ml)	Na$^+$ (mEq/L)	Inulin (mg/100 ml)
Micropunctures of proximal tubules				
11.21	140	209	137	98
Micropunctures of bends of loops of Henle				
9.14	283	583	138	93

Problem 6-1

1. The principle of measuring the filtration rate of a single glomerulus (sGFR) by micropuncture is identical to that used for measuring the GFR of all nephrons combined. Through the inulin clearance (see pp. 49–51), one determines the amount of plasma cleared of inulin by the single glomerulus; the variables, TF_{In}, $\dot{v}$, and P_{In} are analogous to U_{In}, $\dot{V}$, and P_{In} of the usual formula for inulin clearance, $U_{In} \cdot \dot{V}/P_{In}$. Thus,

$$sGFR = \frac{TF_{In} \cdot \dot{v}}{P_{In}}$$

For the micropunctures of the proximal tubules (Table 6-A):

$$sGFR = \frac{209 \text{ mg}}{100 \text{ ml}} \cdot \frac{11.21 \text{ nl}}{\text{min}} \div \frac{98 \text{ mg}}{100 \text{ ml}}$$

$$= \frac{209 \text{ mg}}{100 \text{ ml}} \cdot \frac{11.21 \text{ nl}}{\text{min}} \cdot \frac{100 \text{ ml}}{98 \text{ mg}}$$

$$= 23.9 \text{ nl/min}$$

For the micropunctures of the bends of loops of Henle:

$$sGFR = \frac{583 \text{ mg}}{100 \text{ ml}} \cdot \frac{9.14 \text{ nl}}{\text{min}} \div \frac{93 \text{ mg}}{100 \text{ ml}}$$

$$= 57.3 \text{ nl/min}$$

The difference between the two values reflects the fact that juxtamedullary nephrons have a higher sGFR than do outer cortical nephrons (Table 6-1). The latter nephrons can be micropunctured at the surface of the kidney (Fig. 1-2A) whereas juxtamedullary nephrons, arising deep within the cortex and being surrounded by cortical and medullary tissue, are accessible to micropuncture only at the bend of the loop of Henle. (In this experiment, flow of tubular fluid to the juxtaglomerular apparatus was blocked by oil droplets, and tubuloglomerular feedback was therefore interrupted. Although this fact yields a value for sGFR that is somewhat higher than during punctures of the distal tubule when the feedback loop is intact, differences of the above magnitude have also been demonstrated by other techniques, when the feedback was not abolished.)

2. The fraction is most easily computed by utilizing Equation 3-1. For the proximal tubules:

$$\text{Fraction of filtered water reabsorbed} = 1 - \frac{1}{\text{TF/P inulin}}$$

$$= 1 - \frac{1}{209/98}$$

$$= 1 - 0.47$$

$$= 0.53, \text{ or } 53\%$$

This value is lower than that of approximately two-thirds (or 67%) usually cited for reabsorption in the proximal tubule because the very end of that tubule is located beneath the surface of the kidney and is therefore not available for micropuncture.

By the time that tubular fluid reached the bend of the loop of Henle, $1 - 0.16$, or 84%, of the filtered water had been reabsorbed (see also Answer to Problem 8-2).

One could also calculate the fractions by knowing the amount of tubular fluid flowing at the point of micropuncture (e.g., 11.21 nl per minute for the proximal tubule) and the sGFR of 23.9 nl per minute for that nephron; that is, 11.21/23.9 or 0.47 was flowing at this point, so that $1 - 0.47$, or 53%, must have been reabsorbed. That method, however, involves the rather cumbersome quantitative collection of tubular fluid. It is far easier to obtain the same information by simply measuring the concentration of inulin in simultaneous samples of tubular fluid and plasma.

3. The answer to this question illustrates the utility of the *clearance ratio*. The derivation of that ratio and its reduction to the expression $U_X/P_X \div U_{In}/P_{In}$ are explained in footnote b to Problem 4-1. That expression, which yields the fraction of the filtered load of substance X that is excreted by both kidneys, can be adapted to samples obtained by micropuncture by substituting the concentration of X and inulin in tubular fluid (TF_X and TF_{In}) for those in urine (U_X and U_{In}). Thus, the fraction of filtered Na^+ flowing at the point of micropuncture in the proximal tubule is equal to TF/P for Na^+ divided by TF/P for inulin, i.e., $140/137 \div 209/98$, or 0.48; the fraction of filtered Na^+ reabsorbed up to this point is therefore 0.52, or 52%. For the bend of the loop of Henle,

283/138 ÷ 583/93, or 0.33, was still present, and therefore 0.67, or 67%, had been reabsorbed. Note that this experiment does not tell you where the extra 15% (67% − 52%) of Na^+ was reabsorbed. That could have occurred anywhere between the end of the proximal tubule at the surface of the kidney (belonging to an outer cortical nephron) and the bend of the long loop of Henle (belonging to a juxtamedullary nephron). It is probable that the extra 15% was taken up from the proximal tubule, including its pars recta, as it dips beneath the surface of the kidney (Fig. 1-2A), not from the thin descending limb of Henle.

Problem 7-1

The dietary allotment of Na^+ is commonly quoted as so many "grams per day" without specifying whether the amount refers to sodium or to sodium chloride. The purpose of this question is twofold: (a) to emphasize the importance of specifying whether the amount quoted refers to Na^+ or to NaCl, and (b) to give some ball-park values.

A normal intake for an adult is 6 to 15 g of salt (i.e., NaCl) per day. One millimole of NaCl is equivalent to 58 mg (see Answer to Problem 1-2); therefore:

$$\frac{58 \text{ mg}}{1 \text{ mMole}} = \frac{6,000 \text{ mg}}{X}$$

$$X = 103 \text{ mMoles}$$

Each millimole of NaCl contains 1 mEq of Na^+ and 1 mEq of Cl^-. Thus, the normal daily intake of sodium should be quoted as follows: 6 to 15 g of NaCl (or table salt), or 103 to 259 mMoles of NaCl, or 103 to 259 mEq of Na^+ (Fig. 7-7).

If the use of salt at the table is omitted, the daily intake can be reduced to 4 to 7 g of NaCl, which is 69 to 120 mMoles per day or 69 to 120 mEq of Na^+ per day.

If, besides eliminating salt at the table, added salt during cooking is also omitted, the daily intake is reduced to 3 to 4 g of table salt (52 to 69 mMoles of NaCl or 52 to 69 mEq of Na^+ per day).

A therapeutic low-salt diet (e.g., as prescribed for congestive heart failure) contains about 2 g of table salt per day, that is, 34 mMoles of NaCl or 34 mEq of Na^+. If the intake is reduced below this value, the variety of foods that may be eaten is very limited, and the food becomes unpalatable. Furthermore, the concurrent use of diuretic agents makes such severe restriction unnecessary.

Ball-park values: It is useful to memorize the following average values, realizing that the range of normality is great.

Normal daily intake: 10 g NaCl; 200 mEq Na^+
Low-salt diet: 2 g NaCl; 35 mEq Na^+
One level teaspoon contains: 6 g NaCl; 100 mEq Na^+

The term *normal* is possibly more ambiguous in this context than in most, for it is likely that the intake of sodium by a healthy human is set much more by custom than by need. In fact, there is some suspicion that the amount of salt we eat may be harmful — at least to individuals who are susceptible to certain disorders, such as hypertension.

Problem 7-2   The first impulse might be to reason that since exchangeable Na^+ resides almost exclusively in extracellular fluid (ECW), one calculates the amount needed by multiplying the deficit of 20 mEq per liter by the ECW. But that practice would result in far too little Na^+ being given. The reason is that the infusion of 5% NaCl (which has an osmolality of approximately 1,600 mOsm/kg H_2O; see Answer to Problem 1-2) will raise the osmolality of the extracellular fluid, causing H_2O to shift out of the intracellular space until osmotic equilibrium between the two compartments is re-established (as described in the Answer to Problem 2-3, under Gain of NaCl). In this way, the NaCl that is being added to the extracellular compartment is continuously being "diluted," and therefore much more NaCl must be added than would be calculated on the basis of the ECW. When the new steady-state value of 132 mEq of Na^+ per liter is reached, the intracellular fluid will have the same higher osmolality as the extracellular. That is, the intracellular compartment will have participated fully in the change, but without the addition of intracellular solute. Hence, NaCl must be added *as if it were distributed throughout the intracellular as well as extracellular space,* and the amount that needs to be added is therefore calculated by multiplying the deficit of 20 mEq per liter by the total body water (TBW). If the TBW is estimated as 60% of body weight (Fig. 2-1), then 636 mEq of Na^+ (20 mEq/L · 31.8 liters) needs to be given to the patient.

A solution of 5% NaCl contains 856 mEq of Na^+ per liter (see Answer to Problem 1-2). Therefore, the patient should be given 743 ml of this solution; in practice, one would write an order for 750 ml of 5% saline. Because it is wise to correct imbalances slowly, most physicians might aim to err on the low side by initially prescribing 500 ml of 5% saline.

Problem 8-1 Renal handling of salt, water, and urea in varying diuretic states. The following data were obtained on a healthy medical student, under three conditions: (a) while drinking ad libitum; (b) after 12 hours of thirsting; and (c) within 90 minutes after drinking 1 liter of tap water.

	$\dot{V}$ (ml/min)	U_{in} (mg/ml)	P_{in} (mg/ml)	GFR (ml/min)	U/P Inulin	Proportion of Filtered Water (i.e., of GFR) Reabsorbed (%)
While drinking ad libitum	1.2	15.8	0.151	126	105	99.1
After 12 hours of thirsting	0.75	25.2	0.155	122	163	99.4
Within 90 minutes after drinking 1 liter water	15.0	1.23	0.154	120*	8	87.5*

Lessons: (1) Water diuresis is due to decreased tubular reabsorption of water, not to increased filtration. Yet, even during very marked water diuresis (15 ml/min), nearly 90% of the filtered water is reabsorbed. (2) Note the typical values for U/P inulin in various states of diuresis.

Answer to Problem 8-1 continued on page 287.

Problem 8-1 (Continued)

	P_{Na} (mEq/L)	Filtered Load of Na (mEq/min)	U_{Na} (mEq/L)	Urinary Na Excretion (mEq/min)	Proportion of Filtered Na Reabsorbed (%)
While drinking ad libitum	136	17.1	128	0.154	99.1
After 12 hours of thirsting	144	17.6	192	0.144	99.2
Within 90 minutes after drinking 1 liter water	134	16.1	10.2	0.153	99.1*

*Lesson: Water diuresis significantly decreases the fraction of filtered water that is reabsorbed (i.e., % GFR reabsorbed; see previous page), but not the fraction of filtered sodium that is reabsorbed. That is, by and large, sodium balance and water balance can be regulated independently of each other.

Answer to Problem 8-1 continued on page 288.

Problem 8-1 (Continued)

	U_{Osm} (mOsm/kg)	P_{Osm} (mOsm/kg)	C_{H_2O} (ml/min)	$T^c_{H_2O}$ (ml/min)	$U_{Urea\,N}$[a] (mg/100 ml)	$P_{Urea\,N}$[a] (mg/100 ml)	C_{Urea} (ml/min)	Proportion of Filtered Urea Reabsorbed (%)
While drinking ad libitum	663	290	−1.54	+1.54	480	12	48	62
After 12 hours of thirsting	1,000	300*	−1.75*	+1.75	720	15	36	71*
Within 90 minutes after drinking 1 liter water	100	287*	+9.77*	—*	48	10	72	40*

[a]Concentrations of urea are usually determined by measuring the amount of nitrogen in urea; hence, the expression *urea nitrogen*. The two nitrogen atoms constitute 28/60 of the urea molecule: $CO(NH_2)_2$. The clearance of urea (C_{Urea}) can be calculated without converting "Urea N" to "Urea," since the conversion factors for $U_{Urea\,N}$ and $P_{Urea\,N}$ cancel out.

Lessons: (1) C_{H_2O} has a positive value when the urine is hyposmotic to plasma; it has a negative value when the urine is hyperosmotic to plasma; and C_{H_2O} is zero when the urine has the same osmolality as plasma. (2) C_{H_2O} is converted to $T^c_{H_2O}$ only when C_{H_2O} is negative. (3) There is an inverse relationship between the rate of urine flow and the rate at which urea is reabsorbed (see also Fig. 4-4 and Answer to Problem 4-2). (4) A change in plasma osmolality of just 1 to 3% suffices to fully inhibit secretion of ADH, or to stimulate it maximally.

Answer to Problem 8-1 continued on pages 289–290.

Problem 8-1
(Cont.)

How to compute the fraction of a filtered substance that is reabsorbed. The handling of urea can serve as an example. An inulin clearance of 126 ml per minute means, of course, that 126 ml of plasma were filtered each minute. Hence, the urea contained in 126 ml of plasma was filtered each minute. The fact that the urea clearance was simultaneously 48 ml per minute means that the equivalent of 48 ml of plasma was completely cleared of urea each minute. In other words, the urea contained in 78 ml of plasma (126 − 48) must have been reabsorbed each minute. This amounts to 78/126 = 0.62, or 62%; and the equation for this intuitive fact is

$$\text{Fraction of filtered urea that is reabsorbed} = \frac{C_{In} - C_{Urea}}{C_{In}}$$

$$= \frac{C_{In}}{C_{In}} - \frac{C_{Urea}}{C_{In}}$$

$$= 1 - \frac{C_{Urea}}{C_{In}}$$

$$= 1 - \left(\frac{U_{Urea} \cdot \dot{V}}{P_{Urea}} \cdot \frac{P_{In}}{U_{In} \cdot \dot{V}} \right)$$

$$= 1 - \left(\frac{U_{Urea}}{P_{Urea}} \cdot \frac{P_{In}}{U_{In}} \right)$$

$$\text{Fraction of filtered urea that is reabsorbed} = 1 - \left(\frac{U_{Urea}}{P_{Urea}} \div \frac{U_{In}}{P_{In}} \right) \quad \text{(Answers 8-1)}$$

There is another intuitive way of arriving at the same mathematical expression, through knowledge of the filtered load of urea ($C_{In} \cdot P_{Urea}$) and of the amount of urea excreted ($\dot{V} \cdot U_{Urea}$). The fraction of filtered urea that is excreted, X, can be calculated through the proportionality:

$$\frac{C_{In} \cdot P_{Urea}}{1.00} = \frac{\dot{V} \cdot U_{Urea}}{X}$$

$$\therefore \text{Fraction of filtered urea that is excreted} = \frac{\dot{V} \cdot U_{Urea}}{C_{In} \cdot P_{Urea}}$$

$$= \frac{\dot{V} \cdot U_{Urea}}{\dfrac{U_{In} \cdot \dot{V}}{P_{In}} \cdot P_{Urea}}$$

$$= \frac{\dot{V} \cdot U_{Urea}}{1} \cdot \frac{P_{In}}{U_{In} \cdot \dot{V} \cdot P_{Urea}}$$

$$= \frac{U_{Urea}}{P_{Urea}} \cdot \frac{P_{In}}{U_{In}}$$

Fraction of filtered urea that is excreted $= \frac{U_{Urea}}{P_{Urea}} \div \frac{U_{In}}{P_{In}}$

∴ Fraction of filtered urea that is reabsorbed $= 1 - \left(\frac{U_{Urea}}{P_{Urea}} \div \frac{U_{In}}{P_{In}} \right)$ (Answers 8-1)

For the example cited in the table (while drinking ad libitum):

Fraction of filtered urea that is reabsorbed $= 1 - \left(\frac{480}{12} \div \frac{15.8}{0.151} \right)$

$$= 1 - (40 \div 105)$$

$$= 1 - 0.38$$

$$= 0.62$$

Answers Equation 8-1 is useful because one can compute the fraction without needing accurate urine collections; all that is required is the simultaneous determination of urea and inulin concentrations in urine and plasma. Similarly, one can determine the fraction of the filtered load of a given substance flowing at a point of micropuncture (e.g., see Fig. 11-2) without measuring the flow rate of tubular fluid; all one needs is the concentrations of inulin and of the given substance in the micropuncture sample and in the plasma.

Problem 8-2

(a) Water is probably reabsorbed in appreciable amounts from all parts of the nephron except the ascending limbs of Henle and the early distal tubules (Table 7-1). During the formation of hyperosmotic urine, about 70% of the filtered H_2O is reabsorbed in the proximal tubules, 10 to 20% in the loops of Henle, 10 to 15% in the late distal tubules, and — perhaps surprisingly — only about 1% in the collecting ducts. These figures are based on TF/P and U/P ratios for inulin, obtained through micropuncture (see Chap. 3). They illustrate at least two important points: (1) that the vast majority of filtered H_2O is reabsorbed in the renal cortex, i.e., in the proximal and late distal tubules; and (2) that although the H_2O that is reabsorbed from the collecting ducts is critical to raising the urine osmolality from isosmolality to hyperosmolality (Fig. 8-1A), this process entails the reabsorption of relatively small amounts of H_2O.

(b) The reabsorbed H_2O must be immediately returned to the systemic circulation, lest the kidneys swell and burst. Almost all the reabsorbed H_2O enters the capillary beds, which are found in the cortex and the outer and inner medulla (Fig. 1-2B). Eventually, the reabsorbed H_2O leaves the kidneys via the renal veins. An unknown but probably minimal amount of the H_2O that is reabsorbed from tubules is returned to the systemic circulation through the renal lymphatics.

(c) The answer to this question is based on mass balance for solute: The input of solute to the kidneys must equal the output of solute from them. Solute entering the kidneys is equal to 660 ml/min · 290 mOsm/1,000 ml, or 191.4 mOsm per minute. Solute that leaves the kidneys via the urine is equal to 1 ml/min · 700 mOsm/1,000 ml, or 0.7 mOsm per minute. Therefore, 191.4 − 0.7, or 190.7 mOsm per minute must leave the kidneys via the renal veins (ignoring the very small quantity that leaves through the lymphatics); since this amount will be contained in 659 ml of plasma, the osmolality of renal venous plasma will be 190.7 ÷ 659, or 0.2894 mOsm/ml, which is 289.4 mOsm/kg H_2O. This tiny difference from the osmolality of normal plasma is too small to be detected. Furthermore, the net removal of solute by the kidneys does not result in progressive dilution of plasma because there is net loss of water through other organs. Normally this net loss, known as *insensible water loss* (Table 1-4), occurs from the skin (approximately 500 ml per day in an adult) and through the breath (about 400 ml per day).

Problem 9-1 The data below were obtained on each of four patients.

Normal arterial values from Table 1-2: pH = 7.37 to 7.42; $[HCO_3^-]$ = 23 to 25 mMoles/L; P_{CO_2} = 37 to 43 mm Hg.

Cause of the Disturbance	Arterial Plasma			Type of Disturbance
	pH	P_{CO_2} (mm Hg)	$[HCO_3^-]$ (mM/L)	
Prolonged vomiting	7.55	44	37	Metabolic alkalosis
Ingestion of NH_4Cl[a]	7.18	28	10	Metabolic acidosis
Hysterical hyperventilation	7.57	24	21	Respiratory alkalosis (acute)[b]
Emphysema	7.33	68	34	Respiratory acidosis (chronic)[b]

[a]The net effect of ingesting NH_4Cl is the addition of hydrochloric acid, by the following reaction:

$$2\ NH_4Cl + CO_2 \rightarrow 2\ H^+ + 2\ Cl^- + H_2O + \underset{urea}{CO(NH_2)_2}$$

[b]For an explanation of the difference between acute and chronic respiratory disturbances, see the last paragraph under Compensatory Responses, Chapter 9. A much more detailed discussion is given in: Valtin, H. *Renal Dysfunction: Mechanisms Involved in Fluid and Solute Imbalance.* Boston: Little, Brown, 1979.

Problem 9-2

Respiratory acidosis. When CO_2 is retained, as during alveolar hypoventilation due to barbiturate intoxication, the P_{CO_2} rises. As the CO_2 is hydrated (Eq. 9-1) or hydroxylated (Eq. 9-2), H^+ and HCO_3^- are produced; this H^+ must be buffered by nonbicarbonate buffers (mainly hemoglobin, other proteins, and organic phosphates; Fig. 9-4), and in the process, HCO_3^- rises (Fig. 9-7). Since the primary disturbance is respiratory, the compensatory response will be renal, and it takes days to come to completion. The compensation involves increased reabsorption of HCO_3^- occasioned by the elevated P_{CO_2} (Fig. 10-3B).

Note that here is an instance in which the plasma HCO_3^- concentration rises during acidosis. Inasmuch as HCO_3^- is a major buffer, there is a reflex tendency for the neophyte in acid-base balance to predict a decrease in plasma HCO_3^- during acidosis. The key to understanding why it increases during respiratory acidosis (but decreases during metabolic acidosis) is to remember that the H^+ derived from the processing of CO_2 (Eqs. 9-1 and 9-2) cannot be buffered by the HCO_3^-/CO_2 system.

Metabolic alkalosis. A net loss of H^+ from the body, as occasioned by the loss of gastric HCl during prolonged vomiting, is accompanied by an increase in the plasma HCO_3^- concentration; this fact is evident from Equation 9-11, which will be driven to the left as HCl is withdrawn. The respiratory compensation for this primary metabolic disturbance is a diminution in alveolar ventilation due to the alkalosis and a consequent rise in P_{CO_2}.

Respiratory alkalosis. The primary event in this disturbance of H^+ balance is alveolar hyperventilation and a decline in P_{CO_2}. This change will drive the reactions shown at the top of Figure 9-7 to the left and the plasma HCO_3^- concentration therefore will decrease. The compensatory response by the kidneys — which will begin within hours of the onset of the disturbance but will take days to take full effect — is to decrease the reabsorption of HCO_3^- as a consequence of the lowered P_{CO_2} (Fig. 10-3B).

Arterial pH in mixed disturbances. The reason for this question is to point out that the plasma pH can be predicted only if the two components shift the pH in the same direction. Thus, a mixture of two acidoses will certainly result in an acidotic pH and two alkaloses in an alkalotic pH. When, however, the two components shift the pH in opposite directions (i.e., a mixture of an acidosis and an alkalosis), the plasma pH might be alkalotic, normal, or acidotic, depending on which component predominates.

Problem 10-1   The Henderson-Hasselbalch equation, being an expression of the ionization or dissociation properties of acids and bases, can be utilized to solve this problem.

$$pH = pK + \log \frac{[\text{base; i.e., } H^+ \text{ acceptor}]}{[\text{acid; i.e., } H^+ \text{ donor}]}$$

For phenobarbital,

$$pH = 7.2 + \log \frac{[\text{Ionized form}]}{[\text{Nonionized form}]}$$

Plasma, pH 7.3

$$7.3 = 7.2 + \log \frac{[\text{Ionized form}]}{[\text{Nonionized form}]}$$

$$0.1 = \log \frac{[\text{Ionized form}]}{[\text{Nonionized form}]}$$

$$\therefore \frac{[\text{Ionized form}]}{[\text{Nonionized form}]} = \frac{1.26}{1}$$

The concentration of total unbound phenobarbital is 6.0 mg/100 ml plasma; $\frac{1.26}{2.26}$ of this total exists in the ionized form, and $\frac{1.00}{2.26}$ of the total exists in the nonionized form. Hence:

$$[\text{Ionized form}] \quad = \frac{1.26}{2.26} \cdot 6.0 = 3.3 \text{ mg/100 ml}$$

$$[\text{Nonionized form}] = \frac{1.00}{2.26} \cdot 6.0 = 2.7 \text{ mg/100 ml}$$

Plasma, pH 7.7

$$7.7 = 7.2 + \log \frac{[\text{Ionized form}]}{[\text{Nonionized form}]}$$

$$0.5 = \log \frac{[\text{Ionized form}]}{[\text{Nonionized form}]}$$

$$\therefore \frac{[\text{Ionized form}]}{[\text{Nonionized form}]} = \frac{3.16}{1}$$

$$\therefore [\text{Ionized form}] \quad = \frac{3.16}{4.16} \cdot 6.0 = 4.6 \text{ mg/100 ml plasma}$$

$$[\text{Nonionized form}] = \frac{1.00}{4.16} \cdot 6.0 = 1.4 \text{ mg/100 ml plasma}$$

Urine, pH 5.2

$$5.2 = 7.2 + \log \frac{[\text{Ionized form}]}{[\text{Nonionized form}]}$$

$$-2.0 = \log \frac{[\text{Ionized form}]}{[\text{Nonionized form}]}$$

$$2.0 = \log \frac{[\text{Nonionized form}]}{[\text{Ionized form}]}$$

$$\therefore \frac{[\text{Nonionized form}]}{[\text{Ionized form}]} = \frac{100}{1}$$

i.e., when the reaction of the urine is acid, most of the phenobarbital exists in the nonionized form, which can diffuse across the membranes of tubular cells and hence can be passively reabsorbed.

Urine, pH 8.2

$$8.2 = 7.2 + \log \frac{[\text{Ionized form}]}{[\text{Nonionized form}]}$$

$$1.0 = \log \frac{[\text{Ionized form}]}{[\text{Nonionized form}]}$$

$$\therefore \frac{[\text{Ionized form}]}{[\text{Nonionized form}]} = \frac{10}{1}$$

i.e., when the reaction of the urine is alkaline, most of the phenobarbital exists in the ionized form, to which renal tubular cells are relatively impermeable. Hence, alkalinization of the urine can markedly diminish the reabsorption and thus enhance the renal excretion of a weak acid, such as phenobarbital.

	Total Unbound Phenobarbital in Plasma (mg/100 ml)	Ratio of Unbound Phenobarbital: $\dfrac{[\text{Ionized}]}{[\text{Nonionized}]}$	Plasma Concentration of Unbound Phenobarbital	
			Ionized	Nonionized
			(mg/100 ml)	
Plasma, pH 7.3	6.0	$\dfrac{1.26}{1}$	3.3	2.7
Plasma, pH 7.7	6.0	$\dfrac{3.16}{1}$	4.6	1.4
Urine, pH 5.2	—	$\dfrac{1}{100}$	—	—
Urine, pH 8.2	—	$\dfrac{10}{1}$	—	—

Note that alkalinization may have a further advantage. Giving NaHCO₃ alkalinizes not only the urine but also the plasma (Eq. 9-9). This change reduces the concentration of the nonionized form in plasma. Since this is the form that passes most readily across cell membranes, including those of the brain, alkalinization probably reduces the concentration of phenobarbital in cerebral cells, and thereby hastens recovery from coma.

The beneficial effects of increased urine flow and alkalinization during experimental phenobarbital intoxication were presented in the following paper: Waddell, W. J., and Butler, T. C. The distribution and excretion of phenobarbital. *J. Clin. Invest.* 36:1217, 1957. Two clinical examples, in which the principle of nonionic diffusion was applied to salicylate therapy and intoxication, appear in: Levy, G., et al. *N. Engl. J. Med.* 293:323, 1975; and Hill, J. B. *N. Engl. J. Med.* 288:1110, 1973.

Problem 10-2

It is clear from Figure 10-A that, because the NH_3/NH_4^+ buffer system has a pK of 9.2 (Table 1-3), NH_4Cl cannot be a titratable acid (T.A.). Recall that T.A. is defined as the amount of strong base that must be added to acid urine in order to return the pH of that urine to 7.40. If urine is thus titrated from a minimal pH of 4.4 (the shaded area in Fig. 10-A), very little NH_4^+ will be converted

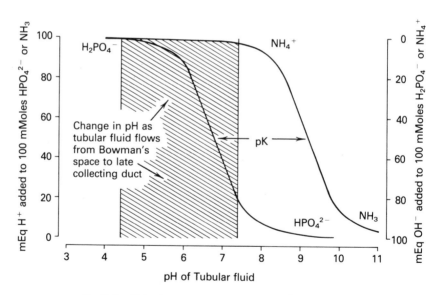

Fig. 10-A : Behavior of the buffer systems, $HPO_4^{2-}/H_2PO_4^-$ and NH_3/NH_4^+, in tubular fluid. Note that, as OH^- is added to acid urine (ordinate on right), most of the phosphate is converted to the HPO_4^{2-} form, whereas the vast majority of the ammonia system remains in the NH_4^+ form. In other words, NH_4^+ salts cannot be appreciably titrated from an acid pH to 7.4, and therefore they are not titratable acids.

to NH_3 — a consequence of the fact that a buffer is most effective within ± 1 pH unit of its pK.

Problem 10-3

Ordinarily, virtually all of the filtered HCO_3^- is reabsorbed (Table 1-1). Suppose that the urinary concentration of HCO_3^- is 1.0 mMole per liter (again, from Table 1-1, a reasonable value, given the numbers for H_2O and HCO_3^- excreted). Then, applying this value and a P_{CO_2} for urine of 40 mm Hg to the Henderson-Hasselbalch equation (Eq. 9-9) yields a urinary pH of approximately 6; and if the urinary HCO_3^- concentration is reduced to 0.1 mMole per liter, the urinary pH will be approximately 5. These calculations show that the urinary pH could be lowered almost to the minimal value merely by reabsorbing virtually all of the filtered HCO_3^-. Even though that happens normally (note that no HCO_3^- is listed for the composition of urine in the Answer to Problem 11-1), nevertheless, the situation is theoretical because titratable acids (mainly NaH_2PO_4) are formed simultaneously, as shown in Figure 10-9.

Problem 11-1

These questions were asked because it is a rather remarkable (though understandable) fact that students can be very sophisticated about renal function, and yet not know the composition of normal urine!

The variation in the normal values is so great that it is almost meaningless to give average figures; hence the ranges are given in Table 11-A. When an individual is in balance (the steady state), the daily output of various substances (both renal and extrarenal) equals the daily production of those substances (both exogenous and endogenous). For a solute such as Na^+, which normally is excreted almost exclusively by the kidneys, the urinary *concentration* therefore depends not only on the intake of Na^+ but also on the intake of water. It is because the intakes of both solute and solvent can vary greatly from day to day that normal urinary concentrations have such wide ranges.

Note that a healthy individual whose diet contains proteins (i.e., a diet that yields fixed acids) excretes urine with an acid pH. Note also that he or she normally excretes urine which is hyperosmotic to plasma.

The major solutes which contribute to the osmolality of normal urine are depicted in Figure 11-A. Quantitatively, the most important electrolytes are Na^+, K^+, NH_4^+, and Cl^- (HCO_3^- is normally "absent"). Urea is the most abundant nonelectrolyte, and it ordinarily constitutes 40 to 50% of the total osmolality. (The reason for the inequality of the columns for cations and anions is given in the legend to Figure 11-A).

Table 11-A : Composition of the urine of a normal adult human whose diet includes protein.

pH	5.0 to 7.0
Osmolality	500 to 800 mOsm/kg H_2O
Na^+	50 to 130 mEq/L
K^+	20 to 70 mEq/L
NH_4^+	30 to 50 mEq/L
Ca^{2+}	5 to 12 mEq/L
Mg^{2+}	2 to 18 mEq/L
Cl^-	50 to 130 mEq/L
$H_2PO_4^-$	20 to 40 mEq/L*
SO_4^{2-}	30 to 45 mEq/L
Organic acids	10 to 25 mM/L*
Urea	200 to 400 mM/L
Creatinine	6 to 20 mM/L

*At an acid urinary pH of 6 or lower, nearly all of the urinary inorganic phosphate exists in the monovalent form (Fig. 10-A). Urinary organic acids (e.g., lactic, uric, citric, pyruvic acids) have different valences; the molar concentration listed assumes an average valence of minus two.

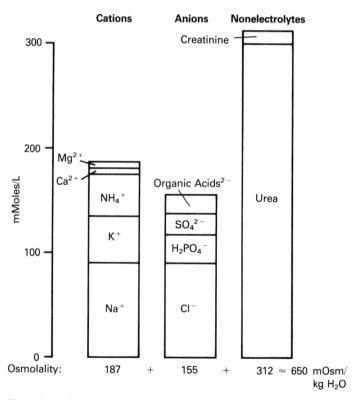

Fig. 11-A : Solute concentrations of normal urine. Note that the concentrations have been expressed as millimoles per liter. Since urine contains more divalent anions than cations, the column for the anions is lower than that for the cations. If the concentrations were given as milliequivalents per liter, the two columns would of course be of equal height.

Index

transport maximum for phosphate and, 68
Passive model, of countercurrent multiplication, 172–175
Pedicels of glomerular capillaries, 48
Penicillin, secretion of, 87
Peritubular capillaries, 3, 5
  blood flow in, ammonia excretion and, 239
  functions of, 3
  sodium intake affecting, 142–143
Peritubular membrane. *See* Membrane(s), cellular
Permeability
  antidiuretic hormone affecting, 132, 161, 171, 184
  filtration coefficient and, 35, 45
  of glomerular capillaries, 45
  of nephron segments, various, 132
  selective, of cell membrane, 29
  to urea, 73
  to water, 132
pH
  arterial, normal values for, 13
  intracellular, 207
  of tubular fluid, 228
pH maintenance, 195–218. *See also* Ammonia; Ammonium; Titratable acid
  buffer systems in, 196–204. *See also* Buffer system(s)
  compensatory responses in, 205–206
  disturbances of, development of, 293
  Henderson-Hasselbalch equation and. *See* Henderson-Hasselbalch equation
  isohydric principle and, 206–207
  kidneys in, role of, 225. *See also* Ammonium; Bicarbonate, filtered, reabsorption of; Titratable acid
  mammalian, problem of, 195–196. *See also* Nonvolatile acid(s); Volatile acid
  metabolic disturbances and, 204–206
  mixed disturbances and, 204–205
  normal values in
    plasma, 13
    cerebrospinal fluid, 14
  physicochemical buffering in, 196–197
  potassium excretion and, 257, 258–260
  primary disturbances in, 204

renal component in, 200–201
respiratory component in, 199, 205
respiratory disturbances and, 204–206
Phenobarbital poisoning, treatment of, nonionic diffusion in, 294–295
Phenolsulfonphthalein (PSP), tubular secretion of, 88
Phlorizin, 65
Phosphate(s)
  clearance of, ratio of, to creatinine clearance, 279. *See also* Clearance ratio
  inorganic
    as buffers
      titratable acid excretion and, 233, 234
      titration curve for, 208, 235
    excretion of, 67, 68, 279
    filtered load of, 66, 279. *See also* Filtered load
    reabsorption of, 67, 68, 279
    transport maximum for, 67–68
  organic
    definition of, 28
    in intracellular fluid, 27, 207
    permeability for, 29
  plasma concentrations of, 13
  titratable acid excretion and. *See* Titratable acid
  transport maximum for, 67–68
Phosphoric acid
  buffering of, replenishment of depleted bicarbonate stores and, 231
  formation of, 196
  pK of, 14
  urinary concentration of, 297, 298
Physicochemical buffering of nonvolatile acids, 196–199
Pituitary gland in antidiuretic hormone secretion, 175–177
pK, 197
  for various compounds, 14
Plasma
  arterial, pH of, in acid-base disturbances, 293
  chloride concentration in, bicarbonate reabsorption and, 230–231
  composition of, compared to interstitial fluid, 27, 29
  glomerular filtration of. *See* Glomerular filtration
  and interstitial fluid, balance between. *See* Starling hypothesis